The Cardiac Catheterization Handbook

The Cardiac Catheterization Handbook

Edited by

MORTON J. KERN, MD

Professor of Medicine
Director
The J. Gerard Mudd Cardiac Catheterization Laboratory
St. Louis University Health Sciences Center
St. Louis, Missouri

Foreword by

William Grossman, MD

FOURTH EDITION

with 496 illustrations

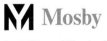

Mosby

An Affiliate of Elsevier Science

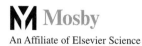 **Mosby**

An Affiliate of Elsevier Science

The Curtis Center
Independence Square West
Philadelphia, Pennsylvania 19106

NOTICE

Cardiac catheterization is an ever-changing field. Standard safety precautions must be
followed, but as new research and clinical experience broaden our knowledge,
changes in treatment and drug therapy may become necessary or appropriate. Readers
are advised to check the most current product information provided by the
manufacturer of each drug to be administered to verify the recommended dose, the
method and duration of administration, and contraindications. It is the responsibility
of the licensed prescriber, relying on experience and knowledge of the patient, to
determine dosages and the best treatment for each individual patient. Neither the
publisher nor the author assumes any liability for any injury and/or damage to
persons or property arising from this publication.

Previous editions copyrighted 1999, 1995, 1991

Library of Congress Cataloging-in-Publication Data

The cardiac catheterization handbook / edited by Morton J. Kern; foreword by William
Grossman.—4th ed.
    p. ; cm.
  Includes bibliographical references and index.
  ISBN 0-323-02247-2
  1. Cardiac catheterization—Handbooks, manuals, etc. I. Kern, Morton J.
  [DNLM: 1. Heart Catheterization. WG 141.5.C2 C2675 2003]
  RC683.5.C25 C39 2003
  616.1'20754—dc21   2002043186

Acquisitions Editor: Anne Lenehan
Developmental Editor: Sarah Cameron
Publishing Services Manager: Patricia Tannian
Project Manager: Sarah Wunderly
Book Design Manager: Gail Morey Hudson
Cover Designer: Jen Brockett

Printed in United States of America

Last digit is the print number: 9   8   7   6   5   4   3   2   1

CONTRIBUTORS

SAAD BITAR, MD
Assistant Professor of Medicine
The J. Gerard Mudd Cardiac Catheterization Laboratory
St. Louis University Health Sciences Center
St. Louis, Missouri

FRANK BLEYER, MD
Assistant Professor of Medicine
St. Louis University Health Sciences Center
St. Louis, Missouri

ANNE BRADLEY
Associate General Counsel
St. Louis University Health Sciences Center
St. Louis, Missouri

TED FELDMAN, MD, FSCAI, FACC
Professor of Medicine
Northwestern Medical School
Director, Cardiac Catheterization Laboratory
Evanston Hospital
Evanston, Illinois

STEVE HERRMANN, MD
Instructor in Medicine
The J. Gerard Mudd Cardiac Catheterization Laboratory
St. Louis University Health Sciences Center
St. Louis, Missouri

DENISE L. JANOSIK, MD
Associate Professor of Medicine, Electrophysiology Laboratory
St. Louis University Health Sciences Center
St. Louis, Missouri

GLENN LEVINE, MD
Assistant Professor of Medicine
University of Texas Health Sciences Center
Houston, Texas

KEVIN LISMAN, MD
Cardiology Fellow
University of Texas Health Sciences Center
Houston, Texas

SANJEEV PURI, MD
Assistant Professor of Medicine
The J. Gerard Mudd Cardiac Catheterization Laboratory
St. Louis University Health Sciences Center
St. Louis, Missouri

ANTONELLA QUATTROMANI, MD
Assistant Professor of Medicine
Electrophysiology Laboratory
St. Louis University Health Sciences Center
St. Louis, Missouri

HASSAN RAJJOUB, MD
Instructor in Medicine
The J. Gerard Mudd Cardiac Catheterization Laboratory
St. Louis University Health Sciences Center
St. Louis, Missouri

ROBERT ROTH, RN
Manager, Cardiovascular Services
St. Louis University Health Sciences Center
St. Louis, Missouri

LISA SCHILLER, MD
Assistant Professor of Medicine
Electrophysiology Laboratory
St. Louis University Health Sciences Center
St. Louis, Missouri

To
Margaret and **Anna Rose**

FOREWORD

The expansion and widespread application of cardiac catheterization throughout the world today could hardly have been imagined by Werner Forssmann when, in 1929, he was the first to pass a catheter into the heart of a living person—himself. For many years, cardiac catheterization remained primarily an investigative tool, but the precise information concerning anatomy and physiology in patients with heart disease that cardiac catheterization procedures yielded made possible the development of open heart surgery. Forssmann's initial intent, as stated in his historic article published in *Klinische Wochenschrift* in 1929, was to use cardiac catheterization as a therapeutic technique. In the last 15 years, cardiac catheterization has amply fulfilled Forssmann's dream, and each month sees the addition of new therapeutic innovations based on advanced catheter technologies.

Cardiac catheterization is practiced in every major university hospital throughout the United States and is rapidly expanding to the point where even moderate-sized community hospitals have active programs of cardiac catheterization and angiography. This expansion of the field has led to increased demands for training of physicians, nurses, and technicians expert in the highly technical and demanding aspects of intravascular catheterization and angiography. *The Cardiac Catheterization Handbook* provides an outstanding teaching manual for these individuals. This is a well-written and clearly focused book. So many aspects of cardiac catheterization and angiography cannot be explained simply through the use of description; this book has many excellent figures and diagrams that help the reader to understand precisely what is meant in the text. Pressure tracings are presented and are most helpful in the identification of specific conditions such as valvular stenosis, constrictive pericarditis, and cardiomyopathy. A chapter on high-risk cardiac catheterization defines the patient subgroups most likely to have complications during cardiac catheterization and angiography and gives helpful suggestions as to how these complications might be avoided. A chapter on interventional techniques provides a highly concise and practical description of state-of-the-art aspects of coronary angioplasty, including illustrations of application of the technique. Balloon valvuloplasty for aortic and mitral stenosis is a relatively new technique that is discussed in clear detail, with practical suggestions for application. The use of thrombolytic agents in dealing with acute thrombotic states is discussed, with practical aspects (including dosages and routes of administration) described in detail. A unique chapter on medicolegal issues in the cardiac catheterization laboratory offers helpful hints as to common failings of documentation and record keeping, which must be avoided by the physician who wishes to protect himself or herself against inappropriate malpractice suits. Finally, there are excellent chapters dealing with the formulas for calculation of angiographic volumes, valve areas, and other hemodynamic parameters.

This handbook has become a valued companion for trainees entering into the cardiac catheterization laboratory. Dr. Kern and his coauthors are to be congratulated on an impressive accomplishment.

William Grossman, MD

Dana Professor of Medicine
Harvard Medical School
Chief, Cardiovascular Division
Beth Israel Hospital
Boston, Massachusetts

PREFACE
to the Fourth Edition

The Cardiac Catheterization Handbook continues to be a valuable tool for health care professionals beginning their experience in cardiac catheterization. This handbook is designed to provide the cardiovascular physician-in-training, noninvasive cardiologist, cardiovascular nurse and technician, related industry personnel, as well as practicing cardiologists unfamiliar with the cardiac catheterization laboratory, with a practical guide and basic introduction to the performance and care of patients undergoing cardiac catheterization.

As with every technique in medicine, cardiac catheterization has undergone continuous evolution from its inception more than 50 years ago. In this fourth edition, in addition to the basic approach to the patient undergoing cardiac catheterization, we highlight conscious sedation, new vascular access techniques, and vascular closure methods. Angiographic techniques are simplified, and angiography for peripheral vascular disease and other systems commonly examined in the catheterization laboratory is discussed. Hemodynamic data study, a lost art in many cardiac catheterization laboratories, is updated. The study of pressure waveforms is important because waveforms remain the underlying standard for the evaluation of many cardiovascular abnormalities, especially those involving cardiac valves or cardiomyopathy. New approaches to common electrophysiologic problems are reviewed. Special techniques involving myocardial biopsy, pericardiocentesis, intraaortic balloon pumping, and foreign body retrieval are updated. High-risk catheterization is discussed in detail, with current ACS guidelines emphasizing preventive measures and management of the patient in extremis.

The handbook also provides practical points of patient care, handling of intravascular equipment, and evaluation of angiographic, electrocardiographic, and hemodynamic data.

Common errors and artifacts in data collection as well as waveform interpretation are emphasized. Pertinent medico-legal aspects of catheterization laboratory documentation and management are summarized by a member of St. Louis University's legal staff. Appropriate angiographic, hemodynamic, and other special methods (IVUS, FFR) and their examples are provided to elucidate confusing problems.

Finally, the chapter on interventional cardiology procedures is updated, describing the current applications of coronary stenting, physiologic methods for lesion assessment, thrombus aspiration, and rotational ablation. As with all areas of cardiology, these methods are rapidly changing with multicenter clinical outcome research.

I remain grateful to the staff of the J.G. Mudd Cardiac Catheterization Laboratory, my coauthors, our cardiology trainees, nurses, administrative staff, and Mary Streif for her secretarial assistance. I also thank my wife, Margaret, and daughter, Anna Rose, who as I mentioned in *Hemodynamic Rounds*, are the systole of my life.

It is my hope that *The Cardiac Catheterization Handbook* will continue as a mainstay of education in the cardiac catheterization laboratory for years to come.

Morton J. Kern, MD

PREFACE
to the Third Edition

The Cardiac Catheterization Handbook has been valued by health care professionals entering the cardiac catheterization laboratory as well as experienced cardiologists wishing to review the fundamentals and new techniques used in catheterization. With this revision we have continued the tradition of providing teaching materials and fundamentals in a basic format for the physician-in-training and cardiovascular nurse/technician professionals working within the cardiac catheterization laboratory. As we have emphasized before, this practical guide and introduction to the invasive practice of cardiology is not an all-inclusive handbook, and the reader should refer to the excellent works of Dr. William Grossman, Dr. Carl Pepine, Dr. Barry Uretsky, and others who have provided full descriptions of the cardiac catheterization methodology.

This edition highlights several of the new advances in the cardiac catheterization laboratory, focusing on radiation safety, new approaches to vascular access and hemostasis, expansion of hemodynamic examples and case results, outcomes for physiologic measurements for interventional procedures, and updates on the interventional methodologies for atherectomy, stenting, and thrombus aspiration. As with all changing techniques, the details regarding new approaches are altered as discoveries have been validated. The fundamentals remain sound and the evolution of invasive approaches is still key to the practice of interventional cardiology.

I am continually grateful to the contributions of the J. Gerard Mudd Cardiac Catheterization Laboratory to my own education and to that of our colleagues. I greatly appreciate the steadfast and diligent work of Donna Sander in making my thoughts come true in text form. Finally, I would like to acknowledge the continued encouragement and support of my wife, Margaret, and my daughter, Anna Rose. We hope the

Cardiac Catheterization Handbook remains a pillar for the teaching of techniques in the cardiac catheterization laboratory.

Morton J. Kern

PREFACE
to the Second Edition

One of the most satisfying events in academic medicine and cardiology is the acceptance of material to teach the fundamentals to individuals-in-training. This goal has been largely achieved in the first edition. We hope to continue the tradition by providing complete information in a basic format for the physician-in-training, noninvasive cardiologist, cardiovascular nurse, and technician within the cardiac catheterization laboratory. As indicated in the preface to the first edition, this practical guide and introductory framework is not intended to be all-inclusive, and the reader is referred to the excellent works of Drs. Grossman and Pepine and others, who provide enhanced detail and in-depth description, background, and methodology for the techniques indicated. This edition is notable for additions in many areas, especially interventional techniques. Catheterization laboratory environmental safety and OSHA precautions are added to Chapter 1. The complications of vascular access and new methods of hemostasis are discussed in Chapter 2. More hemodynamic examples (Chapter 3), an approach to electrophysiologic procedures (Chapter 4), how-to methods for coronary Doppler blood flow (Chapter 6), intra-aortic balloon pump use in high-risk patients (Chapter 8), and descriptions of now standard atherectomy and coronary stent placement (Chapter 9) are also among the updated sections.

Again, I would like to acknowledge the J. Gerard Mudd Cardiac Catheterization Team. The encouragement of my wife, Margaret, and daughter, Anna Rose, was greatly appreciated. I would also like to acknowledge the support of Dr. Frank Hildner in providing a forum for much of the hemodynamic material that has been published in *Catheterization and Cardiovascular Diagnosis* under the continuing series of hemodynamic rounds.

Morton J. Kern

PREFACE
to the First Edition

This handbook is designed to provide the cardiovascular physician-in-training, noninvasive cardiologist, cardiovascular nurse, and other technical personnel unfamiliar with the cardiac catheterization laboratory a practical guide and basic introductory framework for the techniques used and care of the patient undergoing cardiac catheterization.

The handbook is not designed to be all-inclusive. The comprehensive, complete, and detailed works (referenced at the end of Chapter 1) on cardiac catheterization are required reading. The introduction to the cardiac catheterization laboratory presented in this book discusses many seemingly obvious—but often overlooked—important points with regard to approach to the patient and routine angiographic and hemodynamic methodology. Practical points of patient care, handling intravascular equipment, evaluation of angiographic and hemodynamic data, and common errors and artifacts in data collection and interpretation are emphasized. Pertinent medicolegal aspects in catheterization laboratory management are reviewed. Where appropriate, examples are provided to help clarify confusing problems.

The invasive aspects of the practice of cardiology should not be undertaken by the uncommitted and not begun until the basics have been mastered. Although the safety of cardiac catheterization has improved greatly over the years, dedication to technique and patient safety must remain the highest priority of the operator and the cardiac catheterization team.

I want to thank the J. Gerard Mudd Cardiac Catheterization Team, Donna Sander for book preparation, and MMDK, ARDK.

Morton J. Kern

CONTENTS

4   ANGIOGRAPHIC DATA, 217
Saad Bitar and Morton J. Kern

5   ELECTROPHYSIOLOGIC STUDIES AND ABLATION TECHNIQUES, 326
Denise L. Janosik, Antonella Quattromani, and Lisa Schiller

6   RESEARCH TECHNIQUES, 379
Steve Herrmann, Morton J. Kern, and Sanjeev Puri

1

INTRODUCTION TO THE CATHETERIZATION LABORATORY

Morton J. Kern and Robert Roth

Cardiac catheterization is the insertion and passage of small plastic tubes (catheters) into arteries and veins to the heart to obtain x-ray pictures (angiography) of coronary arteries and cardiac chambers and to measure pressures in the heart (hemodynamics). The cardiac catheterization laboratory performs angiography to obtain images not only to diagnose coronary artery disease, but also to look for diseases of the aorta and pulmonary and peripheral vessels. Besides providing diagnostic information, the cardiac catheterization laboratory performs catheter-based interventions (e.g., angioplasty) to treat acute cardiovascular illness. Table 1-1 lists procedures that can be performed with coronary angiography.

INDICATIONS FOR CARDIAC CATHETERIZATION

Cardiac catheterization is used to identify structural cardiac diseases such as atherosclerotic artery disease, abnormalities of heart muscle (infarction or cardiomyopathy), and valvular or congenital heart abnormalities. In adults the procedure is used most commonly to diagnose coronary artery disease. Other indications depend on the history, physical examination, electrocardiogram (ECG), cardiac stress test, echocardiographic results, and chest radiograph. Indications for cardiac catheterization are summarized in Table 1-2.

Elective Procedures

In general, cardiac catheterization is an elective diagnostic procedure and should be deferred if the patient is not prepared either psychologically or physically.

Table 1-1

Procedures That May Accompany Coronary Angiography*

Procedure	Comment
1. Central venous access (femoral, internal jugular, subclavian)	Used as IV access for emergency medications or fluids, temporary pacemaker (pacemaker not mandatory for coronary angiography)
2. Hemodynamic assessment	
a. Left heart pressures (aorta, left ventricle)	Routine for all studies
b. Right and left heart combined pressures	Not routine for coronary artery disease; mandatory for valvular heart disease; routine for congestive heart failure (CHF), right ventricular dysfunction, pericardial diseases, cardiomyopathy, intracardiac shunts, congenital abnormalities
3. Left ventricular angiography	Routine for all studies; may be excluded with high-risk patients, left main coronary or aortic stenosis, severe CHF, renal failure
4. Internal mammary artery selective angiography	Not routine unless used as coronary bypass conduit
5. Pharmacologic studies	
a. Ergonovine	Routine for suspected coronary vasospasm
b. Intracoronary/intravenous/ sublingual nitroglycerin	Routine for all coronary angiography
6. Aortography	Routine for aortic insufficiency, aortic dissection, aortic aneurysm, with or without aortic stenosis, routine to locate bypass grafts not visualized by selective angiography
7. Cardiac pacing and electrophysiologic studies	Arrhythmia evaluation
8. Interventional and special techniques	Coronary angioplasty (e.g., PTCA, stenting) Intracoronary flow-pressure for lesion assessment Balloon catheter valvuloplasty Myocardial biopsy Transseptal or direct left ventricular puncture Conduction tract catheter ablation
9. Arterial closure devices	Available for patients prone to access site bleeding

PTCA, Percutaneous transluminal coronary angioplasty.
*See Table 1-2 for indications.

Table 1-2

Indications for Cardiac Catheterization

Indications	Procedures
1. Suspected or known coronary artery disease	
a. New-onset angina	LV, COR
b. Unstable angina	LV, COR
c. Evaluation before a major surgical procedure	LV, COR
d. Silent ischemia	LV, COR, ERGO
e. Positive exercise tolerance test	LV, COR, ERGO
f. Atypical chest pain or coronary spasm	LV, COR, ERGO
2. Myocardial infarction	
a. Unstable angina postinfarction	LV, COR
b. Failed thrombolysis	LV, COR, RH
c. Shock	LV, COR, RH
d. Mechanical complications (ventricular septal defect, rupture of wall or papillary muscle)	LV, COR, RH
3. Sudden cardiovascular death	LV, COR, R + L
4. Valvular heart disease	LV, COR, R + L, AO
5. Congenital heart disease (before anticipated corrective surgery)	LV, COR, R + L, AO
6. Aortic dissection	AO, COR
7. Pericardial constriction or tamponade	LV, COR, R + L
8. Cardiomyopathy	LV, COR, R + L, BX
9. Initial and follow-up assessment for heart transplant	LV, COR, R + L, BX

AO, aortography; *BX*, endomyocardial biopsy; *COR*, coronary angiography; *ERGO*, ergonovine provocation of coronary spasm; *LV*, left ventriculography; *RH*, right heart oxygen saturations and hemodynamics (e.g., placement of Swan-Ganz catheter); *R + L*, right and left heart hemodynamics.

Urgent Procedures

If the patient's condition is unstable because of a suspected cardiac disorder, such as acute myocardial infarction, catheterization must proceed. In the event of decompensated congestive heart failure, rapid medical management is often needed. A patient must be able to lie flat for easy catheter passage. Such acute cardiac decompensation may benefit more, however, from aggressive management in the catheterization laboratory than from management in an intensive care unit. In the catheterization laboratory, intubation, intraaortic balloon pumping, and vasopressors can be instituted rapidly before angiography and a decision for revascularization.

CONTRAINDICATIONS

Contraindications include fever, anemia, electrolyte imbalance (especially hypokalemia predisposing to arrhythmias), and other systemic illnesses needing stabilization (Box 1-1).

COMPLICATIONS AND RISKS

For diagnostic catheterization, analysis of the complications in more than 200,000 patients indicated the incidence of risks as death, less than 0.2%; myocardial infarction, less than 0.05%; stroke, less than 0.07%; serious ventricular arrhythmia, less than 0.5%; and major vascular complications (thrombosis, bleeding requiring transfusion, or pseudoaneurysm), less than 1% (Box 1-2 and Table 1-3). Vascular complications occurred more frequently when the brachial approach was used. Risks are increased in well-described subgroups (Box 1-3).

CATHETERIZATION LABORATORY DATA

Information gathered during the cardiac catheterization can be divided into two categories: hemodynamic (see Chapter 3) and

---

Box 1-1

Contraindications to Cardiac Catheterization

Absolute Contraindications
Inadequate equipment or catheterization facility

Relative Contraindications
Acute gastrointestinal bleeding or anemia
Anticoagulation (or known, uncontrolled bleeding diathesis)
Electrolyte imbalance
Infection and fever
Medication intoxication (e.g., digitalis, phenothiazine)
Pregnancy
Recent cerebrovascular accident (<1 month)
Renal failure
Uncontrolled congestive heart failure, high blood pressure, arrhythmias
Uncooperative patient

Box 1-2

Complications of Cardiac Catheterization

Major
Cerebrovascular accident
Death
Myocardial infarction
Ventricular tachycardia, fibrillation, or serious arrhythmia

Other
Aortic dissection
Cardiac perforation, tamponade
Congestive heart failure
Contrast reaction (anaphylaxis, nephrotoxicity)
Heart block, asystole
Hemorrhage (local, retroperitoneal, pelvic)
Infection
Protamine reaction
Supraventricular tachyarrhythmia, atrial fibrillation
Thrombosis, embolus, air embolus
Vascular injury, pseudoaneurysm
Vasovagal reaction

Table 1-3

Major Complications of Diagnostic Catheterizations

	Number	Percent
Death	65	0.11
Myocardial infarction	30	0.05
Neurologic	41	0.07
Arrhythmia	229	0.38
Vascular	256	0.43
Contrast	223	0.37
Hemodynamic	158	0.26
Perforation	16	0.03
Other	166	0.28
Total (patients)	*1184*	*1.98*

Modified from Noto TJ, Johnson LW, Krone R, et al: Cardiac catheterization 1990: a report of the Registry of the Society for Cardiac Angiography and Interventions (SCA&I), *Cathet Cardiovasc Diagn* 24:75-83, 1991; in Uretzky BF, Weinert HH: *Cardiac catheterization: concepts, techniques, and applications*, Walden, Mass, 1997, Blackwell Science.

Box 1-3

Conditions of Patients at Higher Risk for Complications of Catheterization*

Acute myocardial infarction
Advanced age (>75 years)
Aortic aneurysm
Aortic stenosis
Congestive heart failure
Diabetes
Extensive three-vessel coronary artery disease
Left ventricular dysfunction (left ventricular ejection fraction <35%)
Obesity
Prior cerebrovascular accident
Renal insufficiency
Suspected or known left main coronary stenosis
Uncontrolled hypertension
Unstable angina

*See also Chapter 8.

cineangiographic (see Chapter 4). The term cineangiography describes the x-ray photography of cardiac structures. Use of this term persists even though the images are now stored electronically on digital computer imaging media (e.g., CD-ROM) rather than on cine film. The cineangiogram provides anatomic information about the chambers of the heart and the coronary arteries. Hemodynamic information is recorded from catheters inside the heart and consists of pressure measurements, cardiac outputs, and blood oxygen saturation measurements.

PREPARATION OF THE PATIENT
Consent for the Procedure

Consent is obtained by the operator or his or her assistant, usually a physician:

1. Explain in simple terms what procedure will take place and for what reason each step of the procedure will occur.
2. Explain the risks for routine cardiac catheterization. Major risks include stroke, myocardial infarction, and death. Minor risks include vascular injury, allergic reaction, bleeding, hematoma, and infection.

3. Explain any portions of the study used for research and the associated risks (e.g., electrophysiologic study—perforation, arrhythmia [<1:500]; pharmacologic study—varies depending on drug and study duration; intracoronary Doppler or pressure wire study—spasm, myocardial infarction, embolus, dissection [<1:500]).
4. Provide the necessary information and explanation, but do not overwhelm the patient.

There is no alternative to coronary angiography. Often the patient's and family's concern about "not knowing" about coronary disease necessitates performing the test.

The decision to undergo the procedure is always the patient's. If the patient is reluctant to have the catheterization, the referring physician should be asked to speak to the patient to clarify why the procedure is necessary. A reluctant patient should never sign the consent. When possible, the family should be present when the procedure is discussed. This approach encourages a cooperative and generally sympathetic appreciation of the procedure and expected outcome.

Communication with Patients: A Nonmedical Person's Understanding

The clinician establishes rapport and builds the patient's confidence by listening and explaining. The procedure should be discussed with the patient in terms he or she can understand. The purpose of the procedure should be clear—"to look at the coronary arteries" and "to examine the heart muscle (ventricular function)." Simple terms are best so that the patient can grasp the concepts. The clinician should explain what small catheters are (plastic tubes similar in size to spaghetti) and that they will be used to put x-ray contrast dye into the arteries supplying blood to the heart. The heart muscle may be weakened (infarcted) in certain areas, and the way to identify this weakness is to take x-ray pictures. This example of a simple, forthright explanation facilitates the operator team–patient relationship so that confidence in the operator and team performing the procedure is established.

Laboratory Atmosphere: The Patient's Confidence Builder

1. In the laboratory a confident, professional attitude should be assumed by all personnel at all times.

Straightforward routine communication should occur quietly and without alarming tones. Patients should be addressed directly, by name, to let them know what their instructions are as opposed to requests or communications to co-workers.

2. The circulating team members should be confident, reassuring, and professional in every respect. The patient feels helpless and is tuned in to all types of stimuli (especially verbal).

3. Extraneous conversation is distracting for the patient and the operators. In the laboratory, all "players" should be in the game; that is, the patient's needs and safety become paramount.

4. Communication with the patient (and family) before, during, and after the procedure ensures a satisfied and well-cared-for individual.

5. Factory worker attitudes of "another coronary" or "another transplant" should be avoided. Each procedure is potentially life threatening and should be undertaken seriously and with concern as if each patient were a family member.

6. Cardiac catheterization is stressful to the patient and the operator team. This stress should be minimized by thoughtful preparation and professional attention to detail.

7. Practical notes for the new operator include the following: Immediately before the catheterization in the laboratory, reexamination of the ECG is essential. A brief reiteration of the history ensures that no interval change has occurred since the last interview. A brief examination of the patient—checking heart sounds, breath sounds, and carotid and peripheral pulses—is also essential immediately before and after cardiac catheterization. No patient should be studied without full understanding of the clinical conditions and results of previous catheterizations and other pertinent laboratory data.

When on the catheterization table, the patient remembers two major potentially painful points of a case: (1) the initial introduction of the local anesthetic and (2) any discomfort experienced after the study has been completed. Such discomfort usually occurs while the operator or nurse is holding the puncture site. If the local anesthetic injection is performed too quickly or the arterial closure-compression after the procedure is difficult or painful, the patient will remember that the physician who performed the catheterization "hurt me." The period between the two events is often forgotten (thanks to premedication). These two points should be kept in mind as the major "take-home" messages. Patients cannot discern the operator's skill or level of accomplishment during the procedure, but they judge the operator (and the team) on the manner and care at the beginning and end of the study. Skill and accomplishment during the procedure are essential, but these are developed during the operator's training period.

8. General catheterization orders are as follows: Before catheterization, preferably the preceding night, pre-catheterization orders should be written. All medications and procedural premedications should be tailored to the patient and timing of the catheterization. If the patient is using long-acting (neutral protamine hagedorn [NPH]) insulin, the dose should be reduced 50%, and the patient should not eat breakfast. The patient should be watched carefully for hypoglycemic reactions (e.g., shaking, confusion, and slurred speech).

9. Patients should wear their glasses and dentures to make communication easier.

In-Laboratory Preparations

The staff of the cardiac catheterization laboratory is responsible for patient preparation before the start of the procedure. On the patient's arrival in the laboratory, a staff member should review a brief checklist to ensure that all preprocedural requirements have been met. A sample checklist follows:

—Check the patient's ID band.
—Check blood pressure and baseline ECG.
—Check baseline peripheral pulses.
—Check known allergies.
—Determine whether the patient has received recent anticoagulation therapy. If so, measure the international normalized ratio and partial thromboplastin time.

—Check whether a female patient has childbearing potential by measuring β-human chorionic gonadotropin levels.

—Assess the patient's understanding of the procedure and answer the patient's questions.

—Verify that the proper paperwork has been copied and filled out for the procedure.

—Check laboratory results (key tests: blood urea nitrogen, creatinine, prothrombin time, partial thromboplastin time, electrolytes).

—Check that the consents for the procedure are signed and in the chart. If not, make arrangements for consent.

—Check that the intravenous (IV) line is patent.

—Check that the patient has ingested nothing by mouth before the procedure.

—Check whether premedications were given as ordered.

—Document the precatheterization condition, and note any physical deficits.

After all precatheterization requirements have been fulfilled, the patient may be taken to the angiographic suite, and the technical preparations can be completed.

Catheterization Suite Preparations

Before the start of the catheterization procedure, the staff performs the following tasks:

1. *Establishes ECG monitoring.* The ECG should be considered first of the two major "lifelines." The heartbeat is monitored for rate and rhythm during the entire procedure. It is the responsibility of the staff to place the electrodes and lead wires in such a fashion that a quality trace is obtained. Care must be taken that the electrodes and lead wires do not interfere with the movement of the x-ray and cineangiographic unit. All leads should be secure, and a good signal should be present before the application of sterile drapes; reaching under the sterile drapes to reattach loose lead wires once the procedure has begun is difficult. Radiolucent leads permit complete 12-lead ECG monitoring but are more prone to breakage than heavier cable leads.

2. *Establishes intravenous (IV) access for emergency medications or sedation.* The second lifeline is the IV access. Emergency drugs to counteract vagal or allergic reactions or other problems are best administered by this route. In

most cases the patient is given an oral or intramuscular sedative as premedication before arriving at the cardiac catheterization laboratory. When the patient is in the laboratory, the nurse or physician may identify the need for additional sedation or analgesia before the start of the procedure. The IV line is also important for hydration after cardiac catheterization.

Caution must be exercised when premedicating elderly patients. If meperidine (Demerol), fentanyl, or morphine is used, a narcotic antagonist such as naloxone (Narcan) should be available. Flumazenil (a benzodiazepine antagonist) should also be available if diazepam (Valium) or midazolam (Versed) is used.

Sterile Preparations

Cardiac catheterization is performed using aseptic technique.

Vascular Access Site Preparation. The most common vascular access site is the right or left groin for the femoral approach or the right (or occasionally left) wrist for the radial artery approach. The usual sterile preparation begins by shaving the area and vigorously applying an antiseptic solution. Shaving should be done carefully to avoid lacerations or abrasions.

During patient preparation the staff should always be aware of the patient's need for privacy. The patient should be kept covered as much as possible. Procedure rooms are typically cold; every effort should be made to keep the patient warm and comfortable.

Sterile Field Preparation and Patient Draping. A staff member assigned to assist the physician in the procedure puts on a hair cover and surgical facemask and washes the hands and forearms as a surgical scrub. He or she then puts on a sterile surgical gown and gloves. A sterile drape is placed over the patient, starting at the patient's upper chest and extending to the foot, covering the entire examination table. An equipment stand is prepared in a sterile fashion to hold all the sterile catheters and other equipment to be used during the procedure. At this time, a circulating staff member hands catheters and necessary equipment not included in the sterile catheter laboratory pack to the scrub nurse or technician.

It is important for all personnel to understand sterile techniques to avoid accidentally contaminating any sterile fields. As a basic rule, no unsterile object may be passed over a sterile field. When moving around a crowded angiographic room, all personnel should be careful to avoid bumping into or passing hands or arms over the sterile tray, table, or patient drapes. Personnel should not walk between the sterile table or equipment tray and the patient. Touching the ends of any catheters, extension tubes, or syringe tips in a sterile field or the power injector syringe tip that is exposed should be avoided.

Observers in the Laboratory. Any observers in the angiographic room should respect the professional atmosphere and keep extraneous conversation to a minimum. Observers should wear a lead apron as protection against secondary and scattered radiation. Usually it is unnecessary for observers to wear gowns. Observers should avoid sterile fields and should be aware of the precautions necessary for protection from blood and body fluids.

No one but catheterization laboratory personnel should ever manipulate or adjust any device, equipment, or medication system in the laboratory. To prevent observers who are not laboratory personnel from becoming overly enthusiastic and attempting to assist the nurses or physicians, they should never be given sterile gloves. This is an important potential liability issue for the laboratory, hospital, and staff.

Conscious Sedation for Invasive Cardiac Procedure

The purpose of conscious sedation is to relieve patient anxiety, discomfort, or pain associated with the procedure.

Definition
The following criteria define conscious sedation:
  1. The patient at no time loses protective reflexes.
  2. The patient retains the ability to maintain an open airway continuously without help.
  3. The patient responds appropriately to verbal and physical stimulation.

When the patient can no longer do the things listed, the sedative technique has evolved to deep sedation or general anesthesia. At this point the monitoring and care of the patient must be elevated to avoid an adverse outcome.

A conscious sedation protocol has four major components: (1) preprocedure baseline assessment, (2) drug dosage and administration, (3) patient monitoring, and (4) postprocedure monitoring and assessment and discharge criteria.

Preprocedure Assessment. Before the administration of sedative agents the patient should have a complete assessment of his or her current physical condition. The clinician should pay particular attention to any preexisting conditions that would put the patient at risk for an adverse outcome if sedatives are administered. A preprocedure evaluation should include a review of the major organ systems, the time and type of the last oral intake, a history of drug and alcohol use, a history of smoking, and a history of previous experience with sedative agents.

Preprocedure Fasting. Sedative agents may impair airway reflexes, placing the patient at increased risk for aspirating gastric contents. For elective procedures these risks can be minimized by allowing sufficient time for gastric emptying before the procedure. The patient should be NPO for solids and nonclear liquids after midnight or at least 8 hours before the start of the procedure. Clear liquids may be appropriate 1 to 3 hours before the procedure, depending on the type and dose of the sedative agent to be used.

Physical Examination and Airway Assessment. An airway assessment should be part of the preprocedure routine. Factors associated with difficult airway management include the following:
1. A history of sleep apnea, snoring, or stridor
2. Dysmorphic jaw or facial features
3. Advanced rheumatoid arthritis
4. A short neck with limited extension caused by obesity, mass, or injury
5. Mouth or jaw irregularities or deformities, including loose or capped teeth or dentures

American Society of Anesthesiologists Physical Status Classification. The American Society of Anesthesiologists Physical Status

Classification (Table 1-4) is helpful in determining the patient's eligibility for conscious sedation. It uses a 1 to 5 classification range, with 1 being a healthy patient and 5 being a moribund patient.

Monitoring Parameters

Level of Consciousness. The patient's level of consciousness should be assessed frequently before and during the procedure. The level of consciousness can be assessed by the patient's response to verbal commands or to light tactile stimulation. Once aroused, the patient should respond appropriately to verbal commands. The nurse or operator can assess this easily by periodically talking to the patient and listening to his or her response. When the patient's only response is reflex withdrawal from painful stimuli, deep sedation is evident, and special care must be taken to ensure patency of the airway, proper ventilation, and hemodynamic stability.

Pulmonary Ventilation. Pulmonary ventilation can be monitored by the observation of spontaneous respiratory activity or, when possible, auscultation of breath sounds. During certain invasive procedures, direct monitoring of the respiratory rate is often difficult because of sterile drapes and equipment.

Table 1-4

American Society of Anesthesiologists Physical Status Classification

Class	Description
1	A healthy patient (e.g., varicose veins in an otherwise healthy patient)
2	A patient with mild systemic disease that in no way interferes with normal activity (e.g., controlled hypertension, controlled diabetes, or chronic bronchitis)
3	A patient with severe systemic disease that is not incapacitating (e.g., insulin-dependent diabetes, angina, pulmonary insufficiency)
4	A patient with severe systemic disease that is a constant threat to life (e.g., cardiac failure, major organ insufficiency)
5	A moribund patient who is not expected to survive for 24 hours with or without surgery (e.g., intracranial hemorrhage in coma)

Oxygenation. Continuous assessment of the patient's blood oxygen saturation by pulse oximetry should be a part of any conscious sedation monitoring and assessment protocol. This monitor is only a tool and not a replacement for direct observation of the patient. There can be a 1-minute delay between the onset of hypoxia and the decrease in the monitor reading.

Hemodynamics. Sedative agents may cause arrhythmias and hypotension. Although continuous ECG monitoring is performed during preprocedure patient preparations, blood pressure should also be monitored frequently at 1- to 2-minute intervals during the onset of sedation and 5- to 10-minute intervals during the procedure. Hemodynamics should return to baseline before discharge.

Aldrete Scoring System. The Aldrete Scoring System (Table 1-5) can be used to assess the effects of sedation on the patient's major systems (neurologic, respiratory, circulatory). A score of 0, 1, or 2 is given for level of activity, level of consciousness, respiratory ability, blood pressure, and color.

Drugs for Conscious Sedation. First-line drugs and dosages for conscious sedation are listed in Table 1-6.

Postprocedure Monitoring and Discharge Criteria. Patients who receive conscious sedation should be monitored for 1 to 2 hours before discharge. During this time the patient should be assessed and monitored with the same parameters used in the preprocedure assessment. When the patient returns to baseline, discharge is appropriate. The following discharge criteria should be met before the patient is sent back to the floor or home:

1. The Aldrete score has returned to baseline (Aldrete score 9 or 10).
2. At least 2 hours has elapsed since the last dose of sedative agents.
3. Vital signs have returned to baseline.
4. Ventilation (respiratory rate and oxygen saturation) has returned to baseline.

Table 1-5

Aldrete Scoring System

Score	Activity	Respiration	Circulation	Consciousness	Color
2	Able to move four extremities	Able to breathe deeply and cough	BP ± 20% of baseline	Fully alert and answers questions	Normal pink
1	Able to move two extremities	Limited respiratory effort (dyspnea)	BP ± 20-50% of baseline	Arousable	Pale, dusky, blotchy
0	Not able to control any extremities	No spontaneous respiratory effort	BP >50% of baseline	Failure to elicit response	Frank cyanosis

BP, blood pressure.

Table 1-6

First-Line Drugs for Conscious Sedation

Drug	Dose	Max	Onset (min)	Duration (min)
Morphine (narcotic analgesic)	1-2 mg	10 mg or 0.15 mg/kg	1-2	30-60
Meperidine (narcotic analgesic)	10-20 mg	100 mg or 1.5 mg/kg	1-2	20-40
Fentanyl (narcotic analgesic)	10 µg	200 3 µg/kg	1	10-15
Midazolam (sedative, amnesic)	0.5-1.0 mg	5-10 mg or 0.1 mg/kg	1-3	15-30

5. The patient is mentally alert, and all protective reflexes are intact.

Outpatients who are being discharged to home should be able to ambulate appropriately for their age and condition. An escort should be available, and the patient should be instructed about not driving a motor vehicle for an appropriate period.

Postcatheterization

Checkup. The operator should check on the patient several hours after the procedure. Vital signs should be stable. Low blood pressure is usually due to diuresis and responds to normal saline. Tachycardia with low blood pressure indicates blood loss until proved otherwise. The arterial access site should be checked for pain and hematoma. The operator should check for loss of distal pulses. Urine output should be greater than 30 ml/hr. Low urine output may reflect unsatisfactory volume replacement or early onset of contrast-induced renal failure. A cool extremity requires immediate assessment to determine whether thrombus, spasm, or vasoconstriction is responsible for arterial occlusion. If thrombus is suspected, aspirin, 325 mg, should be given orally or heparin, 5000 U bolus plus 1000 U/hr, should be started intravenously. Limb ischemia or an enlarging hematoma requires urgent consultation with a vascular surgeon.

Angiogram Review. To provide the patient and family with an understanding of the coronary artery disease or other findings, a preliminary schematic diagram of the heart and coronary arteries can be provided. A similar diagram should be put in the chart to help others understand the findings. A catheterization instruction book is helpful and may contain a blank standard diagram. The booklet explains the catheterization procedure and the possible meaning of various findings on the coronary angiogram. In some cases, reviewing the actual coronary cineangiograms with the patient and family members may be helpful. After discharge the patient may wish to see the angiograms to understand the disease better and to ask questions and receive answers specifically with regard to future treatment (after the operator discusses the findings and plans with the primary care physician). Taking the time to explain the findings by referring directly to the diagram or cineangiographic film is rewarding. "No one ever took time to explain my heart problem this way, and now I understand what is wrong" is a frequent comment. The risk of a patient becoming alarmed or depressed after viewing the cine-angiogram has not been borne out by experience with more than 20,000 patients in our laboratory since the late 1960s. The time commitment by the physician (for whom showing the films is not routine) is an additional burden but is worth the effort. In busy laboratories this approach may not be feasible. The operator should always discuss the findings and possible recommendations with the primary physician first because catheterization is principally a consultative service.

SPECIAL PREPARATIONS

Table 1-7 lists conditions that require special preparations.

Contrast Media Reactions

The Committee on Safety of Contrast Media of the International Society of Radiology reported in more than 300,000 patients that the overall incidence of adverse reaction was 5% or less. Adverse reactions were found in 10% to 12% of patients with a history of allergy and in 15% of patients with reported reaction on previous x-ray examination. From these reports, major reactions do not tend to recur on reexamination, whereas minor reactions are more likely to be repeated.

There are three types of contrast allergies (Box 1-4): (1) cutaneous and mucosal manifestations, (2) smooth muscle and minor anaphylactoid responses, and (3) cardiovascular and major anaphylactoid responses. Management of contrast reactions is summarized in Fig. 1-1.

Major reactions involving laryngeal or pulmonary edema are often accompanied by minor, or less severe, reactions. Although some reactions to a pretest contrast dose may be violent (but rarely life threatening), pretesting has been found to be of no value in determining who will have an adverse reaction.

All procedures using contrast media should be assessed for the risk/benefit ratio. Full emergency resuscitation equipment and a trained team should always be available for any patient receiving contrast media. Nonionic contrast media have replaced ionic contrast media for most patients to minimize the chance of allergic and other adverse contrast reactions.

Table 1-7

Conditions Requiring Special Preparations

Condition	Management

1. Allergy
  a. Prior contrast studies
  b. Iodine, fish
  c. Premedication allergy
  d. Lidocaine
	1. Allergy
	  a. Contrast premedication
	  b. Contrast reaction algorithm
	  c. Hold premedication
	  d. Use Marcain (1 mg/ml)

2. Patients receiving anticoagulation (INR >1.5)	2. Defer procedure
	  a. Vitamin K^+, 10 mEq/hr
	  b. Fresh frozen plasma
	  c. Hold heparin
	  d. Protamine for heparin

3. Diabetes
  a. NPH insulin (protamine reaction)
  b. Renal function (prone to contrast-induced renal failure)
  c. Metformin usage
	3. Hydration to increase urine output >50 ml/hr; metformin held 48 hours; if renal insufficiency postpone catheterization and consider urgency and risks of lactic acidosis

4. Electrolyte imbalance (K^+, Mg^{2+})	4. Defer procedure, replenish or correct electrolytes
5. Arrhythmias	5. Defer procedure, administer antiarrhythmics

6. Anemia	6. Defer procedure
	  a. Control bleeding
	  b. Transfuse

7. Dehydration	7. Hydration

8. Renal failure	8. Limit contrast
	  a. Maintain high urine output
	  b. Hydrate

INR, international normalized ratio.

Patients reporting allergic reactions to contrast media should be premedicated with prednisone and diphenhydramine (Benadryl). The routine for the laboratory may vary, but common dosages include 60 mg of prednisone the night before and 60 mg of prednisone the morning of the procedure, along with 50 mg of oral Benadryl given at the time of call to the catheterization laboratory. Pretreatment with cortico-

Box 1-4

Anaphylactoid Reactions to Contrast Medium

Cutaneous and Mucosal
Angioedema
Flushing
Laryngeal edema
Pruritus
Urticaria

Smooth Muscle
Bronchospasm
Gastrointestinal spasm
Uterine contraction

Cardiovascular
Arrhythmia
Hypotension (shock)
Vasodilation

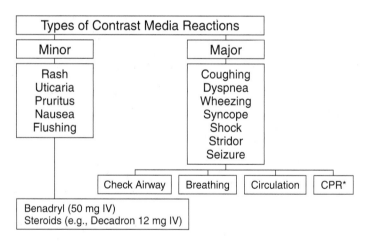

*See CPR algorithm Figure 8-1.

Fig. 1-1.   Types and management of contrast reactions. Before contrast administration, the patient should be asked if he or she has a history of reaction during prior x-ray procedures of artery, kidney, or gallbladder, or has a known allergy to fish. After contrast administration, the patient should be checked if a reaction is suspected; signs include hives, flushing, rash, and low blood pressure.

steroids to alleviate reactions to IV contrast media has been found to be helpful in reducing all types of reactions except those characterized predominantly by hives. Premedication may not completely prevent the occurrence of adverse reactions. Routine treatment of patients with prior allergic reactions with an H_2-blocker (e.g., cimetidine) does not appear to have any benefit. Patients with known prior anaphylactoid reactions to contrast dye should be pretreated with steroids and an H_2-blocker.

Protamine Reactions

Although protamine is used widely for reversing systemic heparinization after cardiac catheterization, major reactions simulating anaphylaxis can occur, albeit rarely. Minor protamine reactions may appear as back and flank pain or flushing with peripheral vasodilation and low blood pressure. Major reactions involve marked facial flushing and vasomotor collapse, which may be fatal. Patients taking NPH insulin have an increased sensitivity to protamine. The incidence of major protamine reactions in NPH insulin–dependent diabetics is 27% compared with 0.5% in patients with no history of insulin use. Diabetic patients receiving NPH insulin and patients with allergies to fish should not be given protamine after cardiac catheterization. If use of protamine is necessary for these patients, it should be administered cautiously in anticipation of a major reaction.

Contrast-Induced Renal Failure (Contrast-Induced Nephropathy)

Patients with diabetes or renal insufficiency or patients who are dehydrated from any cause are at risk for contrast-induced renal failure. Advance preparations to limit contrast-induced renal failure include hydration and maintenance of large-volume urine flow (≥ 200 ml/hr). These patients should be hydrated intravenously the night before the procedure. After the contrast study, IV fluids should be continued liberally unless intravascular volume overload is a problem. Furosemide (Lasix), mannitol, and calcium channel blockers are not helpful in reducing contrast-induced renal failure (Table 1-8). Fenoldopam given intravenously before the procedure is associated with reduced contrast-induced renal failure. After

Table 1-8

Summary of Contrast-Induced Renal Failure Prophylaxis Trials

Beneficial	Deleterious	Conflicting Data	No Effect
IV hydration	Furosemide (without volume replacement)	Calcium channel blockers	Hemodialysis
Forced diuresis	Ionic contrast	Dopamine	Atrial natriuretic peptide
Nonionic contrast	Endothelin receptor blocker	Theophylline	Allopurinol
Acetylcysteine	Mannitol (without volume replacement)	Captopril	
Prostaglandin E_1 Fenoldopam			

From McCullough PA, Mauley HS: Prediction and prevention of contrast nephropathy, *J Intervent Cardiol* 14:547-558, 2001.

the study the patient's urine output should be monitored. If output falls and is not responsive to increased IV fluids, renal insufficiency is probable. A consultation with a nephrologist may be helpful. Different types of contrast agents (ionic, nonionic, or low osmolar) have a similar incidence of contrast-induced nephropathy.

Insulin-Dependent Diabetic Patients

For patients taking subcutaneous insulin (NPH, regular), an overnight fast with their normal dose of insulin would cause hypoglycemia. The dose of NPH insulin should be decreased by 50% for patients coming to the catheterization laboratory when they are NPO in the early morning. Patients receiving NPH insulin are at higher risk for protamine reactions.

Diabetic Patients Using Metformin

Metformin (Glucophage) is an analog of phenformin, an oral antihyperglycemic agent that was withdrawn from the market because of the risk of lactic acidosis. Rare cases of metformin-associated lactic acidosis have been reported in diabetic patients with chronic renal insufficiency.

Contraindications and precautions in the product literature state:

> "Parenteral contrast studies with iodinated materials can lead to acute renal failure and have been associated with lactic acidosis in patients receiving Glucophage. Therefore, in patients in whom any such study is planned, Glucophage should be withheld for at least 48 hours prior to and 48 hours subsequent to the procedure and reinstituted only after renal function has been reevaluated and found to be normal."

Metformin is contraindicated in patients with renal dysfunction, as determined by elevated serum creatinine levels. There is no evidence that withholding metformin for 48 hours before a contrast procedure in patients with normal renal function provides any clinical benefit.

Pathophysiology of Metformin-Associated Lactic Acidosis.
Metformin is excreted unchanged in the urine. Approximately 90% of the absorbed drug is eliminated through the kidneys within the first 24 hours. Metformin is not nephrotoxic. The incidence of metformin-associated lactic acidosis is about 3 cases per 100,000 patient-years, and the mortality rate is about 1.5 cases per 100,000 patient-years. No cases of metformin-associated lactic acidosis occurred during 56,000 patient-years over a 10-year period in Canada. Since metformin became available in Europe in the late 1950s, there have been only 13 published cases of metformin-associated lactic acidosis in patients with acute renal failure precipitated by parenteral administration of iodinated contrast material. Of the 13 patients, 12 had renal impairment before contrast administration. In 10 of the 13 patients metformin administration was continued after the administration of the contrast medium. Metformin-associated lactic acidosis is aerobic and associated with drug accumulation in plasma, red blood cells, and tissue, a situation that should not occur unless the patient is in renal failure. Metformin accumulation cannot occur rapidly. Anaerobic lactic acidosis (e.g., cardiac or septic shock) can occur in diabetic patients who are incidentally taking metformin. Only confirmation of metformin accumulation in plasma and red blood cells proves that metformin lactic acidosis is present.

Guidelines for Use of Metformin and Iodinated Contrast Material*

A. Elective procedures

1. If renal function is normal (serum creatinine <1.5 mg/dl), contrast material may be administered parenterally without discontinuing metformin before the study. The patient should be hydrated.

2. After the study the patient should consult his or her physician before resuming metformin. In most cases the patient may resume metformin after 48 hours unless there is evidence of acute renal failure or the patient is at high risk for renal failure related to the following:

   a. Low cardiac output

   b. Hypovolemia

   c. Contrast administration (<72 hours) or excess contrast load >3 mg/kg

   d. Cyclosporine therapy

   Metformin may be resumed in these patients only after renal function is found to be normal.

3. If renal function is abnormal (serum creatinine ≥1.5 mg/dl), the contrast study should be canceled. The patient should contact his or her physician to discontinue metformin.

B. Emergency procedures

1. If renal function is normal, the study may proceed as with elective procedures.

2. If renal function is abnormal, the relative risks versus benefits must be considered and the following precautions taken.

   a. Discontinue metformin

   b. Hydrate the patient during and after the procedure (IV saline 1 ml/kg/hr)

   c. Increase urine output (if possible)

   d. Minimize the volume of low-osmolality contrast material

   e. Monitor renal function closely after the procedure

---

*Modified from the Society of Cardiac Angiography and Interventions, *Cathet Cardiovasc Diagn* 43:121-123, 1998.

f. If acute renal failure occurs after the procedure, monitor the patient for signs of lactic acidosis (e.g., abdominal pain, obtundation, hypotension, hypercapnia). Arterial blood gas analysis and measurement of plasma lactate, glucose, and ketones (including β-hydroxybutyrate dehydrogenase) confirm the diagnosis. Early hemodialysis may be needed.

TEAM APPROACH TO CARDIAC CATHETERIZATION
Physician Viewpoint

A new person in the cardiac catheterization laboratory should observe the variety of catheterization procedures for at least 10 consecutive cases. This observation period gives the new member of the catheterization team a chance to appreciate the timing, rhythm, and recurrent steps that are required of each member as an integral part of the laboratory. Each laboratory has an individual routine that may vary among operators. No one laboratory routine is best, but learning the routine and joining the team smoothly are important first steps.

The new operator-in-training learns that the attending physician is ultimately responsible for all aspects of the procedure and must check each step of the procedure to ensure accuracy and safety. A similar approach can be recommended for new nurses and technicians.

Learning the "Routine" Overview

1. The patient is seen by a member of the cardiac catheterization team; indications for the procedure are discussed, risks explained, consent obtained, special preparations made, and orders and chart notes written.
2. The patient arrives in the laboratory, is greeted by the nurses, is moved from a holding area into the angiographic suite, and is prepared and draped in a sterile fashion. The physician may or may not participate in the draping with the nurses.
3. Arterial and venous access is obtained depending on the patient's clinical problem and the routine of the laboratory.
4. Right-sided heart catheterization, coronary angiography, and left-sided ventriculography are performed as

indicated by the clinical situation with the appropriate hemodynamic and angiographic measurements. Percutaneous coronary intervention may proceed ad hoc if the patient has consented in advance.

5. At the conclusion of the data collection, angiographic study, and possible intervention, the catheters are removed.

6. The patient is transferred to the holding area, the sheath is pulled, and compression of the puncture site is performed. After an appropriate period of compression (15 to 20 minutes), the patient is returned to his or her room. For sheaths of 5 F to 6 F, recovery usually requires 4 hours or more of bed rest. For procedures using sheaths of 5 F or less or procedures in which vascular access hemostasis is obtained with a vascular closure device, 1 to 2 hours of bed rest with 4 hours of observation before discharge is usually sufficient.

7. Several hours after the procedure a member of the catheterization team checks the patient's arterial access site(s), identifies (and treats) any problems that may have occurred, and presents the preliminary findings again to the patient (and family) after discussion with the referring physician. Unless the operator is also the primary care physician, the catheterization team should discuss results and management options with the patient's primary care physician before taking the patient's treatment into their own hands.

8. Preparations for discharge (that day or the following morning) or for further procedures are made after the cardiac catheterization data have been reviewed by the attending and referring physicians.

Nurse and Technician Viewpoint—the Catheterization Team

The composition of a catheterization team varies among laboratories. The smallest functioning unit would consist of a physician, an assisting physician or nurse, a nurse circulator or recording technician assigned to the laboratory, and a nurse outside the laboratory able to assist. For more specialized procedures the team is increased appropriately.

Personnel are trained specifically to provide technical support necessary for the safe performance of cardiac catheterization procedures. Several disciplines are called on to provide this support. Each member of the team assumes an important role during the procedure.

Personnel and Functions

1. A circulating nurse or technologist must be capable of assisting the physician in all aspects of care of the patient, including routine cardiovascular emergency care.
2. A scrub nurse is needed at the x-ray table to assist the operating physician with all equipment and supplies used in catheterization. The nurse assists in the exchanging of catheters and other specialized maneuvers.
3. A radiologic technologist is trained in x-ray principles related to cardiovascular procedures, cineangiography, fluoroscopy, and the use of power contrast injectors and digital cineangiographic imaging systems.
4. A monitoring and recording technologist is responsible for monitoring and recording the ECG and the hemodynamic data and keeping the physician apprised of changes in cardiac pressures and rhythms. The technician must be able to interpret pressure and ECG waveforms and operate all physiologic recording equipment.

Optimal Staffing. Not every case of coronary arteriography requires all of the above-mentioned people to be present. In most laboratories three assistants are required for most catheterization procedures: one person is scrubbed and assists the physician at the table; one is not scrubbed and circulates in the room, providing patient care and procuring any supplies that are needed during the procedure; and one performs the duties of recording technician and radiologic technologist by selecting proper cineangiographic programs and hemodynamic recording functions as required.

Cross-Training. Cross-training of the individuals in the catheterization laboratory helps in maintaining the morale and confidence in each job described. Cross-training also means that each individual in the laboratory is competent to start up the laboratory and assist in operation on an emergency 24-hour basis when needed.

Cardiopulmonary Resuscitation. All members of the catheterization team should be fully trained in cardiopulmonary resuscitation (CPR) and the use of defibrillators. An algorithm for CPR in the catheterization laboratory is presented in Chapter 8.

Patient Viewpoint

Teaching Before the Procedure. Most patients undergoing cardiac catheterization have vague and often confused ideas of how the procedure is performed. They know little as to what information will be provided about their cardiac status. Procedural patient teaching is important to allay fears and to provide optimal patient care, cooperation, and satisfaction.

The teaching should start at the time the patient enters the hospital. The nurse on the floor should provide information on what the patient can expect while being cared for on the floor before and after the cardiac catheterization. Topics such as the diet, medications, IV therapy, and postprocedural bed rest should be discussed.

The nurse should explain step by step how the procedure is performed, how long it will take, and what the patient should expect regarding sensations and discomfort associated with the procedure. A prepared booklet (sometimes with a videotape) explaining the procedure should be given to the patient to read before the procedure. This booklet reinforces the verbal teaching done by the nurse (e.g., the steps of the catheterization, breath holding, and types of equipment the patient will see). When possible, the nurse should see the patient first. The information given by the nurse may stimulate questions that the patient can ask when the physician arrives to speak to the patient. Some laboratories may not have the resources to send a staff member to do this type of teaching. If that is the case, the floor nurse should be well versed in the catheterization laboratory techniques to provide adequate patient teaching.

The physician's role in patient education should focus on four areas. First, the physician should make clear to the patient the reasons the procedure is being performed. Second, the patient should be told what information the cardiac catheterization will provide. Third, the patient should be told what treatment options are available when a diagnosis is made. Fourth, the physician should discuss the possible risks and potential complications of the procedure. The risks, benefits, and alternatives to cardiac catheterization should be discussed with the patient and family. After this teaching has been done, the physician obtains the written informed consent from the patient. The physician has the final patient responsibility. It is not the nurse's or technician's job to obtain consent.

Teaching in the Laboratory. Teaching should continue when the patient has arrived in the catheterization holding area. The team members should introduce themselves and explain their jobs. A staff member should orient the patient to the x-ray suite and explain briefly the function of the various pieces of equipment. While in the laboratory, the patient should be encouraged to communicate freely with the staff and physician. It is important that the patient inform the staff of any pain or discomfort during the procedure.

Patients are often overwhelmed by the mere thought of such an invasive procedure and may have difficulty digesting all of the information that will be given. Teaching sessions should be limited to 10 to 15 minutes, with important points stressed two or three times. A well-informed patient is less anxious, and this makes the procedure much easier and more comfortable for the patient, the physician, and staff members.

Team Teaching and Conferences

The educational experience of the staff and physician is enhanced by a daily or at least a weekly cardiac catheterization conference. These conferences emphasize to the physicians and technical staff the relationship of clinical data to the hemodynamic and angiographic data. Review of data and discussion of various therapies (e.g., medicine, surgery, angioplasty) provide an excellent opportunity to learn from colleagues who share cases of educational value.

EQUIPMENT IN THE CATHETERIZATION LABORATORY

Figs. 1-2 to 1-4 show the catheterization laboratory and equipment.

Fluoroscopic Imaging System

A high-resolution, image-intensifying television system with digital cineangiographic capabilities is the "eyes" of the

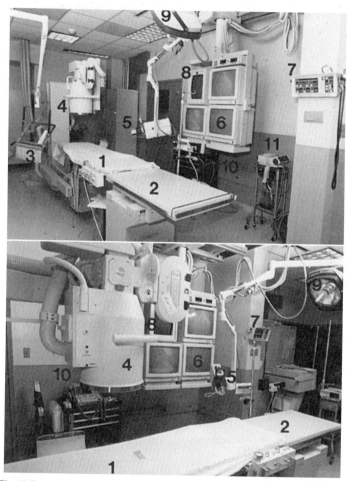

Fig. 1-2.   Two views of the cardiac catheterization suite. *1*, Patient approximately where operator will stand, with C-arm controls on side of table; *2*, movable patient table; *3*, x-ray shield; *4*, C-arm with image intensifier on top and x-ray tube below table; *5*, ceiling-mounted contrast power injector; *6*, fluoroscopic monitors; *7*, control panel for contrast power injector; *8*, physiologic monitor display; *9*, ceiling-mounted operating light; *10*, emergency cart; *11*, cardiac output thermodilution computer.

cardiovascular laboratory. The fluoroscopic image comes from a C-arm, which is a semicircular support with the x-ray tube at one end and the image intensifier at the other. Rotation of the C-arm allows viewing over a wide range of different angles. The patient is placed in the center of the semicircle, which can be

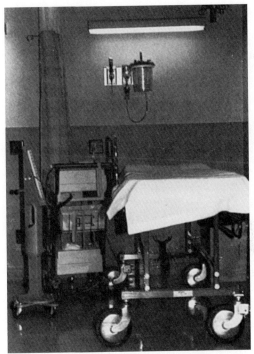

Fig. 1-3.   View of the holding area for cardiac catheterization with an ECG machine, blood pressure sphygmomanometer, and wall suction. The patient can be observed comfortably in this area after the procedure.

moved 180 degrees around the patient as needed to visualize the heart. Two C-arms, side by side, are called biplane and with a double monitoring system can provide visualization of the heart from two different angles at the same time. The fluoroscopic and the physiologic recorders have sets of display television monitors.

Physiologic Recorder

In addition to observation and recording of images of the heart during catheterization, it is necessary to observe and record the ECG and various blood pressures within the cardiovascular system. A reliable ECG and pressure monitoring system is essential for the safety of the patient and collection of hemodynamic information (described in detail in Chapter 3).

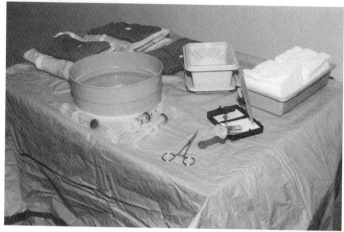

Fig. 1-4.   Sterile supplies: syringes, needles, gauze, waste container (blue box, backstop), injection syringe, gown and gloves, and sterile towels and trays. See text for details.

Contrast Power Injector

A high-pressure contrast media injector is needed to administer a large bolus of contrast media into the left ventricle (10 to 20 ml/sec), pulmonary arteries (10 to 25 ml/sec), or aortic arch (40 to 60 ml/sec). When properly set and flushed, the power injector can be used to inject contrast media into the coronary arteries (3 to 8 ml/sec). Some injector systems also incorporate a pressure transducer and have replaced traditional manifolds with stopcocks. (See Chapter 4 for the Acist injector system.)

Crash Cart and Defibrillator

Every cardiovascular laboratory is equipped with an emergency "crash cart" near the x-ray table. The crash cart contains emergency drugs, oxygen, airways, suction apparatus, and other emergency equipment.

A defibrillator should be charged and ready for use during a procedure. The defibrillator must be tested daily and must be kept at close range for prompt use. Electrode gel, temporary pacemakers, and new electrode patches should be on every cart.

Sterile Equipment and Supplies

The angiographer works from a sterile pack or tray that contains the various supplies needed to perform the procedure. The pack contains syringes and needles, local anesthetic, basins for flushing solutions, small drapes and towels, clamps, scalpels, pressure manifolds, and connecting tubings (see Fig. 1-4). These trays may be made up at the hospital or prepackaged by various suppliers.

Equipment for Sterilization

Most laboratories send reusable items to a central hospital supply area for sterile processing. The three main methods of sterilization are steam, chemical gas, and liquid chemical sterilization. Steam autoclave sterilization uses superheated high-pressure steam to kill organisms. It is effective, but most plastic items, such as catheters and manifolds, cannot withstand the intense heat. Ethylene oxide gas sterilization is the most effective technique for heat-sensitive products. Pressures and temperatures used in the gas sterilizer are much lower than those used in the steam autoclave. Degassing and properly ventilating an object take several hours longer than the steam method. In addition, ethylene oxide is toxic, and special care must be taken when it is used. Chemical sterilization can be performed by several liquid antiseptic solutions. These chemicals are useful for soaking metal instruments or transducers that are reused frequently in the angiographic suite.

TRAINING REQUIREMENTS
Cardiovascular Technologist Training Requirements in Cardiac Catheterization

Cardiovascular technology is a field recognized by the American Medical Association.

Definition. The cardiovascular technologist specializing in invasive cardiovascular technology is a health care professional who, through the use of specific high-technology equipment and at the direction of a qualified physician, performs procedures on patients leading to the diagnosis and treatment of congenital and acquired heart disease and peripheral vascular disease. The technologist is proficient in the use of physiologic analytical equipment during diagnostic and therapeutic procedures. The cardiovascular technologist is trained in advanced life support techniques because the patient population under study is often at increased risk for cardiopulmonary arrest. The technologist, through established methodology of diagnostic examinations, creates a database from which a correct anatomic and physiologic diagnosis may be developed for each patient. The invasive cardiovascular technologist is a highly specialized diagnostician of the various presentations of cardiovascular disease.

Area of Practice. The invasive cardiovascular technologist performs diagnostic procedures involving patients in the invasive cardiovascular laboratory (and coronary care and medical-surgical intensive care environments, if needed). The technologist may also assist a qualified physician in the performance of procedures in specialized clinics. The following are specific diagnostic examinations or procedures but are not all-inclusive (or exclusive) to the invasive cardiovascular technologist's scope of practice. (See Appendix A for specific examinations and procedures.)

Emergency Life Support. The cardiovascular technologist is proficient in basic life support techniques as recommended by the American Heart Association, as follows:

1. Techniques of CPR, cardioversion, or defibrillation
2. Management of airway, including orotracheal and nasotracheal intubation and bag-mask ventilation
3. Proficiency in the preparation and delivery of emergency medications by means of IV line placement and intravenous infusion, including the medications listed in Appendix G, at the request of a qualified physician

Preparation, Inventory, Maintenance, and Sterile Techniques. The invasive cardiovascular technologist is proficient in the preparation of the patient for all procedures and for the maintenance, inventory, stocking, and sterile preparation of all equipment, parts, catheter devices, and room preparations for each procedure, as follows:

1. Information and support to the patient before, during, and after each procedure, including sterile preparation of the patient

2. Cleaning, packaging, and sterilization of all sundry catheterization trays and ancillary area equipment
3. Maintenance of the sterile field during such procedures
4. Preparation, recording, interpretation, and filing of all procedural protocols and reports
5. Ordering of all disposable supplies necessary for each procedure
6. Retrieval of data regarding individual patients and disease entities for clinical and research purposes

Equipment Used in the Invasive Cardiovascular Laboratory. The invasive cardiovascular technologist is proficient in the operation and maintenance of all diagnostic and therapeutic equipment used for procedures, including electrical safety for each piece of equipment. The equipment listed is neither all-inclusive nor exclusive to the various types and brands of equipment used in the cardiovascular laboratory areas.

1. Physiologic equipment
   a. ECG/pressure recorder/analyzer (with or without computer interface)
   b. Pressure transducers
   c. Electrocardiography
2. Radiographic equipment
   a. Cineangiography operations
   b. Image intensifier
   c. Digital interfaces
   d. Videotape recorders
3. Cine film and processing (if still using cine film)
   a. Sensitometer and densitometer for film quality control
   b. Cineangiographic film projector (including computer digitizer with left ventriculography analyzers)
4. Blood gas and oxygen content and saturation analyzer
5. Cardiac output thermodilution computer
6. Contrast media pressure injector
7. Temporary pacemakers
   a. External
   b. Transvenous pacing catheters
   c. Pacemaker driver and connecting cables
8. Intraaortic balloon pumps and consoles
9. Emergency (code) cart equipment, including medications and defibrillator

ENVIRONMENTAL SAFETY IN THE CATHETERIZATION LABORATORY

The cardiac catheterization laboratory is a potentially hazardous area if proper safety measures are not followed. There is the constant risk of exposure to radiation, blood and body fluids, and infectious diseases, such as hepatitis and tuberculosis. Laboratory-specific environmental safety plans reduce the risk associated with this environment.

The invasive cardiovascular technologist is responsible for the radiation protection of patients and laboratory personnel in cooperation with the hospital radiation safety officer. Electrical hazard protection is also maintained through the technologist and the biomedical engineering department. Maintenance of sterility and cleanliness of the procedure equipment and supplies are the technologist's responsibility, including the following:

1. Regular ground-fault checks of all electrical equipment
2. Regular sterile-batch checks
3. Infection control

Blood and Body Fluids

Occupational exposure to blood and body fluids is a serious concern for personnel working in the cardiac catheterization laboratory. The Occupational Safety and Health Administration (OSHA) published the bloodborne pathogen standards in the *Federal Register* in 1991. The standard outlines specific guidelines that must be followed to protect employees from occupational exposure (Box 1-5).

Bloodborne Viruses

Hepatitis B virus (HBV) and human immunodeficiency virus are two bloodborne viruses that pose a risk to health care workers. These viruses have been found in blood, semen, vaginal secretions, tears, saliva, cerebrospinal fluid, amniotic fluid, breast milk, body cavity fluids, and urine. Blood and equipment contaminated with blood and bloody saline flush solutions pose the greatest risk to cardiac catheterization laboratory personnel.

Box 1-5

Highlights of the Occupational Safety and Health Administration (OSHA) Standard

The catheterization laboratory should provide the following:

- Information regarding the OSHA standards and the departmental exposure control plan
- Explanation of bloodborne diseases
- Explanation of the modes of transmission
- Explanation of the employee's risk category
- Explanation of environmental controls—benefits and limitations
- Rationale for selection of protective equipment being used
- Information on the hepatitis B vaccine
- Explanation of how to report an incident of exposure and the proper follow-up procedure

Modes of Transmission by Occupational Exposure

Transmission of bloodborne viruses can occur when contaminated body fluids come in contact with the skin by needles or through an open sore or small cut or contact with the eyes or other mucous membranes.

Universal Precautions

The goal of the exposure control plan is to isolate the health care worker from these hazards. Universal Precautions is an infection control technique in which all blood and body fluids are treated as if they are contaminated. The Universal Precautions technique should be incorporated in the specific exposure control plan for the cardiac catheterization laboratory.

Standard Precautions

In 1996, the Centers for Disease Control and Prevention and the Hospital Infection Control Practices Committee published new guidelines in the *American Journal of Infection Control*. The new guidelines recommend the use of Standard Precautions as the primary strategy for nosocomial infection control. Standard Precautions is designed to reduce the risk of transmission of microorganisms from recognized and unrecognized sources of possible infection.

Standard Precautions incorporates the major features of Universal Precautions for blood and body fluid and body substance isolation, which is designed to reduce the risk of transmission of pathogens from moist body substances. Standard Precautions applies to blood; all body fluids, secretions, and excretions, regardless of whether they contain visible blood; nonintact skin; and mucous membranes.

In addition to Standard Precautions, the guidelines recommend Transmission Based Precautions for patients known or suspected to be infected or colonized with highly transmissible or epidemiologically significant pathogens. The three types of Transmission Based Precautions are (1) airborne precautions, (2) droplet precautions, and (3) contact precautions.

In the past, it was rare to have a patient with a known transmissible disease scheduled for elective catheterization. Interventional procedures have expanded the indications for cardiac procedures, however. In these instances consultation with the hospital's infection control nurse should be considered to initiate Transmission Based Precautions properly.

Environmental Assessment

The working environment should be assessed before an exposure control plan is written. In the catheterization laboratory, procedure-specific hazards exist. Some of these hazards and methods of protection are listed in Tables 1-9 and 1-10.

Table 1-9

Catheterization Laboratory Hazards

Procedure	Exposure
IV therapy	Needle stick, blood-to-skin contact
Local anesthesia administration	Needle stick
Arterial puncture	Needle stick, splashing of blood
Catheter insertion or exchange	Splashing of blood to skin or mucous membrane contact
Catheter flushing	Splashing of blood to skin or mucous membrane contact
Catheter removal and groin compression	Splashing of blood to skin or mucous membrane contact
Contact with soiled linen or equipment	Needle stick, splashing of blood to skin or mucous membrane contact

Table 1-10

Methods of Protection

Eye	Glasses with side shields or goggles
Nose and mouth	Masks
Skin	Gloves, fluid-resistant gowns
Parenteral	Proper methods of sharp instruments storage and disposal; do not recap or resheath needles

Eye, Nose, and Mouth Protection

The eyes and nose should be protected from potential splashing of blood and contaminated fluids. Personnel at most risk are the operators and assistant, the circulating personnel, and the person removing the catheter and sheath and holding arterial puncture site pressure. Personnel performing these high-risk tasks should wear glasses or goggles, a facemask, or a facemask with an incorporated plastic eye shield if glasses or goggles are not worn (Fig. 1-5).

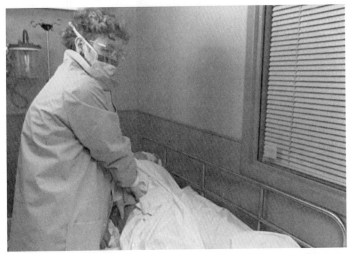

Fig. 1-5. A nurse-technician performing femoral artery compression wears protective gloves, gown, and facemask with shield (satisfying OSHA standards).

Skin Protection

Gloves should be worn anytime personnel are required to handle supplies or samples that are considered contaminated. Anyone involved in the sterile procedure would be wearing sterile gloves. Circulating personnel should wear gloves when accepting items being passed from the sterile field, such as used catheters or wires, syringes containing blood for blood gas and saturation analysis, and biopsy specimens. Gloves should be worn if a pressure transducer is being flushed with saline that has been contaminated with blood during the procedure. This point is of particular concern because the saline may not appear to be contaminated. It may have been aspirated through the same manifold through which blood has passed, however, producing an invisible contamination.

Glove integrity should be monitored. If personnel are reporting holes or tears in gloves, double gloving or higher quality gloves should be considered. Hand lotions containing petroleum products compromise latex glove material and should not be used.

Exposed skin should be covered when removing catheters and sheaths and holding puncture site pressure. An inexpensive disposable gown, such as an isolation gown or a disposable laboratory coat, should be donned first and the gloves pulled over the sleeves. This technique minimizes exposure to the hands and arms. If the protective clothing becomes contaminated with blood or body fluids, it should be removed immediately and the exposed skin should be washed with soap and water. Protective clothing worn during procedures should be removed before personnel leave the department or hospital building.

Equipment Consideration

As awareness of the hazards of bloodborne pathogens increases, a variety of protective equipment and instruments are being made available for use in the cardiac catheterization laboratory. Most companies that make angiographic manifolds offer closed drainage systems. This system incorporates a 1000-ml bag in the manifold system, which allows aspirated blood to be flushed directly into a sealed bag. This system reduces the potential exposure during the procedure and at the end of the procedure during cleanup.

Another product to reduce exposure improves on the conventional waste bowl frequently used on the sterile back table (the Backstop) (Fig. 1-6). The closed bowl design allows bloody, fluid-filled syringes to be emptied into the receptacle and prevents backsplashing by incorporating a diaphragmed slot in which the syringe can be inserted and emptied.

Employer Responsibility

Hepatitis B Virus Vaccination. The OSHA standard states that HBV vaccination must be made available as a prerequisite of employment to all employees with potential for occupational exposure. If the employee declines vaccination, it is mandatory that an HBV vaccine declination is signed.

Risk Category. The OSHA standard requires employers to inform employees of a job's risk category on employment. Table 1-11 outlines the risk categories. Most, if not all, catheterization laboratory staff fall into category I.

Employee Training. The employer must provide proper training to employees regarding bloodborne pathogens and the OSHA

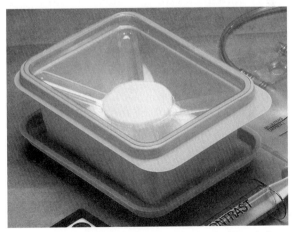

Fig. 1-6.   Blood containment device to prevent splashing during syringe flushing. (Courtesy Merit Medical, Salt Lake City, Utah.)

Table 1-11

Risk Categories

Risk Category	Definition
I	Employment and procedures require exposure to blood and body fluids
II	Employment and procedures may require exposure to blood and body fluids
III	Employment and procedures usually do not require exposure to blood and body fluids

standards. Records must be kept documenting the dates, content, name of person conducting the training, and names of the persons attending the session. These records must be maintained at least 3 years. The training should include safety methods covering the information in Tables 1-9 to 1-11.

Eliminating Careless Practices to Reduce Risks. Often in the cardiac catheterization laboratory employees are exposed as a result of carelessness and lack of attention to procedures. All incidents of employee exposure should be documented properly. A periodic review should be conducted to determine ways to eliminate future exposure. Careless practices that should be avoided in the catheterization laboratory include the following:

1. Vigorous squirting of blood in syringes into the back table waste bowl, resulting in splashing
2. Throwing of bloody gauze across the table into trash receptacles
3. Improper handling of guidewires and catheters, which may spring out of the saline bowl and cause splashing
4. Failing to return needles properly to a needle counter or container on the back table

Extra attention and care in such areas prevent unnecessary exposure of staff.

Radiation Safety

The catheterization laboratory environment should be made as safe as possible for the staff and patient. Because radiation cannot be seen, felt, or heard, it is easy to become lackadaisical about proper protective measures. Standards for radiation protection (from the Society for Cardiac Angiography and Intervention) include four basic principles:

1. The less exposure, the less chance of absorbed energy biologic interaction
2. No known level of ionizing radiation is a permissible dose or absolutely safe
3. Radiation exposure is cumulative. There is no washout phenomenon
4. All participants in the cardiac catheterization laboratory have voluntarily accepted some degree of radiation exposure, but they are obliged to minimize and reduce risks to other personnel and themselves

The source of radiation is the primary x-ray beam emanating from the undertable x-ray tube upward through the patient and onto the image intensifier. Scatter of this beam exposes all subjects to radiation in a dose geometrically inverse to the distance from the source. Radiation scatter is increased when the angle of the tube is set obliquely. A high degree of angulation increases the amount of radiation scatter (see Chapter 4). Acrylic shields and table-mounted lead aprons should be used to reduce the amount of scatter.

Fluoroscopy generates approximately one fifth the x-ray exposure of cineangiography. The increased use of cineangiography for complex catheterization procedures has increased the total exposure and should be a consideration in procedures requiring extensive intracardiac manipulation, such as angioplasty, valvuloplasty, or electrophysiology studies.

Every cardiac catheterization laboratory should have a department-specific radiation safety policy. This policy should include the following:

1. Routine monitoring of personnel radiation exposure
2. Continuing education programs for personnel on radiation safety
3. Program to make personnel aware of the risks associated with radiation exposure
4. Requirement for protective equipment be worn by all personnel
5. Procedures to check safety of all equipment (x-ray dose output, integrity of lead aprons, thyroid shields)

Lead Eyeglasses. A single x-ray exposure of 200 rad (R) can produce cataract formation in humans. Eyeglasses made of 0.5- to 0.75-mm lead-equivalent glass should be worn by personnel exposed to radiation on a daily basis (Fig. 1-7). Glasses containing 0.5 mm of lead offer four times the protection of regular eyeglasses. Glasses with photochromic lenses offer two times the protection of regular eyeglasses. Plastic lenses offer no eye protection from radiation.

Radiation-protective glasses must contain a wraparound side shield. Glasses with proper-fitting side shields not only are good for radiation protection, but also provide protection from blood products splashing into the eyes.

Radiation Badges. All personnel should wear a radiation monitoring badge when in the catheterization laboratory. To ensure accurate readings, a badge should always remain on the person to whom it is assigned. Badges should never be left lying on a counter or attached to a lead apron in an area where there is potential radiation exposure. When badges are not being used, they should be stored in an area away from any potential radiation exposure.

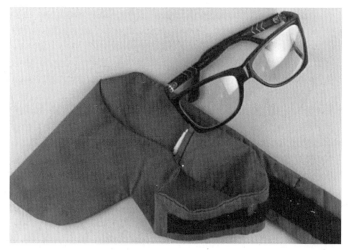

Fig. 1-7.   Radiation safety glasses and thyroid shield should be worn by all personnel inside the catheterization suite.

At the end of each month, exposed badges are collected and sent for analysis. A monthly exposure report indicates each staff member's exposure for that month. This information should be posted in the laboratory so that each staff member can monitor his or her individual exposure. The report should be reviewed each month by the laboratory medical director and the institution's radiation safety officer.

Radiation Dose Limitation. Although no known threshold for radiation exposure exists to define specific risks, the National Council on Radiation Protection and Measurements indicates that no dose of greater than 3 Rem should be allowed over a 3-month period.

Definitions of Radiation Units

1. *Roentgen (R)* is the measure of ionization delivered to a specific point (exposure). One chest radiograph equals 3 to 5 mR.
2. *Radiation absorbed dose (rad)* is the amount of radiation energy deposited per unit mass of tissue. The amount of absorbed dose per given exposure depends on tissue type. For soft tissue, 1 R = 1 rad; for bone, 1 R = 4 rad (i.e., greater absorption).
3. *Radiation equivalent dose in man (Rem)* is used to express the biologic impact of a given exposure. For x-radiation, 1 rad = 1 Rem.

Methods to Limit Exposure

1. Wear leaded aprons (preferably wraparound): 0.5 mm or more thickness provides 80% protection.
2. Limit the fluoroscopic or cineangiographic time (cineangiographic time produces much greater exposure than fluoroscopic time).
3. Use collimators.
4. Reduce the distance between the x-ray source and the patient.
5. Maximize the distance between the x-ray source and the operator and assistants.
6. Limit the milliamperes per kilovolts as much as possible for an adequate image.

7. Use slower panning, and provide good initial angiographic setup. Angled views almost double the radiation.
8. Keep the image magnification as low as possible.
9. Use extra shielding (leaded thyroid guards, lead glasses, and protective table shields).

Radiation exposure is greater during angioplasty than during diagnostic catheterization. If the protective shields are used carefully, the radiation exposure for single- and double-vessel angioplasty compared with diagnostic catheterization may be comparable. Radiation exposures are generally higher for these procedures, however, especially when biplane angiography is performed.

Lead Aprons. Lead aprons should contain 0.5-mm-thick lead lining. When properly cared for, an apron can provide years of service. The lead lining can crack or tear, however; this is usually caused by careless handling or improper storage. Aprons should be placed on an appropriate hanger or in a storage rack after use (Fig. 1-8). Repeatedly throwing an apron over a chair or stretcher may damage the lead lining.

To assess the integrity of the lead, aprons should be examined under fluoroscopy at least once a year. Documentation should be kept regarding the integrity of each apron. To do this, each apron should contain some sort of identification (e.g., number, color, name).

Because of the nature of work in the catheterization laboratory, personnel are not always able to maintain a frontal position to the x-ray beam. Wraparound lead aprons should be considered. Aprons should be long enough to cover the long bones (femur) and should extend to the knee or just below the knee. Because proper fit is important, many companies take measurements to ensure a proper fit. A hanging rack for the lead aprons should be used to prevent cracking resulting from excessive folding of aprons left lying over chairs or benches.

Thyroid Shields. Because the thyroid gland is particularly sensitive to ionizing radiation, a lead thyroid shield should be worn in the presence of ionizing radiation. Similar to aprons, thyroid shields should be stored properly and the lead periodically checked radiographically.

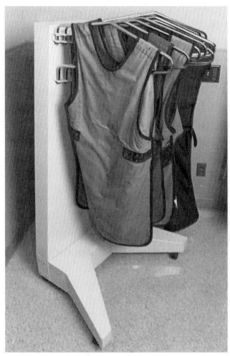

Fig. 1-8.   One proper storage method to prevent lead aprons from developing cracks, which reduce radiation protection. All aprons should be hung up when not in use.

Responsibilities of Laboratory Management Personnel

Responsibilities of management personnel are as follows:
1. Perform budget and finance functions
2. Develop policies and procedures
3. Establish laboratory standards
4. Develop quality assurance programs
5. Keep records
6. Develop training and continuing education programs

Physician Training Requirements in Cardiac Catheterization

Diagnostic Catheterization in Adults.   The following are the proposed physician requirements for certification in the performance of cardiac catheterization. The physician should spend a minimum of 12 months in the cardiac catheterization laboratory. The trainee acquires a clear understanding of the indications, limitations, complications, and medical and surgical implications of the findings of cardiac catheterization and angiography. This background includes an understanding of the pathophysiology and the ability to interpret a wide variety of hemodynamic and angiographic data in adults. (Pediatric catheterization requires a special training track.) All trainees receive basic instruction in radiation safety, use of fluoroscopy, and radiologic anatomy. The trainee learns to perform catheterization of the right and left sides of the heart by the cutdown and percutaneous routes. Temporary right ventricular pacing, endomyocardial biopsy, pericardiocentesis, and standard ventriculography and coronary angiography are performed. A working knowledge of catheterization laboratory equipment, including physiologic recorders, pressure transducers, blood gas analyzers, image intensifiers and other x-ray equipment, and angiographic image processing is emphasized for trainees seeking advanced catheterization laboratory experience.

Trainees are exposed to adult patients with valvular, congenital, cardiomyopathic, pericardial, and ischemic heart disease. Studies of acutely ill patients (cardiogenic shock, acute myocardial infarction, or unstable angina) are currently a routine part of invasive cardiology. Techniques of myocardial biopsy, transseptal catheterization, and intraaortic balloon counterpulsation require advanced, specialized training. At the end of the cardiac catheterization training period, a trainee should have performed at least 300 catheterization procedures; in 150 of them, the trainee should have been the primary operator.

Interventional Cardiology (Percutaneous Coronary and Peripheral Vascular Interventions, Valvuloplasty). Because the potential for harm is greater with interventional techniques, only physicians highly skilled and thoroughly trained in the fundamentals of diagnostic catheterization should undertake this course of specialized training. To meet the proposed training standards of the Society for Cardiac Angiography and of the Task Force of the American College of Cardiology for advanced cardiac catheterization procedures such as angioplasty, the physician must have at least 1 year of additional training in the cardiac catheterization laboratory before American Board of Internal Medicine certification eligibility.

Suggested Readings

American Heart Association: Basic life support techniques: guidelines (1992 standards), *JAMA* 268:2184-2198, 1992.

American Hospital Association: *OSHA's final bloodborne pathogens standard: a special briefing*, Chicago, 1992, American Hospital Association, Item No. 155904.

Bailey CJ, Turner RC: Metformin, *N Engl J Med* 334:574-579, 1996.

Baim DS, Grossman W, editors: *Grossman's cardiac catheterization, angiography, and intervention*, ed 6, Philadelphia, 2000, Lippincott Williams & Wilkins.

Bakalyar DM, Castellani MD, Safian RD: Radiation exposure to patients undergoing diagnostic and interventional cardiac catheterization procedures, *Cathet Cardiovasc Diagn* 42:121-125, 1997.

Bashore TM, Bates ER, Kern MJ, et al (writing committee members): American College of Cardiology/Society for Cardiac Angiography and Interventions clinical expert consensus document on cardiac catheterization laboratory standards: a report of the American College of Cardiology task force on clinical expert consensus documents, *J Am Coll Cardiol* 37:2170-2174, 2001.

Cohen MC, Eagle KA: Expert opinion regarding indications for coronary angiography before noncardiac surgery, *Am Heart J* 134:321-329, 1997.

Forssmann-Falck R: Werner Forssmann: A pioneer of cardiology, *Am J Cardiol* 79:651-660, 1997.

Greenberger PA, Patterson R, Simon R, et al: Pretreatment of high-risk patients requiring radiographic contrast media studies, *J Allergy Clin Immunol* 67:185-187, 1981.

Grossman W, editor: *Cardiac catheterization and angiography*, ed 4, Philadelphia, 1998, Lea & Febiger.

Hazinski MF, Crimmins RO, editors: *American Heart Association 1996 handbook of emergency cardiac care for health care providers*, St Louis, 1996, Mosby.

Hildner FJ: Ten basic instructions and axioms for new students of cardiac catheterization, *Cathet Cardiovasc Diagn* 22:307-309, 1991.

Hirshfeld JW, Banas JS, Cowley M, et al: American College of Cardiology training statement on recommendations for the structure of an optimal adult interventional cardiology training program: a report of the American College of Cardiology task force on clinical expert consensus documents endorsed by the Society for Cardiac Angiography and Interventions and the Diagnostic and

Interventional Catheterization Committee of the Council on Clinical Cardiology, American Heart Association, *J Am Coll Cardiol* 34: 2141-2147, 1999.

Hirshfeld JW, Ellis SG, Faxon DP, et al: Recommendations for the assessment and maintenance of proficiency in coronary interventional procedures statement of the American College of Cardiology, *J Am Coll Cardiol* 31:722-743, 1998.

Holmes DR, Hirshfeld J, Faxon D, et al: ACC expert consensus document on coronary artery stents, *J Am Coll Cardiol* 32:1471-1482, 1998.

Johnson LW, Moore RJ, Balter S: Reviews of radiation safety in the cardiac catheterization laboratory, *Cardiac Cath Cardiovasc Diagn* 25:186-194, 1992.

Kern MJ: *Interventional cardiac catheterization handbook*, St Louis, 1996, Mosby.

Krone J, Morton MJ, editors: *Complications of cardiac catheterization and angiography: prevention and management*, Mount Kisco, NY, 1989, Futura Publishing.

Limacher MC, Douglas PS, Germano G, et al: ACC expert consensus document on radiation safety in the practice of cardiology, *J Am Coll Cardiol* 31:892-913, 1998.

Mueller HS, Chatterjee K, Davis KB, et al: Present use of bedside right heart catheterization in patients with cardiac disease, *J Am Coll Cardiol* 32:840-864, 1998.

Mudd JG: Should coronary angiograms be reviewed with patients?, *Am J Cardiol* 57:501, 1986.

Nissen SE, Pepine CJ, Bashore TM, et al: American College of Cardiology position statement. Cardiac angiography without cine film: erecting a "tower of Babel" in the cardiac catheterization laboratory, *J Am Coll Cardiol* 24:834-837, 1994.

OSHA standards, Friday, Dec 6, 1991, 29 CER Part 1910.1030 Occupational exposure to bloodborne pathogens; final rule, *Fed Reg* 45:64175-64182, 1991.

Pepine CJ: *Diagnostic and therapeutic cardiac catheterization*, Baltimore, 1994, Williams & Wilkins.

Pinkney-Atkinson VJ: Conscious sedation clinical guideline. Conscious Sedation Working Group, Medical Association of South Africa, *S Afr Med J* 87:484-492, 1997.

Practice guidelines for sedation and analgesia by non-anesthesiologists. American Society of Anesthesiologists, *Anesthesiology* 84:459-471, 1996.

Recommended practices for managing the patient receiving conscious sedation/analgesia, *AORN J* 65:129-134, 1997.

Ritchie JL, Nissen SE, Douglas JS, et al: American College of Cardiology position statement use of nonionic or low osmolar contrast agents in cardiovascular procedures, *J Am Coll Cardiol* 21:269-73, 1993.

Scanlon PJ, Faxon DP, Audet AM, et al (committee members); Ritchie JL, Gibbons RJ, Cheitlin MD, et al (task force members): ACC/AHA guidelines for coronary angiography: executive summary and recommendations: a report of the American College of Cardiology/ American Heart Association task force on practice guidelines (committee on coronary angiography) developed in collaboration with the Society for Cardiac Angiography and Interventions, *Circulation* 99:2345-2357, 1999.

Schwab SJ, Hlatky MA, Pieper KS, et al: Contrast nephrotoxicity: a randomized controlled trial of a nonionic and an ionic radiographic contrast agent, *N Engl J Med* 320:149-153, 1989.

Smith SC, Dove JT, Jacobs AK, et al: ACC/AHA guidelines for percutaneous coronary intervention (revision of the 1993 PTCA guidelines): a report of the American College of Cardiology/ American Heart Association Task Force on Practice Guidelines (committee to revise the 1993 guidelines for percutaneous transluminal coronary angioplasty) endorsed by the Society for Cardiac Angiography and Interventions, *Circulation* 103:3019-3041, 2001.

Standards for acquisition, measurement and reporting of intravascular ultrasound studies (IVUS), *J Am Coll Cardiol* 37:1478-1492, 2001.

Uretsky BF: *Cardiac catheterization: concepts, techniques and applications*, Malden, Mass, 1997, Blackwell Science.

Watson RM: Radiation exposure: clueless in the cath lab, or sayonara ALARA, *Cathet Cardiovasc Diagn* 42:126-127, 1997.

2

ARTERIAL AND VENOUS ACCESS

Saad Bitar, Morton J. Kern, and Frank Bleyer

The most common catheterization problem involves the initial access to the circulation. Although often relegated to the novice, this important step deserves full study. Because most aspects of cardiac catheterization are learned through apprentice-type experience, watching, reading, and doing under supervision are the keys to success.

Some of the key points of vascular access may not seem important to the uninitiated but are crucial to the safety and success of the procedure. Entry into the circulation is generally the only painful part of the catheterization procedure. For best patient response, adequate generous local anesthesia should be administered using a gentle approach. Pain during entry into the vessel may cause a vagal reaction or spasm, prolonging the procedure and potentially causing more significant complications.

The site and location of access are determined by the planned investigation and anticipated anatomic and pathologic conditions of the patient. If possible, previous procedures and any difficulties encountered should be reviewed from old reports. Preprocedural assessment of the quality of all peripheral pulses is mandatory.

PERCUTANEOUS FEMORAL APPROACH
Percutaneous Femoral Artery Puncture

Percutaneous femoral arterial catheterization is the most widely used technique. In patients with a significant history of claudication, signs of chronic arterial insufficiency, diminished or absent pulses, or bruits over the iliofemoral area, the physician should use an alternate entry site to avoid the risk of further impairment of the arterial circulation in the legs (Box 2-1.) The presence of arterial conduit grafts or previous balloon angioplasty of the iliofemoral system is not an absolute contraindication to the percutaneous technique. Prosthetic graft puncture has been shown to be safe if small-diameter sheaths are used. An alternative route should be strongly considered, however.

In patients with diminished pedal pulses the femoral arterial approach using small (<6 F) sheaths and catheters is possible. However, even partial occlusion of the femoral artery may cause a significant drop in distal perfusion pressure and blood supply to the already compromised foot. A small embolus in a patient with diminished pedal pulses may not be tolerated as well as in patients with patent distal vessels.

Artery Location. The femoral arterial entry is usually begun using the patient's right femoral artery with the operator standing at the right side of the patient. The inguinal (groin) skin crease is located. The inguinal ligament, which usually lies directly beneath the inguinal skin crease parallel with a line from the iliac crest to the pubis, is palpated. In obese patients the inguinal skin crease may be lower than the inguinal

---

Box 2-1

Indications for Alternative Routes to Femoral Arterial Catheterization

Claudication
Absent dorsalis pedis and posterior tibialis pulses
Absent popliteal pulses
Femoral bruits
Absent femoral pulses
Prior femoral artery graft surgery
Extensive inguinal scarring from radiation therapy, surgery, or prior catheterization
Excessively tortuous or diseased iliac arteries
Severe back pain, inability to lie flat
Patient request
Morbid obesity

ligament, and there may be several skin folds below and above the inguinal ligament, making it important to locate the inguinal ligament. A metal clamp can be laid over the proposed entry site. The correct arterial entry (not skin entry) should have the tip of the clamp near the medial edge of the middle of the head of the femur (Figs. 2-1 and 2-2).

The femoral artery crosses the inguinal ligament at an imaginary point that divides the ligament into one third medial and two thirds lateral portions. To follow the artery course, the practitioner should think of the femoral artery as a tube approximately 1 cm in diameter running across the

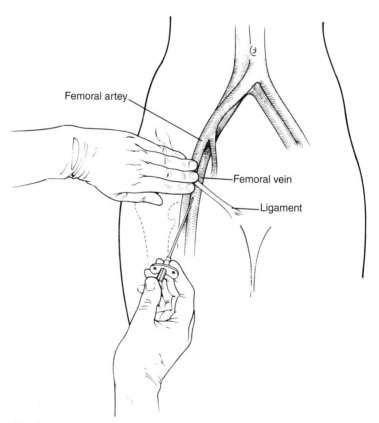

Fig. 2-1   Femoral vein puncture with needle at a 30- to 45-degree angle aiming medially toward the umbilicus. (From Tilkian AG, Daily EK: *Cardiovascular procedures: diagnostic techniques and therapeutic procedures,* St Louis, 1986, Mosby.)

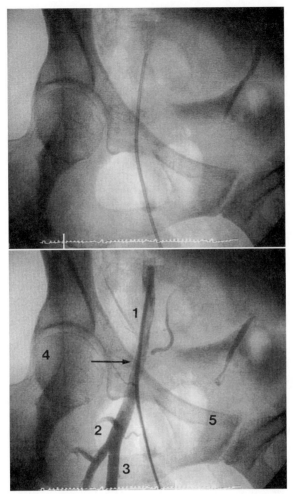

Fig. 2-2   Femoral artery landmarks. Top, Angiogram of sheath in femoral artery in anteroposterior projection. Bottom, Correct positioning is seen relative to angiographic landmarks. *1*, Common femoral artery; *2*, bifurcation of profunda; *3*, superficial femoral artery; *4*, midpoint of femoral head; *5*, iliac-symphysis pubis ridge (inguinal ligament line).

inguinal ligament. As in any tube the center line is the highest point with the edges of the tube lower on each side. The femoral artery pulse is located with the middle and index fingers placed parallel to the long axis of the femoral artery. The index finger palpates the artery 1 to 2 cm below the inguinal ligament, the site of actual arterial entry with the needle (see Fig. 2-1).

Local Anesthesia. With a 25-gauge needle the skin is infiltrated superficially with 2 to 3 ml of 1% lidocaine 1 to 2 cm below (caudal to) where the index finger is placed as described previously. This point is the skin entry site. In obese patients with thick subcutaneous tissue the entry site should be slightly lower to ensure a needle entry angle of 45 degrees or less. Because large amounts of lidocaine may obscure the pulse, small amounts should be injected repeatedly instead of a large bolus. Next, with a 22-gauge needle, 10 to 15 ml of 1% lidocaine is introduced into deep tissue planes on each side of the artery. During lidocaine infiltration, the operator should palpate the arterial pulse with the left middle and index fingers to avoid accidental puncture of the artery and to ensure infiltration of tissue above and around the artery.

Gentle aspiration before the injection of lidocaine is essential to ensure that the needle tip is not in a blood vessel. Inserting the needle first to the deepest level desired, then continuing infiltration at several more shallow layers may decrease the patient's discomfort. Local anesthesia should cover the whole depth of the expected skin-to-artery path. Sufficient lidocaine (about 20 ml of a 1% solution) should be given 2 to 3 minutes for the full anesthetic effect to take place. Hint: Lidocaine should be given early, and while the anesthetic is taking effect, other preparations, such as connecting tubing and flushing catheters, can be completed. The operator should listen to the heart rate monitor for slowing of the rate as an early warning of vagal reaction. Alternatives to lidocaine are shown in Box 2-2.

Skin Entry. Some operators perform a small skin incision before inserting a Seldinger needle. Other operators prefer to nick the skin over the entry needle or guidewire after the puncture. The latter approach usually results in only one nick if the operator does not obtain access on the first attempt. With the left-hand fingers placed over the artery as described previously, the operator makes a skin incision of 2 to 3 mm with a #11 scalpel blade, holding the blade perpendicular to the skin and penetrating 2 to 3 mm into the subcutaneous tissue.

Box 2-2

Anesthetic Alternatives to Lidocaine

Group I
Procaine (ester prototype)
Benoxinate (Dorsacaine)
Butylaminobenzoate (Butesin)
Benzocaine
Butacaine (Butyn)
Butethamine (Monocaine)
Chloroprocaine (Nesacaine)
Procaine (Novocain)
Tetracaine (Pontocaine)

Group II
Lidocaine (amide prototype)
Amydricaine (Alypin)
Bupivacaine (Marcaine)
Cyclomethycaine (Surfacaine)
Dibucaine (Nupercaine)
Dimethisoquin (Quotane)
Diperodon (Diothane)
Dyclonine (Dyclone)
Etidocaine (Duranest)
Hexylcaine (Cyclaine)
Mepivacaine (Carbocaine)
Oxethazaine (Oxaine)
Phenacaine (Holocaine)
Piperocaine (Metycaine)
Pramoxine (Tronothane)
Prilocaine (Citanest)
Proparacaine (Ophthaine)
Pyrrocaine (Endocaine)

From Tilkian AG, Daily EK: *Cardiovascular procedures: diagnostic techniques and therapeutic procedures,* St Louis, 1986, Mosby.

Subcutaneous Tunnel. For large-diameter sheaths (and for anticipated large-diameter vascular closure devices), a subcutaneous tunnel is made with blunt dissection using straight forceps. This channel makes the catheter and sheath entry easier and, more important, permits blood to drain to the outside of the leg if the puncture site opens after the catheters have been removed. It is important to avoid extensive disruption of skin and subcutaneous tissue while creating the channel because these are the natural barriers to infection.

Arterial Puncture. The single anterior arterial wall entry technique is preferred for arterial puncture (Fig. 2-3). This is especially important in patients being treated with anticoagulants (e.g., heparin), antiplatelet agents, or thrombolytic agents. The original Seldinger double-wall puncture technique is not explained here. The single-wall technique begins with the operator's left-hand fingers positioned over the femoral artery as described previously. The arterial needle (without an obturator) is held between the index and middle fingers of the right hand (as if holding a pencil) with the tip bevel directed upward. The needle is introduced through the skin and advanced slowly toward the artery at a 30- to 45-degree angle to the horizontal plane. An entry into the artery that is too vertical creates problems in advancing the guidewire and promotes sheath and catheter kinking. Pulsation may be felt when the needle contacts the arterial wall. A slight resistance to the needle can be felt as it passes through the arterial wall. At this point a jet of blood from the needle hub confirms arterial puncture. The immediate, strong spurt of pulsatile arterial blood should be maintained by holding the needle hub stable with the left-hand fingers. Resting the left wrist on the patient's thigh is helpful. The J-tipped guidewire is straightened and introduced into the needle with the right hand. The wire should be introduced only when good pulsatile blood flow is present.

Guidewire Insertion. The guidewire is advanced gently into the artery. A soft J-tipped guidewire is the safest. Although straight-tipped guidewires have been used, the potential for subintimal dissection or tearing of the blood vessel wall is high. The wire should move without resistance. If resistance is encountered, the wire is pulled out and pulsatile blood return is confirmed. Fluoroscopy should be used frequently to check wire movement. Repositioning of the needle may be necessary if the wire cannot be advanced freely. Sometimes the needle tip partially penetrates the posterior wall. In this case there is good blood return but the wire cannot be advanced because it is directed

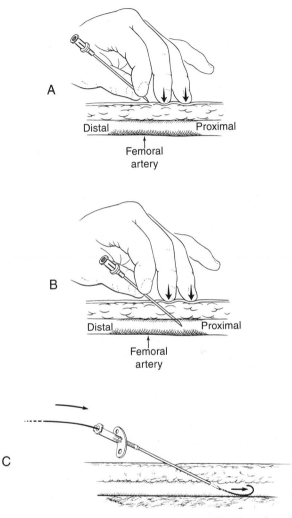

Fig. 2-3   A and **B,** Femoral artery has been entered by a large-bore needle with backflow of blood. Note the operator's finger positions. As soon as the needle passes into the vessel through the anterior wall, brisk pulsatile flow occurs. This technique is called the "front wall stick." It prevents occult bleeding through the posterior wall. **C,** The flexible tip of the guidewire is passed through the needle into the vessel.   *Continued*

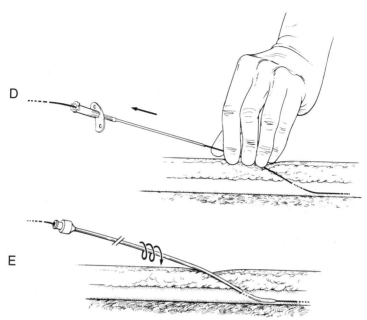

Fig. 2-3, cont'd **D** and **E,** Introducing a valve sheath into the artery. **D,** The needle is withdrawn, the artery is compressed, and the wire is pinched and fixed. **E,** The valve sheath is advanced over a guidewire. (From Uretsky B, editor: *Cardiac catheterization: concepts, techniques, and applications,* Walden, Mass, 1997, Blackwell Science.)

into the posterior wall of the artery rather than the arterial lumen. Withdrawing the needle 1 to 2 mm usually solves this problem. The needle hub is moved a few millimeters laterally or medially, after which the guidewire is slowly readvanced. It is important not to move the needle hub excessively in either direction, which could slice the arterial lumen. In the case of a too-vertical (>45-degree angle) entry into the artery, as is sometimes encountered in obese patients, lowering the needle hub several millimeters may improve the artery and needle tip alignment and permit easier guidewire passage. The operator should attempt to puncture the artery close to the midline of the anterior wall. Puncturing the lateral arterial wall may create a problem in advancing the guidewire or, worse, controlling bleeding after the procedure.

If it is not possible to advance the wire or if the needle comes out of the artery, the needle is withdrawn from the skin and pressure is applied over the puncture site for 2 minutes to ensure hemostasis. The procedure is repeated using a slightly different angle or direction. If the artery is not encountered, the needle is completely withdrawn again and advanced in a different direction. Because of the sharp edge of the needle used for single-wall entry, the direction of the needle generally should not be changed when the needle tip is in the sub-cutaneous tissue. If the artery cannot be located by palpation, a Doppler-tipped needle can be used to localize and enter the artery.

From Guidewire to Catheter Insertion. If no resistance is encountered, the operator advances the guidewire several centimeters at first, then advances it farther into the abdominal aorta using fluoroscopy. Fluoroscopy of the guidewire moving through the iliac artery identifies large arterial plaques and excessive tortuosity, which complicates later catheter manipulation. As noted earlier, use of a J-tipped, soft-spring guidewire is recommended because a straight wire may pass under a plaque, resulting in dissection. After the guidewire is well positioned in the aorta (at the level of the renal arteries), the arterial needle can be removed. Firm pressure is applied over the puncture site (to control bleeding) with the last three left-hand fingers while the operator removes the needle from the skin and maintains puncture site pressure. The guidewire is pinched firmly with the left index finger and thumb to avoid accidental wire removal as the needle is taken off the guidewire from the artery. An assistant may help at this point to withdraw the needle over the wire and wipe the wire clean with wet gauze.

Use of a Sheath Assembly. A catheter sheath is used in nearly all laboratories (Fig. 2-4). The advantages of a sheath include single arterial entry with increased patient comfort and the limitation of arterial damage by several catheter exchanges through the artery. The sheath also maintains constant arterial access, so that an accidental removal of the guidewire does not result in loss of arterial access. Arterial access may be maintained for alternative procedures or later therapeutic

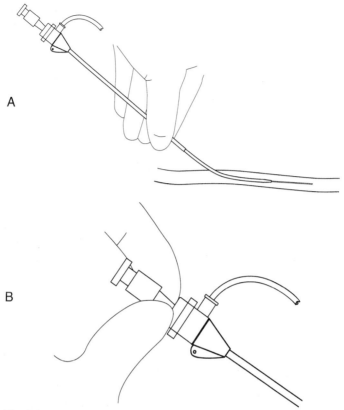

Fig. 2-4   Method of introducing the valve sheath into the artery. **A,** The valve sheath is advanced over a guidewire. **B** and **C,** The obturator is removed from the valve.
Continued

interventions (e.g., percutaneous transluminal coronary angioplasty). The incidence of complications and hematoma with or without a sheath seems to be similar, but the patient's comfort is greater with the sheath.

The sheath-dilator assembly has a valved end with a side arm. Unvalved sheaths should not be used because they leak, and arterial pressure around a catheter cannot be measured through the side arm. A catheter one French size smaller than the sheath size is necessary for satisfactory side arm pressure recording. After guidewire insertion into the artery, the

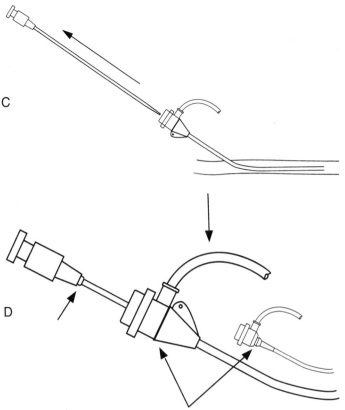

Fig. 2-4, cont'd **D,** The stylet can be inserted to plug the valve after procedure. Arrows indicate position of sewing rings to attach valve to skin should prolonged insertion be required. (Courtesy of Cordis Corporation, Miami, Fla.)

operator advances the sheath-dilator assembly over the wire while holding the guidewire straight and stable. The operator introduces the sheath-dilator assembly into the artery by firmly holding it close to the tip, making clockwise and counter-clockwise half-rotations, and applying firm advancing pressure. (Rotational motion reduces forward friction.) The sheath should not be advanced if significant resistance is encountered, as may occur through scar tissue. In this case serial dilators of bigger sizes are needed before the final sheath is positioned.

The guidewire should be held straight and taut because it may otherwise kink at the site of the sheath tip. After the sheath is inserted completely, the operator holds the sheath hub firmly in place and removes the dilator and guidewire together. The operator aspirates 2 to 3 ml of blood from the side arm of the sheath and flushes the sheath with heparinized saline solution. The arterial pressure can be checked immediately by connection of a pressure manifold to the side arm of the sheath. The sheath should be aspirated and flushed after each catheter removal.

Patient Awareness. Three steps may be associated with pain and vagal reaction: (1) initial administration of lidocaine, (2) arterial needle insertion, and (3) sheath assembly advancement. The operator should listen to the heart rate monitor and feel the strength of the arterial pulse to detect early vagal responses. A vasovagal reaction can occur with no change in heart rate, most commonly in elderly patients.

Ultrasound-Facilitated Arterial and Venous Access. Standard access may be difficult to obtain in patients who have altered anatomy, obesity, or scarring caused by prior surgical procedures (e.g., peripheral vascular surgery, multiple prior catheterizations, or prior intraaortic balloon pumps or support cannulae). Arterial and venous access may be achieved with ultrasonic direct visualization transducer (SiteRite) or with Doppler needle (Smart Needle which differentiates the high-pitched (arterial) or low-pitched (venous) flow velocity sounds.

Hemostasis After Catheter and Sheath Removal. After the catheterization has been completed, the patient's blood pressure is monitored and the catheter is removed. The sheath is aspirated and flushed to clear any thrombi. The patient is transferred to the holding area on a stretcher. If heparin has been given during the procedure, an activated clotting time is obtained, and if it is greater than 200 seconds protamine sulfate (about 30 to 50 mg of protamine reverses 10,000 U of heparin) may be given before sheath removal. Protamine should be administered slowly (at least 5 minutes). Caution should be used in giving protamine to patients receiving NPH insulin, who may be at higher risk for a protamine reaction (see Chapter 1). A protamine reaction may include any or all of the following:

1. Shaking
2. Flushing
3. Chills
4. Back, chest, or flank pain
5. Vasomotor collapse

Treatment for Protamine Reaction. Treatment for protamine reactions involves symptom management with morphine (2 mg intravenously [IV]) or meperidine (Demerol) (25 mg IV), sedation with diphenhydramine (Benadryl) (25 to 50 mg IV), saline administration, and support of low blood pressure. Protamine reactions are usually self-limited, lasting less than 1 hour.

Sheath Removal. To remove the sheath, the operator places his or her left-hand fingers over the femoral artery. Because the actual puncture site is more cranial (toward the patient's head) than the skin incision, the operator's fingers should be placed over the femoral artery *above the skin puncture site*. The operator applies gentle pressure and removes the sheath from the leg, taking care not to crush the sheath and "strip" clot into the distal artery. When a small spurt of blood purges the arterial site of retained thrombi, the operator should apply firm downward pressure. Manual pressure is held firmly for 15 to 20 minutes (5 minutes of full pressure, 5 minutes of 75% pressure, 5 minutes of 50% pressure, and 5 minutes of 25% pressure). In patients receiving antiplatelet treatment (e.g., aspirin or clopidogrel), 20 to 30 minutes of puncture site compression may be necessary. During pressure application the pedal pulses are checked every 2 to 3 minutes. A diminished pulse is acceptable during brief full-pressure application, but the distal pulses should not be obliterated completely. If the pedal pulse is absent during compression, the pressure over the artery should be decreased slightly periodically to allow distal circulation.

Pressure dressings are generally ineffective in preventing bleeding, and they obscure the puncture site so that early hematoma formation may be missed. A small sterile dressing is preferred to a large tape covering.

External Compression and Vascular Closure Devices

Mechanical Clamps. Some laboratories employ mechanical C-type clamps to assist in puncture site hemostasis. The clamp is effective, but it must be applied carefully by a trained individual and the patient must be monitored frequently for misalignment of the clamp and puncture site, bleeding, or excessive pressure with limb ischemia (Fig. 2-5).

Femo-Stop Pressure System. The Femo-Stop (Fig. 2-6) is an air-filled clear plastic compression bubble that molds to skin contours. It is held in place by straps passing around the hip. The amount of applied pressure is controlled with a sphygmomanometer gauge. The clear plastic dome allows the operator to see the puncture site. The Femo-Stop is used most often for patients in whom prolonged compression is anticipated or whose bleeding persists despite prolonged manual or C-clamp compression.

The duration of Femo-Stop compression and time to removal of the device varies depending on the patient and staff protocols. In some hospitals the time from application to removal may be less than 30 minutes. In other patients in whom hemostasis is required, the device may be left at lower pressures for a longer duration.

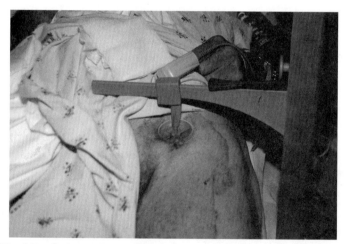

Fig. 2-5   C-clamp (Compressor System, Instromedix, Hillsboro, Ore.) applied to femoral puncture site.

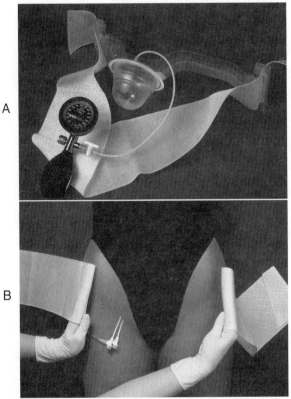

Fig. 2-6   A, The Femo-Stop Pressure System. Use of the Femo-Stop. Before proceeding: (1) Examine puncture site carefully. (2) Note and mark edges of any hematoma. (3) Record patient's current blood pressure.
B, Step 1: Position belt. The belt should be aligned with the puncture site equally across both hips.   *Continued*

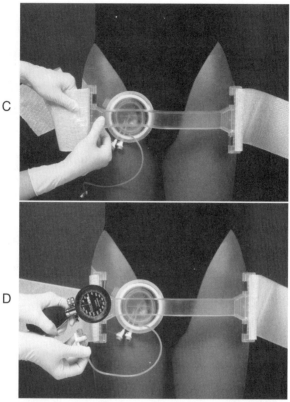

Fig. 2-6, cont'd   **C,** Step 2: Center the dome and adjust belt. The dome should be centered over the arterial puncture site above and slightly toward the midline of the skin incision. The sheath valve should be below the rim of the pressure dome. Attach belt to ensure a snug fit. The center arch bar should be perpendicular to the body.

D, Step 3: Connect dome pressure pump.
Continued

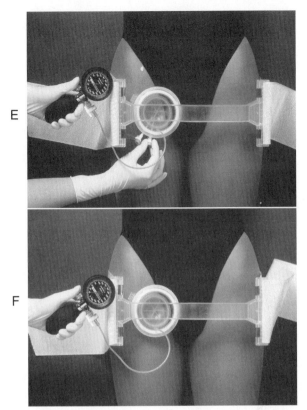

Fig. 2-6, cont'd   E, Step 4: For a venous sheath, inflate dome to 20 or 30 mm Hg and remove sheath. To minimize formation of arteriovenous fistula, obtain venous hemostasis before the arterial sheath is removed.
Step 5: For the arterial sheath, pressurize dome to 60 to 80 mm Hg, and remove sheath and increase pressure in dome to 10 to 20 mm Hg above systolic arterial pressure.
F, Step 6: Maintain full compression for 3 minutes. Reduce pressure in dome by 10 to 20 mm Hg every few minutes until 0 mm Hg. Check arterial pulse. Observe for bleeding. After hemostasis is obtained, remove Femo-Stop and dress wound. (Courtesy RADI Medical Systems, Inc, Reading, Mass.)

Arterial Closure Devices. Four vascular closure devices are currently available. These devices reduce the time to obtain hemostasis. Collagen, either plugs (VasoSeal and Angio-Seal) or liquid (Duett), can be delivered directly to the arterial puncture site through special sheath systems (VasoSeal or Duett) or anchored inside the vessel (Angio-Seal) (Fig. 2-7). A

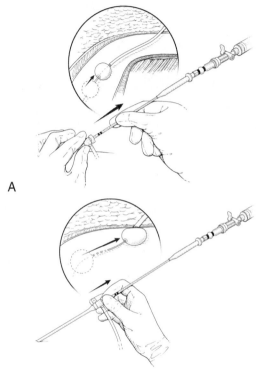

Fig. 2-7   A, Duett vascular closure device. *Top,* A small balloon is inserted through the sheath used for the angiogram. *Bottom,* Balloon is pulled to the end of the sheath.   *Continued*

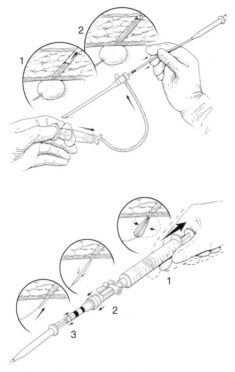

Fig. 2-7, A—cont'd   *Top,* sheath and balloon are pulled back to tamponade the puncture site. The sheath is pulled back from inside of the artery, it is aspirated to confirm the sheath is out of the artery, and a liquid collagen-thrombin mixture is injected to seal the outside of the artery. *Bottom,* Balloon is deflated, and the sheath-balloon assembly is removed. Manual compression is maintained for 5 minutes. (Courtesy of Vascular Solutions, Inc., Minneapolis, Minn.)   *Continued*

B

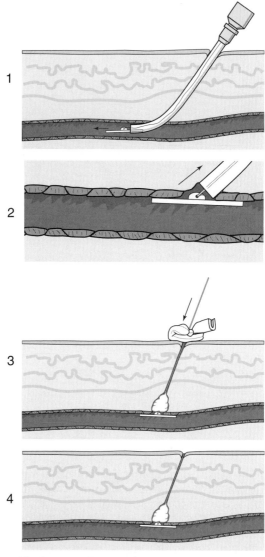

Fig. 2-7—cont'd   B, Angio-Seal hemostasis system. *1,* The AngioSeal sheath assembly preloaded with the anchor and collagen plug is advanced into the vessel. *2,* The anchor is deployed, and retraction on the system secures the anchor against the vessel wall while the sheath is removed, and *3,* the collagen plug is deployed outside the artery. *4,* Tampig of the suture compresses the collagen plug over the vessel. The suture is cut at the skin line, leaving the subcutaneous vascular closure components hidden. (Courtesy of St. Jude Medical, Minneapolis, Minn.)   *Continued*

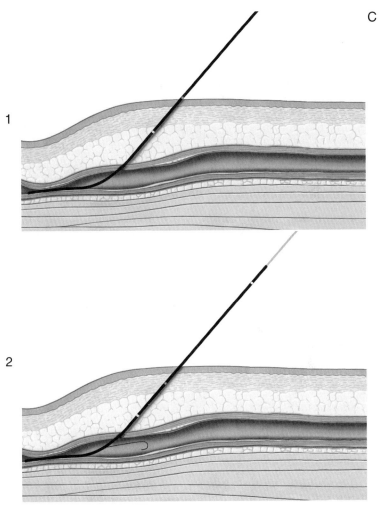

C

1

2

Fig. 2-7—cont'd   C, VasoSeal vascular closure device. *1,* A special introducing catheter with an antegrade J-tipped wire, *2,* is used to mark the artery.   *Continued*

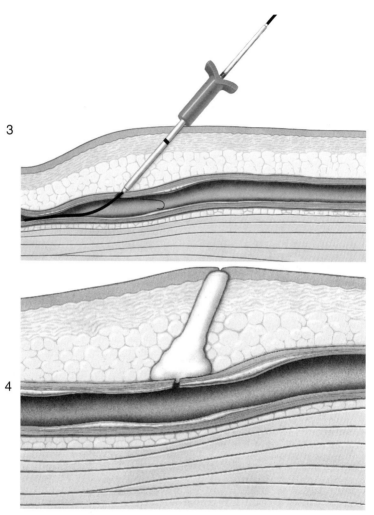

Fig. 2-7, C—cont'd   *3,* Dilator, then sheath, is placed on top of the artery. *4,* A collagen plug is inserted to achieve hemostasis. (Courtesy of Datascope, Fairfield, N.J.)

percutaneous vascular suture delivery system (Perclose) also provides hemostasis and permits early ambulation (Fig. 2-8). These devices may be especially helpful in anticoagulated patients and in patients who have back pain or cannot lie flat.

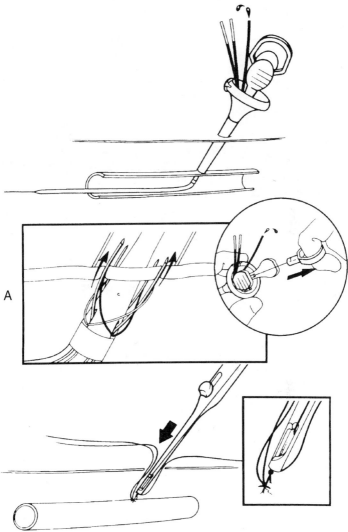

Fig. 2-8   A, The Perclose multiple intravascular suture device permits deployment of suture needles from within the vessel and closure of the suture from the surface of the skin. *Top and middle,* The Perclose device is inserted to the level of the vessel. The fine suture needles are deployed and come through the vessel and out of the device. *Bottom,* The knot pusher secures the knots on top of the vessel in the subcutaneous tissue.

Continued

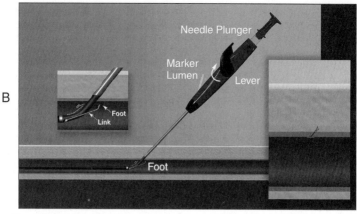

Fig. 2-8, cont'd   B, New suture closure device. (**A** and **B,** Courtesy of Abbot Vascular Devices, Redwood City, Calif.)

Table 2-1

Vascular Closure Devices

Device	Mechanism	Advantages and Limitations
Angio-Seal	Collagen Seal	Secure hemostasis Anchor may catch on side branch
Duett	Collagen Thrombin	Stronger collagen-thrombin seal Intraarterial injection of collagen-thrombin
Perclose	Sutures	Secure hemostasis of suture Device failure may require surgical repair
VasoSeal	Collagen Plug	No intraarterial components Positioning wire may catch on side branch

The advantages and disadvantages of the various arterial closure devices are summarized in Table 2-1.

All vascular closure devices should be used with caution in patients with peripheral vascular disease or low arterial puncture (at or below the femoral bifurcation). In many cases femoral angiography with an oblique angle shows the puncture site and any artery disease. Fig. 2-9 shows an anteroposterior and right anterior oblique view of the femoral artery.

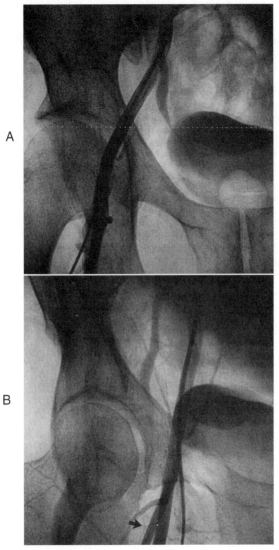

Fig. 2-9 Femoral angiograms. **A,** Anteroposterior projection. **B,** Right anterior oblique projection. Bifurcation of femoral artery is now visible *(arrow).*

Only the right anterior oblique view displays the bifurcation (*arrow*) of the profunda and superficial femoral branches.

Hematoma Monitoring. After 15 to 20 minutes of manual pressure the operator's hand is removed slowly and the area is inspected for hematoma or bleeding. Hemostasis may be difficult to secure in obese, hypertensive, or elderly female patients or in patients with aortic insufficiency. In some patients (e.g., patients who are obese or who have large thighs), greater than 500 ml of blood can be lost before the patient or nurse identifies the problem. For this reason a large opaque occlusive dressing over the puncture site is not recommended. Patients at high risk for groin hematoma and arterial complications who may need longer pressure application or who may benefit from the use of a vascular closure device include the following:

1. Obese patients
2. Patients with hypertension
3. Elderly patients
4. Women
5. Patients with aortic insufficiency
6. Patients who have undergone prior arterial puncture
7. Patients with advanced peripheral atherosclerosis
8. Patients who have coagulopathy or who are receiving anticoagulant or antiplatelet agents

Firm three-finger pressure should control most femoral bleeding. A rolled gauze pack may be placed over the artery to the groin, and pressure applied with the palm of the hand. Standing on a short stool permits the operator's upper body weight to be used for pressure application.

In patients with low cardiac output, mitral stenosis, or cardiomyopathy with a small pulse pressure, the femoral artery can easily be obliterated. In these patients the distal pulses should be checked more frequently and less pressure should be applied to the groin.

After hemostasis is obtained, the puncture area is cleaned with an antiseptic solution. A sterile tape or clear porous dressing is applied. Large pressure dressings or sandbags are not routinely used. A large occlusive dressing obscures bleeding and possibly delays identification of a growing hematoma. During the time pressure is being applied to the puncture site, the physician can discuss the clinical findings and review the postcatheterization instructions with the patient.

If the femoral artery and vein are used in the procedure, the operator should ensure arterial hemostasis first, and then remove the venous sheath to decrease the risk of arteriovenous fistula formation. Preservation of venous access for the first 15 minutes of arterial compression may provide a useful means of treating a vagal reaction should the peripheral IV inadvertently be lost.

Postcatheterization Patient Instructions. Depending on the catheter and sheath size, the patient is kept at bed rest for 2 to 6 hours after femoral artery puncture. With small-diameter catheters (i.e., ≤5 F), shorter times (<2 hours) can be used. The patient is given the following instructions:

1. Keep the head down
2. Hold the groin site when coughing
3. Keep the punctured leg straight
4. Stay in bed
5. Drink fluids
6. Call a nurse for assistance if there is bleeding, leg numbness or pain, or chest pain

Percutaneous Femoral Vein Puncture

The femoral arterial pulse is the landmark for the femoral vein. The femoral vein is located approximately 1 cm medial to the femoral artery; sometimes it is located partially behind the artery. The procedure for femoral vein percutaneous entry involves the following steps.

Femoral Vein Location. The femoral arterial pulse is located as described previously. If arterial and venous puncture is planned, the area infiltrated by lidocaine must be wide enough to provide adequate anesthesia to both puncture sites.

Skin Entry. The skin is entered 0.5 to 1 cm medial and 0.5 cm slightly caudal (toward the foot) to the arterial entry site. Because vein puncture may be successful only after several attempts, the skin incision may be made after the needle has been placed in the vein.

Vein Puncture. Because venous pressure is low, it may be difficult to see unassisted back bleeding from the needle on entry. A 10- or 20-ml syringe with 5 ml of saline can be attached to the Seldinger needle and gently aspirated during needle advancement. The operator inserts the needle medially through the skin at a 30- to 45-degree angle to the horizontal plane while palpating the femoral arterial pulse with the left-hand fingers (*remember: N-A-V = nerve, artery, vein*, from outside in, i.e., lateral to medial). If arterial pulsations are felt at the tip of the needle, the needle is withdrawn and redirected at a slightly more medial angle. A small amount of saline is injected to clear tissue or fat from the needle, and a gentle suction is created with the syringe. If the vein has been entered, venous (nonpulsatile) dark blood fills the syringe. Blood should come easily and without application of much negative pressure. If the vein has not been entered, the same gentle flush–aspiration cycle is repeated while the needle is with-drawn a few millimeters at a time. If the attempt is unsuc-cessful, the needle is flushed and reintroduced in a slightly more lateral or medial direction. If the artery is entered and not used, the needle is removed and firm manual pressure is applied over the artery for 3 minutes. Another attempt to enter the vein can be made after the bleeding has stopped. Several attempts may be needed to puncture the vein. Sometimes it may be necessary to direct the needle close to the artery because the vein may be located partially under the artery.

A vein that has been entered mistakenly during a femoral artery puncture attempt should be used only if the needle tip did not puncture both walls of the artery and go into the vein behind it. Placing a sheath through the artery into the vein may create an arteriovenous fistula or cause uncontrolled bleeding from a large hole in the posterior wall of the femoral artery. The remainder of the venous sheath placement is completed in the same fashion as described for the femoral arterial sheath insertion.

After the catheterization is completed, finger pressure is applied over the vein as described for femoral artery sheath removal. After percutaneous femoral vein puncture, 5 to 10 minutes is usually enough time to obtain adequate hemostasis.

ARM APPROACH
Radial Artery Catheterization

The radial approach for coronary angiography was first described by Campeau in 1989. The technique has gained widespread acceptance around the world. In the Netherlands, Kiemeneij also pioneered the radial approach for coronary interventions, increasing the success rate, improving patient comfort, and providing a method for excellent hemostasis in the fully anticoagulated patient who must remain so after an intervention.

The radial approach has several distinct advantages: (1) the radial artery is easily accessible in most patients and is not located near significant veins or nerves, (2) the superficial location of the radial artery enables easy access and control of bleeding, (3) no significant clinical sequelae after radial artery occlusion occur in patients with a normal Allen's test because of the collateral flow to the hand through the ulnar artery, (4) patient comfort is enhanced by the ability to sit up and walk immediately after the procedure.

Use of Allen's Test. A requirement for the radial procedure is the performance of the Allen's test. The Allen's test assesses ulnar flow and is performed as follows: the radial and ulnar arteries are occluded simultaneously while the patient makes a fist. When the hand is opened, it appears blanched. Release of the ulnar artery should result in return of hand color within 8 to 10 seconds. Satisfactory ulnar flow can also be documented by pulse oximetry.

Patient Selection. Patients with a normal Allen's test are candidates for the radial approach with 5 F and 6 F sheaths and catheters. Small female patients are more likely to have spasm of the radial artery, but this can be treated effectively with the use of intraarterial nitroglycerin or verapamil. Specially coated hydrophilic sheaths are also helpful to reduce spasm on sheath insertion and removal.

Patient Preparation. The patient should be well sedated and comfortably positioned. The arm is abducted at a 70-degree angle on an arm board for sheath insertion. A movable arm board allows the arm to be positioned at the patient's side during the procedure. A roll of sterile towels is used to support the wrist in a hyperextended position. A topical anesthetic helps to decrease the amount of lidocaine needed for local infiltration over the radial pulse. Large amounts of lidocaine may obscure the pulse and make cannulation more difficult. Before complete sheath introduction, use of a vasodilator (nitroglycerin, verapamil) and intraarterial lidocaine reduces artery spasm and improves patient comfort.

Equipment Selection. Arterial puncture is best achieved with a short 20-gauge needle and a 0.025-inch guidewire. A radial artery sheath system of 24 cm with a graduated dilator system over the 0.025-inch guidewire is available. The long sheath technique is advocated for patient comfort and facilitates catheter manipulation. Radial artery spasm may make catheter movement difficult or impossible when a short sheath is used, and patient discomfort is more common. In some patients a longer sheath may diminish ulnar flow during the procedure. Careful catheter selection for the radial approach is important. Box 2-3 lists the most commonly used catheters. The standard preformed diagnostic Judkins or Amplatz catheter shapes may be used but require more manipulation for selective engagement of the coronary ostia. For selective engagement of the left coronary ostium a Judkins left 3.5 catheter is typically used.

Box 2-3

Most Commonly Used Catheters for Radial Coronary Angiography

Right Coronary Artery
Judkins right catheter
Multipurpose catheter
Amplatz right catheter
Amplatz left catheter

Left Coronary Artery
Judkins left catheter (typically 3.5-cm)
Multipurpose catheter
Amplatz left catheter

Vein Grafts
Multipurpose catheter
Amplatz left catheter
Judkins right catheter

Use of the left radial artery approach provides easier manipulation of the standard preformed Judkins shapes with minimal effort. The left arm should be brought over the abdomen so that the operator can work from his or her usual position on the right of the patient.

Adjunctive Medications for Radial Artery Catheterization. After half of the arterial sheath has been inserted, a "cocktail" consisting of 5000 U of heparin, 2 ml of 1% lidocaine, and 200 mg of nitroglycerin is given (Box 2-4). Lidocaine improves patient comfort during catheter manipulation. An additional vasodilator, such as diltiazem, verapamil, papaverine, or adenosine, may be necessary to minimize spasm of the radial artery. Intraarterial injection of 1 to 2 mg of verapamil through the sheath reduces painful vasospasm. Verapamil in doses of 5 mg have been given without unwanted side effects, such as hypotension or bradycardia.

Sheath Removal and Postprocedure Care. Before sheath removal, 1 mg of verapamil is given through the sheath to minimize spasm of the radial artery. A plastic bracelet with a pressure pad is placed around the wrist (Fig. 2-10). Gauze is wrapped around the plastic strap to prevent skin injury when the bracelet is tightened. Another folded gauze is placed under

---

Box 2-4

Medical Regimen for Radial Catheterization

Before the Procedure
Topical anesthetic cream over the radial artery (optional)

Through the Sheath (before catheter insertion)
Heparin, 2000 to 5000 U
Verapamil, 1 to 2 mg, or nitroglycerin, 200 to 400 mg
1% lidocaine, 1 to 2 ml

After the Procedure and Before Sheath Removal
Verapamil, 1 mg (optional)

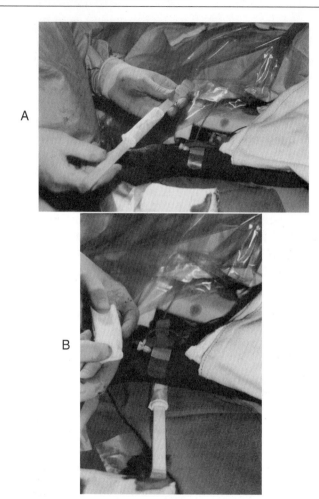

Fig. 2-10   A, The operator holds the plastic bracelet with gauze covering the edges. **B,** The bracelet has been placed under the wrist. Another gauze pack is folded to be placed over the radial sheath beneath the pressure pad.

Continued

the pressure pad over the sheath insertion site. While the operator presses the pad over the puncture site, the sheath is withdrawn gently and the bracelet is tightened. The pad is pressed down and locked over the puncture by tightening of the bracelet bracket. The bracelet should be tight enough to

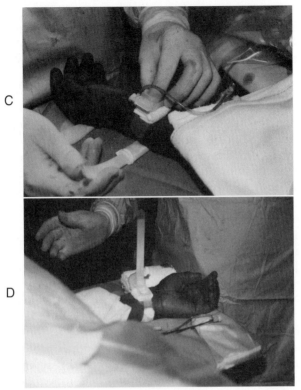

Fig. 2-10, cont'd C, The bracelet is engaged to hold the pad over the puncture site, and the sheath is removed as pressure is applied. **D,** The bracelet is tightened and secured over the radial puncture site. The hand should be checked for adequate perfusion.

ensure hemostasis but not occlude the flow to the hand. The patient is checked 1 to 2 hours later, and the bracelet is loosened. The patient can be discharged 2 hours later and the bracelet removed at home. The patient is given instructions about puncture site compression with the fingers if late bleeding occurs.

Percutaneous Brachial Artery Puncture

The percutaneous brachial arterial entry, favored over the brachial artery cutdown, should be reserved for patients in whom the radial artery cannot be used as access. Percutaneous brachial arterial puncture is a safe and effective alternative to brachial arterial cutdown. Although similar to femoral arterial puncture, there are several important differences. The brachial artery is smaller (3 to 5 mm in diameter) than the femoral artery. Because of the relatively loose subcutaneous tissues the course of the brachial artery may change considerably. Spasm can occur easily with considerable decrease in pulse amplitude, making the puncture more difficult. The artery is more mobile than the femoral artery. Care should be taken to puncture the artery successfully on the first attempt. Because of the smaller space in the arm, uncontrolled hematoma formation here can readily cause compression syndrome with ischemia of the forearm and hand. The median nerve lies immediately medial to the artery. Accidental touching of the median nerve causes a peculiar electrical shock sensation in the hand.

The operator should check the brachial and radial pulses before attempting brachial arterial puncture. They should be strong and equal in both arms. The patency of the ulnar artery and palmar arcus is checked by the Allen's test. Radial and ulnar arteries should be checked separately.

In patients in which femoral access is not possible because of severe atherosclerosis, vascular surgery, or an intraaortic balloon pump, the same type of atherosclerotic disease may exist in the subclavian arterial system. The subclavian-axillary artery system should be auscultated carefully for bruits above and below the clavicula.

Anesthesia Administration. The maximum point of brachial arterial pulse is located 1 to 2 cm above the elbow crease. With a 25-gauge needle the skin and subcutaneous tissue are infiltrated with 2 to 3 ml of 1% lidocaine. Injection of excessive amounts of local anesthetic may make palpation of the artery difficult or obscure the pulse completely.

Puncture of the Artery and Introduction of the Guidewire. An 18-gauge needle with plastic cannula (Medicut or Angiocath) is used to puncture the brachial artery, entering the skin at a 45-degree angle. To facilitate the arterial puncture, the operator can stabilize the artery with the index and middle fingers placed below and above the puncture point. Arterial entry is confirmed by brisk bleeding from the needle. At this point the needle is removed as the plastic outer sheath is advanced slowly into the artery. After removal of the needle the sheath is held stable with the operator's left-hand fingers and a 0.032-inch, small-curve, J-tipped guidewire is advanced into the artery, around the shoulder, and into the aorta under fluoroscopic control.

Sheath Introduction. Firm pressure is maintained over the arterial puncture site, the wire is held (pinched with index fingers and thumb), and the plastic sheath is removed from the wire. The wire is wiped clean with wet gauze.

Additional lidocaine can be applied to the deeper tissue planes. The tip of a no. 11 scalpel blade is used to make a small shallow skin incision at the entry point of the guidewire. The sheath-dilator assembly is advanced over the wire into the artery as described for femoral arterial sheath insertion. After removal of the guidewire and dilator the sheath is aspirated and flushed and the patient's blood pressure is checked.

Sheath Selection. The brachial artery can accommodate up to size 8 F sheaths in large men. In most patients, especially smaller men and women, smaller sheaths (e.g., ≤6 F) are preferred.

Heparin Administration. Heparin (3000 to 5000 U) is given through the sheath or intravenously. If the heparin is given through the sheath, the patient should be warned that it causes a temporary burning sensation in the hand.

Catheter Selection. Standard right and left Judkins, Amplatz, or multipurpose catheters can be manipulated easily from the right arm.

Hemostasis After Percutaneous Brachial Artery Catheterization. A board can be placed behind the patient's elbow to facilitate pressure application. The radial pulse is checked before sheath removal. If the pulse is weak or absent, 0.2 to 0.4 mg of nitroglycerin can be delivered into the artery through the sheath. Intravenous protamine, as for femoral artery hemostasis, is optional.

The sheath is removed while firm finger pressure is applied over the puncture site. A small amount of bleeding is allowed to purge possible clots. The operator should not "strip" the sheath, pushing thrombus into the artery. The radial pulse is palpated continuously with the operator's right hand, and the amount of pressure applied over the artery with the left hand is adjusted to stop bleeding without completely obliterating the radial pulse.

After 15 to 20 minutes the pressure is released slowly. The patient's radial pulse is checked and recorded. The arm circumference at the site of puncture is measured to facilitate the detection of hematoma formation. The patient is instructed to keep the arm in a relaxed but straight position for 4 to 6 hours. Sitting up in bed is permitted, but ambulation is restricted until after the hemostasis period (4 to 6 hours).

Percutaneous Brachial Vein Puncture

Because the antecubital vein anatomy varies greatly among patients, a successful vein puncture depends on visual identification of an adequately sized medial antecubital vein. The veins located on the lateral antecubital area should not be used because of their course through the cephalic venous system over the deltoid muscles, which makes advancing a catheter through the relatively sharp turns in the shoulder area difficult. Application of a tourniquet several centimeters above the elbow may facilitate the identification of a suitable vein. The entry into the vein and placement of a sheath are accomplished through the same steps as described for brachial arterial entry. Heparin injection is not necessary. Because of the low blood flow in the vein, only gentle aspiration should be applied to the sheath before flushing.

Brachial Artery Cutdown Technique

The brachial artery and superficial antecubital or brachial veins can be accessed by the direct cutdown technique as described elsewhere (see Baim and Grossman: *Grossman's Cardiac Catheterization, Angiography, and Intervention*).

Other Vascular Access. Access to the patient's circulatory system is not limited to the previously mentioned techniques (Box 2-5). Techniques that are used rarely in the catheteri-

---

Box 2-5

Possible Vascular Access Routes

Arterial
Axillary
Brachial
Femoral
Radial
Subclavian—*not* used for cardiac catheterization
Translumbar—*not* used for cardiac catheterization

Venous
Brachial
Femoral
Internal jugular
Subclavian

---

zation laboratory, such as axillary artery puncture, should be attempted only by experienced operators. Percutaneous subclavian vein puncture techniques are not explained here because they are not used for routine cardiac catheterization.

Internal Jugular Vein Access. The internal jugular vein is lateral to the carotid artery, medial to the external jugular vein, and usually just lateral to the outer edge of the medial head of the sternocleidomastoid muscle. To identify landmarks, the operator instructs the patient to lie supine without a pillow under the head and, in the case of the right internal jugular, with the head turned 30 degrees to the left. Patients with low venous pressures may be placed in the Trendelenburg (head lower than feet) position.

Several reasonable approaches to internal jugular vein access exist. Some physicians have used ultrasound to guide access to the internal jugular vein. A high anterior approach from the top of the triangle formed by the two heads of the sternocleidomastoid muscle and clavicle is recommended. This location moves the puncture site away from the upper lung tip. The triangle can be difficult to localize correctly in obese patients. In these patients, it is helpful to put a finger in the suprasternal recess and move the finger to the right (for right internal jugular access). The first elevation palpated is the medial head of the sternocleidomastoid muscle. The finger should move over the medial head and follow the edge superiorly until the top of the triangle is palpated.

After the skin is infiltrated with lidocaine, the needle is inserted through the skin, pointing slightly toward the ipsilateral nipple. When blood is aspirated, the guidewire is inserted, followed by the sheath using standard Seldinger technique. The external jugular vein, which crosses the same area superficially, should *not* be cut.

Vascular Access Through Synthetic Graft Conduits. Access through synthetic peripheral vascular grafts should be avoided if possible. Limited experience indicates that when grafts were at least 6 months old, complications were less than 2% if 5 F to 9 F sheaths were used for diagnostic but not interventional procedures.

USE OF HEPARIN DURING CARDIAC CATHETERIZATION

The appropriate doses of heparin and measurement of satisfactory anticoagulation are controversial. An intravenous (5000 U) bolus dose can achieve therapeutic anticoagulation status in 94% of patients. A heparin dose of 3000 U provides measurable anticoagulant effect for most patients undergoing standard catheterization of short duration, with low likelihood of prolonged anticoagulant effect that requires therapeutic reversal. Heparin is recommended for patients in whom a prolonged (>20 minutes arterial time) catheterization procedure is anticipated or in whom prior clinical indications for use of heparin exist (e.g., thrombotic tendency, known severe peripheral vascular disease, embolic phenomenon on previous study). In most medical centers additional heparin (beyond that included in heparinized flush solutions) is omitted from routine left-sided heart catheterization when the procedure is performed in a timely manner.

Heparin reversal with protamine sulfate should be selected for patients in whom fish allergy or previous use of NPH insulin is not a concomitant factor (see Chapter 1). Low-molecular-weight heparin has replaced unfractionated heparin in some circumstances.

PROBLEMS OF VASCULAR ACCESS

"Save time: do it right the first time." A thoughtful and systematic approach to the catheterization procedure decreases problems of access. The order of arterial or venous access is often a matter of personal preference. For novice operators whose stereotactic "view" through their fingers needs refinement, attempts at femoral venous entry before arterial sheath insertion are recommended for the following reason: if the arterial sheath is inserted first, firm palpation to establish the landmarks for venous entry may cause the formation of a generous hematoma that may crimp the arterial sheath. This rapidly forming hematoma makes venous location more difficult. If the artery is punctured inadvertently during venous access attempts, the arterial sheath can be inserted as long as the precautions described in the section on the percutaneous femoral approach are observed.

When the arterial entry is established, difficulties next may be encountered traversing a tortuous iliac or abdominal aortic region or in selectively cannulating the coronary arteries, vein grafts, or left ventricle. For readers unfamiliar with catheterization tools, a review of guidewires and catheters to be used is provided later in this chapter. A special needle equipped with a disposable Doppler transducer (Smart Needle) helps in case the operator has difficulty locating the artery or vein.

Vessel Tortuosity

The most frequently encountered difficulty in advancing the guidewires or catheters into the aorta is tortuosity of the iliac or subclavian vessels, a condition often found in elderly patients. The steerable 0.035-inch Wholey guidewire has excellent characteristics for negotiating a tortuous vessel. Its flexible, relatively atraumatic curved tip is steerable and increases safety. In cases of extreme tortuosity, it might be necessary to advance a catheter close to the guidewire tip (within several centimeters) to increase the torque control and the pushability of the guidewire. A right Judkins coronary catheter can be used to change the direction of the guidewire tip.

In patients with tortuous iliac vessels, a long (20-cm) sheath may be used, recognizing the tradeoff of multiple friction points for some straightening of the vessel. Catheter exchanges over a long (300-cm) exchange guidewire may be required to avoid undue prolongation of the procedure by repeated attempts to advance catheters across tortuous atherosclerotic segments.

In patients with extreme tortuosity in the iliac or subclavian system, the torque control of the catheter is markedly decreased. Use of a preshaped catheter is preferred in these cases because it often requires only minimal manipulation to engage the coronary arteries. In addition, advancing a pigtail catheter into the left ventricle of these patients may be difficult and involve loss of catheter length and control in the tortuous segments. This problem may be partially overcome by inserting a 0.038-inch J-tipped guidewire into the catheter and advancing and manipulating the catheter with the wire in place. In some cases, an extra-stiff (Amplatz-type) guidewire can straighten tortuous vessels, but tissue kinking at the curves may cause pain.

Remember: Wire contact with blood forms thrombi despite anticoagulation. The operator should limit wire-loaded catheter manipulations to 2 to 3 minutes and use a meticulous flush technique.

Complications of Arterial Access

The most common complication of femoral cardiac catheterization is hemorrhage and local hematoma formation, which increases in frequency with the increasing size of the sheath, the amount of anticoagulation, and the obesity of the patient. Other common complications (in order of decreasing frequency) include retroperitoneal hematoma, pseudoaneurysm, arteriovenous fistula formation, arterial thrombosis secondary to intimal dissection, stroke, sepsis with or without abscess formation, and cholesterol or air embolization. The frequency of these complications is increased in high-risk procedures; in critically ill, elderly patients with extensive atheromatous disease; in patients receiving anticoagulation, antiplatelet, and fibrinolytic therapies; and in concomitant interventional procedures. Compared with the femoral approach, the brachial (but not radial) approach has a slightly higher risk of vascular complications.

Infections are more common in patients who undergo repeat ipsilateral (same site) femoral punctures or prolonged femoral sheath maintenance (within 1 to 5 days). Cholesterol embolism manifesting with abdominal pain or headache (from mesenteric or central nervous system ischemia), skin mottling ("blue toes"), renal insufficiency, or lung hemorrhage may be a clinical finding in 30% of high-risk patients.

A retroperitoneal hematoma should be suspected in patients with hypotension, tachycardia, pallor, a rapidly falling postcatheterization hematocrit, lower abdominal or back pain, or neurologic changes in the leg in which the puncture was made. This complication is associated with *high femoral arterial puncture and full anticoagulation*. Pseudoaneurysm is associated with *low femoral arterial puncture* (usually below the head of the femur).

In the past, all femoral pseudoaneurysms were routinely repaired by the vascular surgeon to avoid further neurovascular complication or rupture. With ultrasound imaging techniques these false channels can be easily identified and nonsurgical closure selected. Manual compression of the expansile growing mass guided by Doppler ultrasound with or without thrombin or collagen injection is an acceptable therapy for femoral pseudoaneurysm (Fig. 2-11).

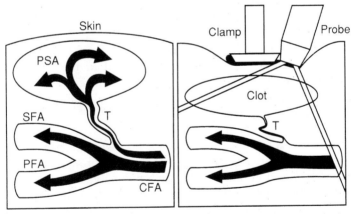

Fig. 2-11 Noninvasive technique for closure of a femoral artery pseudoaneurysm (PSA) by external compression. Arrows represent the course and direction of blood flow. *Left panel,* Blood is shown flowing from the common femoral artery *(CFA)* into a large PSA through a large tract *(T). Right panel,* External application of pressure using a vascular clamp guided by Doppler ultrasound color flow probe results in obliteration of the tract and clot formation in the pseudoaneurysm. *PFA,* Profunda femoris artery; *SFA,* superficial femoral artery. (Redrawn from Agrawal SK, Pinheiro L, Roubin GS, et al: *J Am Coll Cardiol* 20:610-615, 1992.)

Common Problems in Accessing and Cannulating Coronary Arteries and Grafts

Left Coronary Artery

Short Left Main, Separate Ostia for Left Anterior Descending, and Circumflex Arteries. It may be necessary to cannulate the left anterior descending (LAD) and circumflex arteries separately. Slightly advancing the left Judkins catheter or using a left Judkins catheter that is one size smaller (i.e., 3.5 cm from 4 cm) permits cannulation of the LAD artery. Slight withdrawal and clockwise rotation of the catheter or use of a left Judkins catheter that is one size larger permits cannulation of the circumflex artery. An Amplatz-type catheter is especially useful to cannulate the circumflex artery separately but must be used with care to avoid dissection of arteries.

High Left Coronary Artery Takeoff. An unusually high origin of the left main coronary artery from the aorta can usually be cannulated by use of a multipurpose catheter or an Amplatz-type catheter (e.g., AL 2). A long, tapered-tip, multipurpose catheter may be used to cannulate the high-origin left main trunk through the brachial approach.

Wide Aortic Root. In patients with a relatively horizontal and wide aortic root with upward takeoff of the left main coronary artery, a large-curve left Judkins catheter (5 or 6 cm), an Amplatz-type left coronary catheter, or a multipurpose catheter may be required.

Right Coronary Artery. The origin of the right coronary artery shows more variation than that of the left coronary artery. A contrast injection low into the right coronary cusp shows the origin of the right coronary artery and helps direct the catheter. If the right coronary artery is not seen with this injection, it may be totally occluded or may originate anteriorly on the aorta or from the left sinus of Valsalva. In this case the orifice is usually located above the sinotubular ridge. A left Amplatz catheter or a left bypass graft catheter can be used successfully to engage the right coronary artery orifice located anteriorly or in the left cusp. Minimal anterior displacement of the right coronary artery from the right coronary sinus is more common. In this case the right Judkins catheter tip may not be directed toward the right but looks foreshortened in the familiar left anterior oblique view. Directing the catheter tip to the right in the usual fashion using the lateral view permits easy cannulation of the anteriorly directed right coronary orifice. Rarely, an aortogram is needed to confirm the presence of the right coronary artery.

Wide Aortic Root. In a patient with a horizontal and wide aortic root, cannulation of the right coronary orifice and right coronary cusp may require an Amplatz or multipurpose catheter.

High Right Coronary Artery Takeoff. A relatively high origin of the right coronary artery may require a left or right (modified) Amplatz-type catheter. The most common coronary anomaly (see later) is the circumflex artery originating from the right coronary artery or right coronary cusp and coursing posteriorly and downward. This location may be cannulated easily by use of a right Amplatz catheter.

Bypass Grafts. In patients with previous coronary bypass surgery the operative and prior catheterization records and previous angiograms should be reviewed for helpful remarks. The number and type of grafts (i.e., sequential or Y grafts and mammary artery grafts) should be known before the procedure. Special care must be taken to visualize all grafts and native vessels. An aortic root injection may be necessary to document the occlusion of an aortic anastomosis of a vein graft. Metallic markers placed during the operation are helpful in locating the aortic anastomosis site but do not always pinpoint the graft ostia.

In general, vein bypass grafts are anastomosed to the anterior wall of the ascending aorta. The right coronary artery graft is usually anastomosed a few centimeters above and anterior to the right coronary orifice. LAD and diagonal grafts are usually anastomosed higher and slightly to the left. Obtuse marginal grafts are usually the highest and farthest left (Figs. 2-12 and 2-13).

Right Coronary Bypass Vein Graft Catheterization. The right coronary vein graft usually can be entered using a 4-cm right Judkins-type catheter (see Fig. 2-13). In some patients

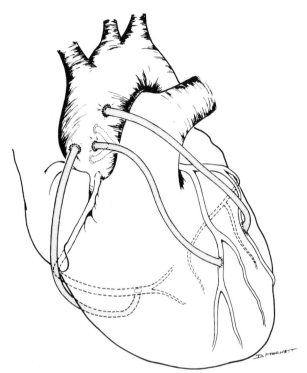

Fig. 2-12 Usual insertion sites of vein grafts to coronary arteries. The proximal (aortic) anastomosis site of the graft to the right coronary artery is most anterior and usually the lowest. Grafts to the branches of the left coronary artery usually are inserted in a progressively higher and more posterolateral position. Variations frequently occur. (From Tilkian AG, Daily EK: *Cardiovascular procedures: diagnostic techniques and therapeutic procedures*, St Louis, 1986, Mosby.)

simple pullback of the catheter from the right coronary orifice, after the right coronary angiogram has been completed, is enough to engage the right coronary vein graft ostium. In other patients the right coronary catheter is placed in the ascending aorta at a level that is slightly higher than the expected level of the right coronary vein graft orifice, and the catheter is rotated clockwise for 45 to 90 degrees. This rotation causes the catheter tip to move along the left border of the ascending aortic silhouette in the left anterior oblique (LAO) position. Advancement or withdrawal while the catheter tip is rotated might be

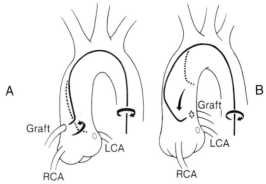

Fig. 2-13 Use of the Judkins right and left vein bypass catheters. **A,** For right coronary artery *(RCA)* grafts, the catheter is rotated clockwise in the left anterior oblique projection until the tip is superior to the graft orifice. It is then advanced down the aortic wall to the orifice of the graft. **B,** For left coronary artery *(LCA)* grafts, clockwise rotation is applied in the left or right anterior oblique projection. (From Tilkian AG, Daily EK: *Cardiovascular procedures: diagnostic techniques and therapeutic procedures,* St Louis, 1986, Mosby.)

necessary for graft engagement. In a patient with a right vein graft with a vertical or downgoing takeoff, the right coronary Judkins catheter tip may be directed toward the wall instead of into the lumen, making adequate opacification of the vein graft unsatisfactory. A right coronary bypass vein graft catheter should be used in these patients. Because of the wider primary curve, the right vein graft catheter tip usually points downward and more parallel to the axis of the graft. Sometimes this catheter may have a tendency to move deeply into the right coronary vein graft. A right (modified) Amplatz catheter also can be used for horizontal or vertical takeoff vein grafts.

Left Anterior Descending Vein Graft Catheterization. Often an LAD vein graft can be entered easily by simply pulling back the right Judkins catheter after right coronary vein graft injection has been completed. Alternatively the right Judkins catheter is placed at a level slightly higher than the expected level of the LAD vein graft orifice, and 30 to 45 degrees clockwise rotation is applied. The catheter tip appears foreshortened in the LAO view and points toward the right border of the ascending aorta silhouette in the right anterior oblique (RAO) view. In some patients it may be necessary to use a left coronary vein graft catheter or left Amplatz catheter. A slight clockwise rotation of the catheter at the level of the expected aortic anastomosis site of the LAD graft engages the catheter into the ostium.

Circumflex Vein Graft Catheterization. A circumflex graft is usually located above the LAD vein graft site. It can be engaged by simply withdrawing the right Judkins catheter from the LAD graft orifice or by repeating the same maneuver described for LAD vein graft cannulation, using right Judkins or left vein graft catheters.

There are many alternative catheters for vein grafts. In some cases it may be necessary to search the whole anterior ascending aortic wall in the LAO and RAO projections systematically by injecting small amounts of contrast media. In a patient with a large ectatic ascending aorta it may be necessary to use a curved multipurpose catheter or a left Amplatz catheter.

The operator should avoid unnecessary manipulation of catheters in vein grafts, especially in old grafts that may contain friable atherosclerotic material with a potential risk of embolization. If a coronary vein graft orifice cannot be entered, an aortic root injection should be performed to document the patency of the graft and to assist in further cannulation attempts.

Internal Mammary Artery Graft Cannulation. The left internal mammary artery originates anteriorly from the caudal wall of the subclavian artery distal to the vertebral artery origin (Fig. 2-14). The left subclavian artery can be entered with use of a right Judkins catheter, but a more sharply angled catheter tip on the mammary artery catheter is preferred. The right Judkins or left mammary artery (LMA) catheter is advanced into the aortic arch up to the level of the right brachiocephalic truncus with the tip directed caudally. Subsequently the catheter is withdrawn slowly and rotated counterclockwise. The catheter tip is deflected cranially, usually engaging the left subclavian artery at the top of the aortic knob in the anteroposterior projection. There are many variations in the shape of the aortic arch and origin and direction of the subclavian

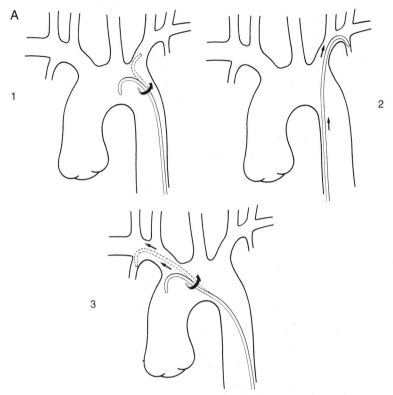

Fig. 2-14   A, Catheterization of the internal mammary arteries. *1,* To catheterize the left internal mammary artery, the catheter is located in the aortic arch in a neutral position, with its tip pointing downward. The catheter is rotated counterclockwise until it falls into the left subclavian artery. *2,* The catheter is advanced with a slight anterior rotation until it engages the origin of the left internal mammary artery. *3,* The right internal mammary artery is entered by counterclockwise rotation of the catheter at the origin of the right innominate artery and advanced until the origin of the internal mammary artery is engaged. (From Tilkian AG, Daily EK: *Cardiovascular procedures: diagnostic techniques and therapeutic procedures,* St Louis, 1986, Mosby.)

Continued

artery. More than one attempt is often necessary to engage the subclavian artery. When the subclavian artery is engaged the catheter is advanced over a guidewire beyond the internal mammary orifice. We recommend a J-tipped guidewire or a Wholey guidewire to guide the catheter into the subclavian

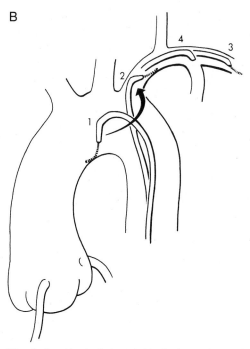

Fig. 2-14, cont'd   **B,** A guidewire is inserted in the internal mammary graft catheter until it is passed into the left subclavian artery. It is removed and withdrawn into the internal mammary artery. (From King SB, Douglas JS Jr: *Coronary arteriography and angioplasty,* New York, 1985, McGraw-Hill.)

artery. In some patients the proximal portion of the subclavian artery can be straightened and the angle between the aortic arch and the subclavian artery can be improved by removing the pillows under the patient's head and hyperextending the neck to the right. When the catheter has been advanced beyond the internal mammary artery takeoff, it is withdrawn slowly and small contrast injections are administered to visualize the internal mammary artery orifice. The catheter tip should be directed caudally. At the level of the internal mammary orifice, slight counterclockwise rotation and advancement may be necessary to cannulate the artery.

Vigorous manipulation of the catheter and deep intubation of the internal mammary artery should be avoided because of the risk of dissection. During internal mammary artery injections the patient should be warned about a painful, burning sensation in the shoulder and anterior chest wall (nonionic contrast media are less painful). In patients with a vertically directed internal mammary artery, an internal mammary artery catheter and a more acute tip angle can be used. Sometimes this catheter cannot be introduced into the subclavian artery because of the tip angle. In this case the subclavian artery can be entered by use of a right Judkins catheter (as described previously), which is then exchanged for an internal mammary artery catheter over an exchange guidewire. Because of the peculiar tip configuration the internal mammary curve catheter, and especially the C-type internal mammary artery catheter, usually engage the internal mammary artery ostium without much difficulty.

Right Internal Mammary Artery Graft Cannulation. Right internal mammary artery cannulation is less common and more difficult than left internal mammary artery cannulation. The right brachiocephalic truncus is entered with use of a right Judkins catheter by deflecting the tip with a counterclockwise rotation at the level of the brachiocephalic truncus. The catheter is advanced into the subclavian artery. The rest of the manipulation is similar to that described for left internal mammary artery graft cannulation.

In patients for whom cannulation of the internal mammary artery is not possible because of excessive tortuosity or obstructive lesions, an internal mammary artery catheter can be introduced through the ipsilateral radial artery. The catheter is advanced beyond the mammary artery orifice over a guidewire. To engage the catheter, the operator withdraws it slowly and administers frequent, small contrast media injections. A technique for cannulation of contralateral internal mammary from the arm approach with use of a Simmons catheter has also been described.

ARTERIAL AND VENOUS ACCESS: NURSE-TECHNICIAN VIEWPOINT

The nursing and technical staff play an integral part in obtaining safe and successful arterial and venous access. Their knowledge of anatomy, patient positioning, and equipment needed for access is essential to provide patient care and support during the access phase of the procedure.

Precatheterization Assessment

Vascular trauma may occur as a result of the access procedure. Before the procedure the staff member should discuss with the patient what sensations the patient might experience while the physician is obtaining vascular access. On the patient's arrival in the cardiac catheterization laboratory the nursing and technical staff must (1) assess the patient's baseline peripheral vascular status, (2) position the patient properly on the procedure table for the femoral or brachial approach, and (3) prepare the access site in a manner that facilitates vascular access by the physician. Alternative access sites also may need to be prepared in advance for unanticipated entry problems. All pulses should be palpated, or, when necessary, Doppler assessment should be performed. Information concerning the presence and stability of the pulse must be conveyed to the physician. Even the uninvolved lower extremity may have loss of pulse from a central embolus or dissection.

Baseline Vascular Assessment

The patient's preprocedure peripheral vascular status (i.e., pulse quality) should be assessed and documented on the catheterization chart before the start of the procedure. In some laboratories the assessment is the responsibility of the nurse, whereas in other laboratories all personnel share this duty. It is a good idea for the person responsible for postcatheterization care to perform the initial assessment so that any changes in vascular status can be recognized easily. Many laboratories are set up so that the entry, preparation, and recovery areas are managed by the same staff members. This setup is ideal because the staff member responsible for precatheterization assessment and postcatheterization care can easily assess any change in the patient's baseline status.

If the femoral approach is used, the femoral artery, dorsalis pedis artery (top of the foot just below the ankle), and posterior tibial artery (inside behind ankle) pulses should be assessed, graded, and recorded on a scale of 0 to 4+ (4 being maximal or a bounding pulse). It is helpful to use a marking pen to indicate the location and grade of the pulse on the patient's foot to facilitate postcatheterization assessment.

If the radial arterial approach is used, a precatheterization assessment of the radial and ulnar pulses must be performed.

The location should be marked and the grade documented on the chart.

Patient Positioning

Femoral Approach. Proper positioning of the patient on the catheterization table by laboratory personnel is important to facilitate arterial and venous access. For the femoral approach the patient should be in the supine position. The x-ray table being used may dictate placement of the patient's arms. In some laboratories the patient's arms are placed behind the head. This placement ensures that the hands and arms are away from the sterile field and will not be in the way of the C-arm of the x-ray unit. The problem with placement of the arms above the head is that the patient will become uncomfortable (and fatigued) during a long procedure. Positioning the arms at the patient's side is probably the most common method. Patients should be instructed to keep their arms as close to the body as possible and under the sterile drape at all times. Instructing patients to *tuck their hands under their hips* may help remind them to keep the arms at the sides and aid in maintaining a comfortable position during the procedure. Positioning of patients' arms at their sides causes the arms to appear in the x-ray field and compromises angiography performed in the severe oblique (angled) projections. For a lateral projection the arms should be raised and placed behind the head.

Patients should be positioned with their legs spread slightly so that their knees are 8 to 12 inches apart. This position facilitates access to the groin by pulling the skin folds apart at the inguinal crease, a landmark for access.

The patient should be positioned as far toward the head of the catheterization table as possible. This positioning allows travel of the C-arm of the x-ray unit to cover the inguinal area and fluoroscopic landmarks (e.g., the femoral head). If access is difficult because of vessel obstruction or tortuosity, it may be necessary to use the fluoroscope over the insertion site. If the patient is positioned too far toward the foot of the x-ray table, fluoroscopic visualization of this area may be impossible.

Special Positioning Problems.

Obese Patient for the Femoral Approach. Obese patients present a challenge to the staff in terms of positioning and site preparation. The first problem encountered is that most catheterization tables are narrow, which leaves no room for comfortable positioning of the patients' arms. A thermoplastic (Plexiglas) arm retainer gives some support and helps keep the patients' arms at the sides. Positioning the arms above the head for short procedures is recommended for obese patients.

The second challenge is that of groin preparation. The protruding abdomen and panniculus of the obese patient usually extend and rest over the groin area, presenting an obstacle to access. The abdomen can be retracted toward the chest and retained in this position by using 3- to 4-inch-wide tape. The tape can be criss-crossed over the retracted abdomen and secured to the sides of the catheterization table. When the abdominal folds are retracted, the groin can be prepared in the usual fashion. Because excessive skin folds in the obese patient may result in higher than normal amounts of skin bacteria, extra care should be taken when cleaning the skin and applying antiseptic solutions. The radial approach should be strongly considered for obese patients.

Positioning for Brachial or Radial Artery Approach. For the brachial or radial artery approach, the arm should be positioned on an arm board to stabilize the position of the wrist. Proper orientation of radial and brachial arteries occurs if the arm is placed on the arm board with the hand secured in the palm-up position. Most x-ray tables have accessory arm boards that mount on the side of the x-ray table. After vascular access has been obtained, the arm should be placed at a 45- to 60-degree angle to the body. Less than 45 degrees or greater than 60 degrees may hinder catheter movement at the entrance to the subclavian artery. The arm board must be allowed to move freely should the physician need to redirect the arm position to aid in catheter manipulation.

EQUIPMENT AND INSTRUMENTS USED FOR ACCESS

A variety of needles, guidewires, vessel dilators, and introducer sheaths are available for use in obtaining vascular access (Figs. 2-15 and 2-16). Because the components necessary for access come in many different sizes, staff members must be knowledgeable regarding compatibility of the different components. Certain needles accept only certain sized guidewires. The same is true for compatibility among wires, catheters, and

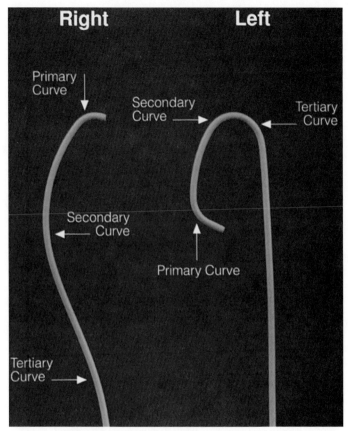

Fig. 2-15   Right and left Judkins catheters, identifying primary, secondary, and tertiary curves of each catheter. These curves are designed to facilitate entry into the ostia of each coronary artery. (Courtesy of Cordis Corporation, Miami, Fla.)

introducer sheaths. Component package inserts contain information regarding size and component compatibility.

The catheterization team members should understand the anatomy of the vascular system for access and catheter placement. Femoral and radial arterial entry gives access to the aorta and left side of the heart, whereas femoral, brachial, or internal jugular venous entry gives access to the right side of the heart. Depending on the clinical presentation, the patient may be scheduled for a right-sided heart catheterization, left-

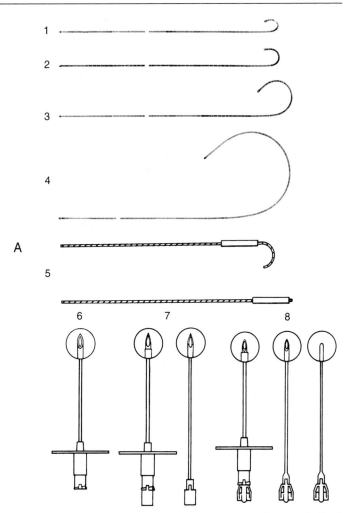

Fig. 2-16 A, Various-size curves of the J-curve guidewire. *1,* Small (1.5-mm) curve. *2,* 3-mm curve. *3,* 6-mm curve. *4,* Large (15-mm) curve. *5,* The curve of the J-curve guidewire is straightened out before vascular entry by sliding the accompanying plastic sleeve over the distal wire tip. *6* through *8,* Three types of percutaneous vascular entry needles. *6,* One-part needle. *7,* Two-part needle consisting of an inner beveled stylet and an outer cannula of metal or plastic. *8,* Three-part needle consisting of an inner beveled stylet, outer cannula, and rounded obturator (note the two cutting edges of the needle tip). (From Tilkian AG, Daily EK: *Cardiovascular procedures: diagnostic techniques and therapeutic procedures,* St Louis, 1986, Mosby.)

Continued

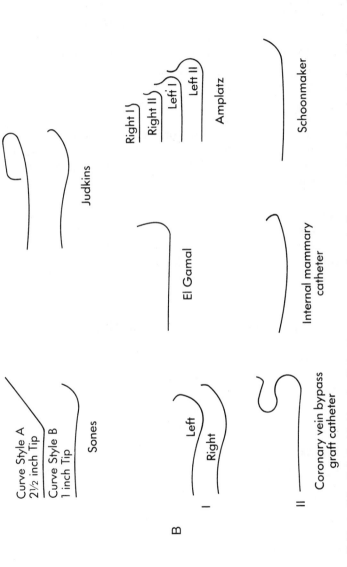

Curve Style A
2½ inch Tip

Curve Style B
1 inch Tip

Sones

Judkins

Right I
Right II
Left I
Left II

Amplatz

Schoonmaker

El Gamal

Internal mammary
catheter

B

Left
Right

I

II

Coronary vein bypass
graft catheter

Fig. 2-16, cont'd   B, Left-sided heart catheters in common use for selective coronary arteriography and ventriculography.

sided heart catheterization, or combined right- and left-sided heart catheterization (see Chapter 3).

Guidewires

Spring Guide. A guidewire is a wrapped spring coil over a central straight core wire, hence the name spring guide (see Fig. 2-16). It looks like a thin, tightly coiled spring when viewed from the outside and is usually made of stainless steel with a coating.

Proximal Tip. The end of the wire that extends outside the patient's body is called the proximal tip. The physician manipulates this end of the wire. It is the end that is nearest, or proximal, to the physician. It is straight and stiff and never goes into the patient.

Distal Tip. The end of the wire that enters the patient and passes through the vessels is called the distal tip. It is farthest away from, or distal to, the physician. This tip is smooth and flexible because of the spring without a segment of a core wire. A J-tip is most commonly used because it bounces over any plaques on the artery wall.

Core Wire. Guidewires are constructed with an inner wire surrounded by a coiled spring–like wire. The inner wire is called the core wire. Core wire may also be called a mandrel. The core wire gives the guidewire body a variable stiffness so that it can be advanced and remain flexible at the same time. This requirement provides safety to the patient. Different core wires allow different degrees of flexibility.

Safety Ribbon. The core wire is attached to the proximal end of the guidewire but not to the distal end. The distal end of the wire is just a flexible spring. If this spring were to break off, it could be lost in the patient's bloodstream, so a thin safety ribbon is attached to the end of the spring.

Fixed-Core Guide. A fixed-core guide is a type of guidewire with a rigid core that is fixed at the proximal end of the wire but is usually unattached at the distal end. The fixed core runs almost the full length of the guidewire. It stops about 3 to 5 cm from the distal tip, leaving an end that is merely a spring without a core. This end is more flexible than the part of the wire that has a core.

Movable-Core Guide. A movable-core guide is a type of guidewire that has a rigid core that is not fixed at either end of the wire. The core can be attached to a handle at the proximal end of the wire. The handle is a similar but separate segment of spring bonded to the proximal end. The physician can extend the core closer to the distal tip of the wire or pull it farther away from the distal tip by manipulating the handle. This manipulation adjusts the length of the flexible spring at the distal tip to suit the physician's needs.

Dagger Effect. In some guidewires, it is possible that, with severe kinking, the core (whether fixed or movable) will separate the coils of the spring wire and poke through them. This is called a dagger effect and could damage the vessel.

J-Tipped Spring Guides. Guidewires that have a curve in the distal tip, usually with a radius of 3, 6, or 15 mm, are called J-tipped spring guides. A J-tipped guidewire easily follows the twisting path of a torturous vessel. A straight wire may catch or dislodge plaques.

Coronary Angiographic Catheters

The Judkins femoral arterial catheterization technique is highly successful because of the simplicity of using preshaped catheters compared with the arm technique, in which the operator must use more manipulation to position the catheter in the coronary ostia. A multipurpose-style catheter is still used and taught, but its devotees are few.

All catheters are inserted with a J-tipped guidewire. The J-tipped guidewire is advanced into the ascending thoracic aorta under fluoroscopic guidance and is followed by the catheter. When the catheter tip has reached the desired location in the aorta, the guidewire is removed and the catheter is aspirated (2 to 3 ml of blood), flushed, and connected to the pressure manifold. The operator should always see the guidewire or catheter tip on the fluoroscopy screen when the catheter or guidewire is manipulated.

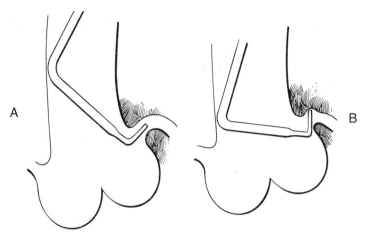

Fig. 2-17   Left Judkins coronary catheter position. **A,** Correct alignment. **B,** Incorrect position and overinsertion. (From King SB, Douglas JS Jr: *Coronary arteriography and angioplasty,* New York, 1985, McGraw-Hill.)

Except in cases involving known severe atherosclerotic disease or the presence of thrombi in the aortoiliac system, the catheters can be removed without a guidewire.

Judkins-Type Coronary Catheters.   Coronary angiography can be completed using Judkins catheters from the femoral approach in more than 90% of patients. Judkins catheters have special preshaped curves and tapered end-hole tips. The Judkins left coronary catheter has a double curve. The length of the segment between the primary and secondary curve determines the size of the catheter (i.e., 3.5, 4, 5, or 6 cm). The proper size of the left Judkins catheter is selected depending on the length and width of the ascending aorta. In a small person with a small aorta a 3.5-cm catheter is appropriate, whereas in a large person or in an individual with an enlarged or dilated ascending aorta (e.g., as a result of aortic stenosis, regurgitation, or Marfan's syndrome), a 5- or 6-cm catheter may be required (Figs. 2-17 and 2-18).

The ingenious design of the left Judkins catheter permits cannulation of the left coronary artery without any major catheter manipulation except the slow advance of the catheter under fluoroscopic control. The catheter tip follows the

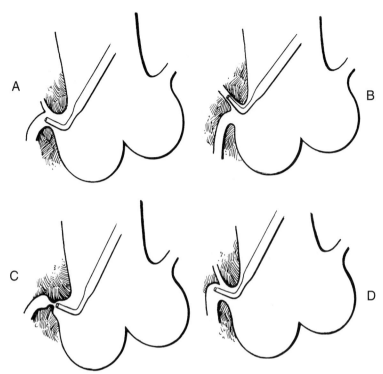

Fig. 2-18   Right Judkins coronary catheter position. **A,** Correct alignment. **B,** Tip subselectively in conus artery. **C,** Tip wedged in proximal stenosis. **D,** Tip impinging on lateral vessel wall. (From King SB, Douglas JS Jr: *Coronary arteriography and angioplasty,* New York, 1985, McGraw-Hill.)

ascending aortic border and falls into the left main coronary ostium, often with an abrupt jump. In the words of its inventor, "the [Judkins] catheter knows where to go if not thwarted by the operator."

A left 4-cm Judkins catheter fits in most adults. When catheter size is adequate, the catheter tip is aligned with the long axis of the left main coronary trunk. A smaller (3.5 cm) catheter in the same patient tips upward and a larger (5 cm) catheter tips downward into the coronary cusp. When the coronary orifice is not cannulated appropriately, the catheter should be replaced with a better-fitting catheter rather than manipulated into the coronary artery (see Fig. 2-17). A slight counterclockwise rotation of the catheter may be necessary to improve alignment of the catheter tip with the left main coronary trunk.

The Judkins right coronary catheter is sized by the length of the secondary curve and comes in 3.5-, 4-, and 5-cm sizes. The 4-cm catheter is adequate in most cases. The right Judkins catheter is advanced into the ascending aorta (usually with LAO projection) with the tip directed caudally (see Fig. 2-17). The right coronary artery can be entered in most cases by one of two maneuvers:

1. The catheter is advanced into the right coronary cusp. The catheter is rotated 45 to 90 degrees clockwise as the tip is pulled back 2 to 3 cm. Rotation of the tip toward the right coronary cusp and downward motion of the catheter are seen on the fluoroscope as the right coronary orifice is engaged.

2. The catheter tip is advanced to 2 to 4 cm above the valve. When the catheter is rotated clockwise for 45 to 90 degrees, the tip rotates toward the right cusp and descends approximately 1 to 2 cm, engaging the right coronary ostium from above.

If the coronary ostium is not engaged, the maneuvers are repeated starting at a slightly different level each time. A brief contrast media injection into the right coronary cusp may show the right coronary artery orifice and help the operator direct the catheter. A slight but firm push and pull on the catheter is necessary to translate rotational motion at the hub down to the tip.

If stored rotational energy is not released by a small counterrotation after seating, the catheter may spring out of the right coronary ostium when the patient takes a deep breath. After seating, the operator checks for pressure damping associated with ostial stenosis or conus branch cannulation (see Fig. 2-18).

Amplatz-Type Catheters. The left Amplatz-type catheter is a preshaped half-circle with the tapered tip extending perpendicular to the curve (Fig. 2-19). Amplatz catheter sizes (left 1, 2, and 3 and right 1 and 2) indicate the diameter of the tip curve. In most normal-sized adults, no. 2 left and no. 1 right (modified) Amplatz catheters give satisfactory results. In the LAO projection the tip is advanced into the left aortic cusp.

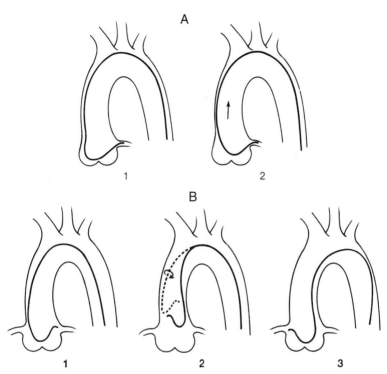

Fig. 2-19   Catheterization of the coronary arteries (Amplatz technique, left anterior oblique projection). **A,** Catheterization of the left coronary artery. *1,* The left coronary catheter is advanced until the secondary curve rests in the noncoronary posterior aortic cusp and its tip points to the left coronary ostium. *2,* The catheter is gently advanced and retracted until the left coronary ostium is engaged. **B,** Catheterization of the right coronary artery. *1,* The right coronary catheter initially may point to the left coronary sinus. *2,* It is withdrawn slightly and rotated clockwise until the tip points toward the right coronary artery, and the secondary curve rests against the left aortic cusp. *3,* The right coronary artery is engaged as the catheter is advanced and withdrawn. (From Tilkian AG, Daily EK: *Cardiovascular procedures: diagnostic techniques and therapeutic procedures,* St Louis, 1986, Mosby.)

Further advancement of the catheter causes the tip to move upward into the left main aortic trunk. It is necessary to push Amplatz catheters slightly to disengage by backing the catheter tip upward and out of the left main ostium. If the catheter is pulled instead of first being advanced, the tip moves downward and into the left main or circumflex artery. Unwanted deep cannulation of the circumflex artery might tear this branch or the left main aortic trunk. The incidence of coronary dissection is higher with Amplatz catheters than with Judkins-type catheters.

The right (modified) Amplatz catheter has a smaller but similar hook-shaped curve. The catheter is advanced into the right coronary cusp. As with Judkins right catheters, the catheter is rotated clockwise for 45 to 90 degrees. The same maneuver is repeated at different levels until the right coronary artery is entered. After coronary injections the catheter may be pulled, advanced, or rotated out of the coronary artery.

Multipurpose Catheters. Multipurpose catheters are catheters that are primarily straight with an end hole and two side holes placed close to the tapered tip. Preshaped, mildly angled configurations are also available. The multipurpose catheter can be used for left and right coronary injections and left ventriculography. (For a description of manipulation, see the section on Sones catheterization later in the chapter.)

Special Purpose Femoral Angiography Catheters. The right coronary vein graft catheter is similar to a right Judkins catheter but has a wider, more open primary curve that allows cannulation of a vertically oriented coronary artery vein graft. The left coronary vein graft catheter is similar to the right Judkins catheter but has a smaller and sharper secondary curve that allows easy cannulation of LAD and left circumflex vein grafts, which usually are placed higher and more anterior than right coronary grafts with a relatively horizontal and upward takeoff from the aorta.

The internal mammary artery graft catheter has a peculiar hook-shaped tip configuration that facilitates the engagement of internal mammary artery grafts, especially in patients with a vertical origin of the internal mammary artery.

Ventriculography Catheters. For the femoral approach, two catheters are generally used:
1. The pigtail catheter has a tapered tip, preshaped to make a full circle, 1 cm in diameter. There are 5 to 12 side holes on the straight portion of the catheter above the

curve. To enter the left ventricle, the pigtail catheter is advanced to the aortic valve. The loop is positioned to the left in the RAO projection, and the catheter is pushed against the valve to make a U shape that facilitates entry into the ventricle during deep inspiration. The catheter is placed in front of the mitral valve with the loop directed away from the valve (in the RAO position). A slight rotation, advancement, or withdrawal may be necessary to find a "quiet" position (one that does not cause frequent premature ventricular contractions) in the ventricle (Fig. 2-20). An angled (145 degrees) pigtail catheter may be helpful for this purpose, especially for horizontally oriented hearts.

A novel 5 F catheter with a helical tip with inward-directed side holes (Halo catheter) seems to produce equivalent left ventriculograms with minimal ectopy (Fig. 2-21). It is excellent to measure distal left ventricular chamber pressure in hypertrophic cardiomyopathy because, in contrast to a pigtail catheter, there are no holes along the shaft to create a falsely low distal pressure.

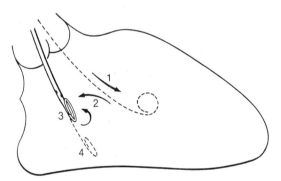

Fig. 2-20 Judkins method of left ventricular catheterization. *1,* Having crossed the aortic valve, the pigtail catheter is in position. *2,* The catheter is withdrawn 2 to 3 cm and rotated 70 to 90 degrees counterclockwise. *3,* The coiled loop is in the inflow tract of the mitral valve. *4,* If the catheter moves excessively in this position, it should be advanced until it is stable. (From Judkins MP, Judkins E: Coronary arteriography and left ventriculography: Judkins technique. In King SB III, Douglas JS Jr, editors: *Coronary arteriography and angioplasty,* New York, 1985, McGraw-Hill.)

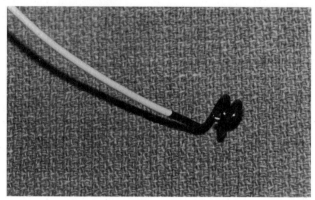

Fig. 2-21   Halo ventriculography catheter. Side holes are contained only within the spiral, which is directed inward to reduce premature ventricular contractions.

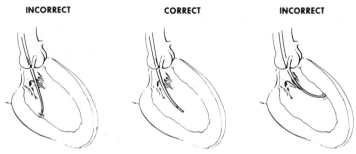

Fig. 2-22   Catheterization of the left ventricle in 35-degree right anterior oblique projection. When positioned correctly *(center)*, the catheter tip should be near the tip of the papillary muscles, aiming toward the apex. If it is touching the inferior or inferolateral wall *(left)*, it should be rotated clockwise. If it is touching the anteroseptal wall *(right)*, it should be rotated counterclockwise. (From King SB, Douglas JS Jr: *Coronary arteriography and angioplasty,* New York, 1985, McGraw-Hill.)

2. The multipurpose catheter can be used for femoral ventriculography. It is advanced across the aortic valve directly or, after making an upward loop with slight rotation, falls into the ventricle. This catheter should be positioned freely in the left ventricular chamber so that the high-pressure contrast jet does not produce ventricular tachycardia, contrast injection in the myocardial tissue (contrast staining), or perforation (Fig. 2-22).

The pigtail catheter (and Halo) produces less ectopy than the multipurpose catheter, and it rarely causes myocardial contrast staining or perforation.

Multipurpose Catheters for the Radial Artery Technique. Sones of the Cleveland Clinic used the straight tapered catheter from the open brachial artery. The Sones catheter, now replaced by the multipurpose catheter, is introduced into the brachial or radial artery and advanced over a guidewire into the subclavian artery under fluoroscopic guidance.

There may be a sharp caudal turn near the origin of the carotid artery that usually requires a J-tipped guidewire for passage. An inexperienced operator manipulating the catheter in this area may dissect or perforate the subclavian artery. To decrease the kinking and tortuosity of brachiocephalic vessels, the operator should instruct the patient to turn his or her head to the left, with the chin extended (as if trying to see the ceiling corner), and to inspire deeply. The operator also may pull the patient's arm straight and extend it toward the head at a 90-degree angle with the chest wall.

Cannulation of the left coronary artery using a Sones or multipurpose catheter is performed in the LAO projection (Fig. 2-23, *A*). The catheter tip is advanced against the aortic valve and pushed to form a U-shaped loop with upward movement of the tip toward the left main aortic trunk. The tip position is verified with small contrast media injections. When the catheter tip is near the left main coronary artery orifice, a slight counterclockwise rotation of the catheter brings the tip into the left main artery. Slightly withdrawing the catheter causes the tip to seat in the left main artery and achieve a more stable angiographic position. Because the catheter moves considerably with breathing, the operator ensures stability by advancing or withdrawing the catheter slightly as needed.

Cannulation of the right coronary artery is also performed in the LAO projection (Fig. 2-23, *B*). A smaller U-shaped curve can be formed in the right cusp with the tip directed to the left coronary orifice. The operator rotates the catheter clockwise into the right cusp keeping the shortened U-shaped loop. When the tip is engaged, the catheter has a tendency to go deeply into the right coronary artery, which requires catheter adjustments during respiratory cycles. In patients with a

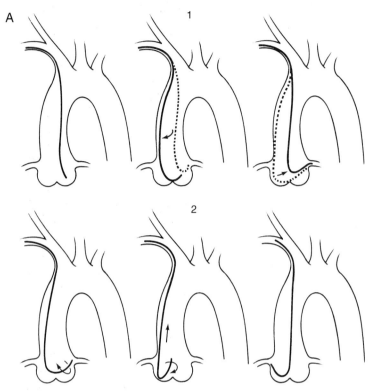

Fig. 2-23 A, Catheterization of the *1,* left and *2,* right coronary arteries in the left anterior oblique projection using the Sones technique. See text for details. *Continued*

vertically originating right coronary artery, the Sones catheter may go directly into the right coronary artery when it is first advanced through the right arm.

Preshaped Coronary Catheters from the Radial Artery Approach. Judkins left and right coronary catheters can be used through the left or right arm with satisfactory results. Compared with the femoral technique, a left Judkins catheter of smaller curve may be necessary with the left radial technique. The preshaped catheter should be introduced and advanced over the J-tipped guidewire. An Amplatz catheter can be used effectively from either the right or the left arm. This catheter is manipulated in a fashion similar to that described for the femoral approach.

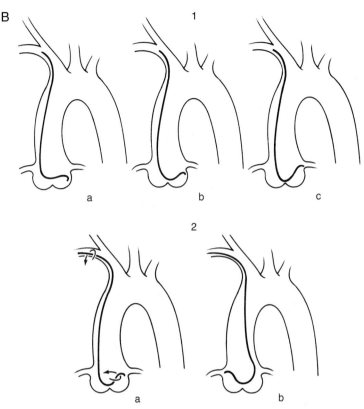

Fig. 2-23, cont'd   B, Castillo modification of the Amplatz technique. *1,* Catheterization of the left coronary artery. *a,* The Castillo catheter is advanced until the secondary curve rests in the noncoronary posterior aortic cusp and its tip points to the left coronary ostium. *b* and *c,* The catheter is gently advanced and retracted until the left coronary ostium is engaged. *2,* Catheterization of the right coronary artery. *a,* Initially the catheter points to the left coronary sinus. *b,* It is withdrawn slightly and rotated until the tip points toward the right coronary artery. The right coronary ostium is engaged as the catheter is advanced and withdrawn. (From Tilkian AG, Daily EK: *Cardiovascular procedures: diagnostic techniques and therapeutic procedures,* St Louis, 1986, Mosby.)

Although the preshaped coronary catheters can be removed without a guidewire, a pigtail ventriculography catheter should be removed over a guidewire to straighten the pigtail loop and prevent it from kinking or lodging in the subclavian or axillary artery.

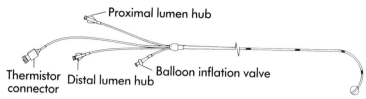

Fig. 2-24 Multilumen balloon-tipped pulmonary artery catheter for hemodynamic measurements of the right side of the heart. (From Tilkian AG, Daily EK: *Cardiovascular procedures: diagnostic techniques and therapeutic procedures,* St Louis, 1986, Mosby.)

Catheters for Right-Sided Heart Catheterization

Hemodynamic Measurements. A balloon-tipped flotation catheter (Fig. 2-24)—originally designed by Swan and Ganz— is the most widely used catheter for right-sided heart hemodynamics. The balloon tip allows the catheter to float through the right side of the heart safely and easily in most cases. The balloon "wedges" in the distal pulmonary artery to measure pressure (reflecting left atrial and ventricular filling pressures). Thermodilution cardiac output measurements are routine and are exclusive to this type of catheter. The balloon-tipped catheter can be introduced through any venous access route. The balloon is inflated with room air. Carbon dioxide may be used if passage to the arterial circulation is anticipated.

Balloon Catheter Technique for Traversing the Right Side of the Heart. From the femoral approach, two techniques can be used to traverse the right side of the heart:

1. The catheter tip is passed directly (medially) across the tricuspid valve and allowed to float just beyond the tricuspid valve in the right ventricle. Then the catheter is pulled back slightly, and a clockwise rotation is applied. When the balloon tip is deflected upward toward the right ventricular outflow tract, the catheter is advanced quickly into the pulmonary artery well beyond the pulmonary valve (Fig. 2-25).

2. The catheter is directed toward the lateral wall of the right atrium. A loop is made with the tip directed in a circle and under the catheter and across to the tricuspid valve. As it is advanced, the catheter floats across the

tricuspid valve, up through the right ventricle, and into the pulmonary artery.

Balloon-tipped catheters do not provide good torque control, making catheterization of the pulmonary artery in patients with right atrial or ventricular enlargement, pulmonary hypertension, or tricuspid regurgitation difficult from the

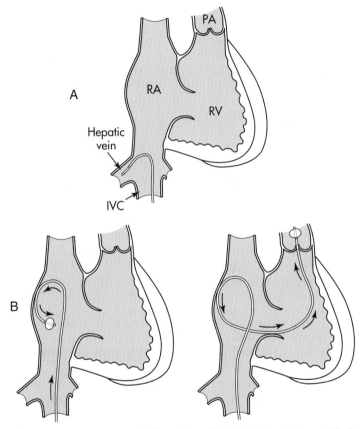

Fig. 2-25   Techniques to facilitate the catheter into the right ventricle in difficult cases. **A,** Directing the catheter into the hepatic vein produces a curve that, when advanced, may direct the catheter tip across the tricuspid valve. **B,** The balloon is deflated, with the catheter directed toward the lateral wall and advanced until a loop has been developed with the catheter tip pointing toward the tricuspid valve. The balloon is inflated, and the catheter is advanced across the tricuspid valve. The catheter usually can be advanced to the pulmonary artery *(PA)* without difficulty.   *Continued*

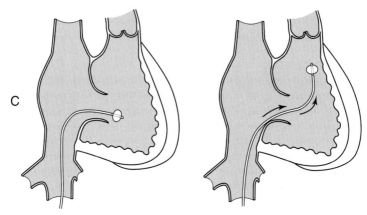

C

Fig. 2-25, cont'd   C, When in the right ventricle *(RV)*, the catheter can be rotated in a clockwise manner. The loop is enlarged with the maneuver, so the catheter should be retracted gently to maintain the same loop size. As the catheter tip points upward in the outflow tract, the catheter should be advanced across the pulmonary valve. *RA,* Right atrium; *IVC,* inferior vena cava. (From Uretzky BF: *Cardiac catheterization: concepts, techniques, and applications,* Walden, Mass, 1997, Blackwell Science.)

femoral approach. In cases in which a guidewire (0.025-inch) does not add control to catheter manipulations, the catheter can be introduced through the antecubital or internal jugular vein (Box 2-6). A Mullins-type long sheath may help the operator to direct the catheter tip toward the lateral right atrial wall and across the tricuspid valve by forming a large loop.

Box 2-6

Conditions of Patients in Whom Superior Vena Caval Approach for Right-Sided Heart Catheterization Is Preferred

Pulmonary hypertension
Right ventricular hypertension
Tricuspid regurgitation/stenosis
Massive right atrial dilation
Massive right ventricular dilation
Anomalous inferior vena cava
Inferior vena cava filter (for pulmonary embolism)
Suspected femoral/iliac vein thrombus (may precipitate pulmonary embolus)
Renal vein thrombosis

When the catheter is in the pulmonary artery, the tip (with the inflated balloon) is advanced to obtain a pulmonary artery wedge pressure (see Chapter 3).

Pulmonary Capillary Wedge Pressure. Pulmonary capillary wedge pressure can be identified from adequate pressure waveforms (see Chapter 3). Correct wedge position can be confirmed with oximetry. In cases in which a critical measure of the mitral valvular gradient is required, transseptal left atrial pressure is used. Adequate pulmonary capillary oxygen saturation is difficult to obtain with the balloon inflated. Advancement of the catheter tip with the balloon deflated into the deep wedge position may yield a confirmatory oxygen saturation. The best location of the pulmonary wedge pressure has been questioned, but for practical purposes any of the four locations (left or right upper lobes or left or right lower lobes) within the pulmonary tree are generally acceptable. The right lower lobe is the most common location for positioning of the pulmonary artery balloon-tipped catheter. In patients with high pulmonary artery pressures (>50 mm Hg), an inflated balloon should not be left in place for more than 10 minutes because prolonged balloon inflation may cause pulmonary infarction or damage to the pulmonary artery. The balloon can be inflated for longer periods in other patients. The operator should be careful not to inflate a balloon vigorously in distal portions of the lung where the balloon may tear a small pulmonary vessel. Complications of pulmonary artery catheterization are listed in Box 2-7.

Several other types of catheters provide high-quality right-sided heart pressure measurement and permit rapid aspiration of blood samples for oxygen saturation measurements but do

---

Box 2-7

Complications of Pulmonary Artery Catheterization

Complications of vascular access
Pulmonary infarction
Pulmonary artery rupture
Injury to chordae in right ventricle
Tricuspid regurgitation
Right bundle-branch block
Dislodgement of pacemaker leads

not have thermodilution cardiac output capability. Multipurpose catheters can be introduced through the femoral or brachial veins and manipulated in a fashion similar to the balloon-tipped catheter method described here. A catheter with an end-hole design allows wedge pressure measurement when the catheter is advanced deeply into the pulmonary artery. Deep inspiration by the patient and simultaneous catheter advancement as the patient coughs facilitate wedge placement with these catheters. A balloon-tipped, blind-end catheter (Berman) for angiography also is available and makes blood sampling easy.

Catheters for Right-Sided Heart Angiography. The Berman catheter is a large-lumen, balloon-tipped angiographic catheter with no end hole and with side holes placed proximal to the balloon. It is easily introduced into the right side of the heart and can be used to measure pulmonary artery pressures. Keeping the balloon inflated increases catheter stability during angiography. This catheter allows flow rates as high as a pigtail catheter. A regular pigtail catheter or one with a special obtuse angle (Grollman) can also be used for right ventriculography.

A comprehensive discussion of all available catheter types and techniques is beyond the scope of this handbook. The new operator should concentrate on mastering a few types of catheters and gain extensive experience in using them effectively.

Suggested Readings

Baim DS, Grossman W, editors: *Grossman's cardiac catheterization, angiography, and intervention*, Philadelphia, 2000, Lippincott Williams & Wilkins.

Baim DS, Knopf WD, Hinohara T, et al: Suture-mediated closure of the femoral access site after cardiac catheterization: results of the suture to ambulate and discharge (STAND I and STAND II) trials, *Am J Cardiol* 85:864-869, 2000.

Campeau L: Percutaneous radial artery approach for coronary angiography, *Cathet Cardiovasc Diagn* 16:3-7, 1989.

Carey D, Martin JR, Moore CA, et al: Complications of femoral artery closure devices, *Cathet Cardiovasc Intervent* 52:3-7, 2001.

Chamberlin JR, Lardi AB, McKeever LS, et al: Safety of femoral closure devices (VasoSeal and Perclose) vs. associated manual compression (FemoStop) in transcatheter coronary interventions requiring abciximab (ReoPro), *Cathet Cardiovasc Intervent* 47:143-147, 1999.

Ellis SG, Mooney M, Talley JD, et al: DUETT femoral artery closure device vs. manual compression after diagnostic or interventional catheterization: results of the SEAL trial, *Circulation* 100:I-513, 1999.

Ernst SM, Tjonjoegin RM, Schrader R, et al: Immediate sealing of arterial puncture sites after cardiac catheterization and coronary angioplasty using a biodegradable collagen plug: results of an international registry, *J Am Coll Cardiol* 21:851-855, 1993.

Kern MJ, Cohen M, Talley JD, et al: Early ambulation after 5 F diagnostic catheterization: results of a multicenter trial, *J Am Coll Cardiol* 15:1475-1483, 1990.

Kiemeneij F, Laarman GJ: Percutaneous transradial artery approach for coronary Palmaz-Schatz stent implantation, *Am Heart J* 128:167-174, 1994.

Kiemeneij F, Laarman GJ, de Melker E: Transradial artery coronary angioplasty, *Am Heart J* 129:1-7, 1995.

Kim D, Orron DE, Skillman JJ, et al: Role of superficial femoral artery puncture in the development of pseudoaneurysm and arteriovenous fistula complicating percutaneous transfemoral cardiac catheterization, *Cathet Cardiovasc Diagn* 25:91-97, 1992.

Kussmaul WG, Buchbinder M, Whitlow PL, et al: Rapid arterial hemostasis and decreased access site complications after cardiac catheterization and angioplasty: results of a randomized trial of a novel hemostasis device, *J Am Coll Cardiol* 25:1685-1692, 1995.

Lesnefsky EJ, Carrea FP, Groves BM: Safety of cardiac catheterization via peripheral vascular grafts, *Cathet Cardiovasc Diagn* 29:113-116, 1993.

Matthay MA, Chatterjee K: Bedside catheterization of the pulmonary artery: risks compared with benefits, *Ann Intern Med* 109:826-834, 1988.

Sanborn TA, Gibbs HH, Brinker JA, et al: A multicenter randomized trial comparing a percutaneous collagen hemostasis device with conventional manual compression after diagnostic angiography and angioplasty, *J Am Coll Cardiol* 22:1273-1279, 1993.

Shrake KL: Comparison of major complication rates associated with four methods of arterial closure, *Am J Cardiol* 85:1024-1025, 2000.

Silber S: Rapid hemostasis of arterial puncture sites with collagen in patients undergoing diagnostic and interventional cardiac catheterization, *Clin Cardiol* 20:981-992, 1997.

Tilkian AG, Daily EK: *Cardiovascular procedures: diagnostic techniques and therapeutic procedures*, St Louis, 1986, Mosby.

Uretsky B, editor: *Cardiac catheterization: concepts, techniques, and applications*, Walden, Mass, 1997, Blackwell Science.

3

HEMODYNAMIC DATA

Morton J. Kern, Ted Feldman, and Saad Bitar

Cardiac catheterization (Fig. 3-1) provides anatomic information through cineangiograms and equally important physiologic information through the recording of hemodynamic
data, including pressure measurements, cardiac output (CO)
determinations, and blood oximetry.

PRESSURE WAVES IN THE HEART

Blood within the heart or vessels exerts pressure. A pressure
wave is created by cardiac muscular contraction and is transmitted from the vessel or chamber along a closed, fluid-filled
column (catheter) to a pressure transducer, which converts the
mechanical pressure to an electrical signal that is displayed on
a video monitor. Cardiac pressure waveforms are cyclical,
repeating the pressure change from the onset of one cardiac
contraction (systole) to the onset of the next contraction. The
complete description of the physiology of heart function is
beyond the scope of this book, but an examination of the
diagram of the cardiac cycle and corresponding pressures
(Figs. 3-2 and 3-3) provides an understanding of basic
hemodynamics in the cardiac catheterization laboratory.

The collection of hemodynamic data for cardiac catheterization is an integral part of every protocol. Even complex
hemodynamic data recording can be accomplished accurately
and rapidly if an efficient and consistently used method is
established in the laboratory. The measurement sequence used
in our laboratory (Boxes 3-1 through 3-3) is an example of one
method. This sequence facilitates simultaneous pressure
measurements across the heart, concentrating on the aortic
and mitral valves, which are affected most commonly by
disease. Of all hemodynamic questions, 90% can be answered

126

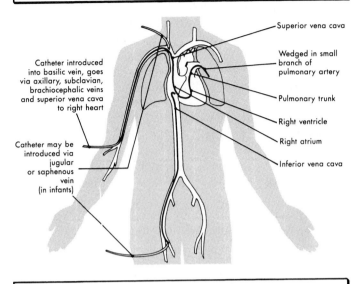

RIGHT HEART CATHETERIZATION

Catheter introduced into basilic vein, goes via axillary, subclavian, brachiocephalic veins and superior vena cava to right heart

Catheter may be introduced via jugular or saphenous vein (in infants)

Superior vena cava

Wedged in small branch of pulmonary artery

Pulmonary trunk

Right ventricle

Right atrium

Inferior vena cava

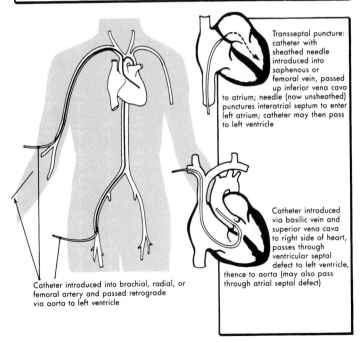

LEFT HEART CATHETERIZATION

Transseptal puncture: catheter with sheathed needle introduced into saphenous or femoral vein, passed up inferior vena cava to atrium; needle (now unsheathed) punctures interatrial septum to enter left atrium; catheter may then pass to left ventricle

Catheter introduced via basilic vein and superior vena cava to right side of heart, passes through ventricular septal defect to left ventricle, thence to aorta (may also pass through atrial septal defect)

Catheter introduced into brachial, radial, or femoral artery and passed retrograde via aorta to left ventricle

Fig. 3-1   Heart catheterization of the right and left sides of the heart from the brachial, radial, and femoral approaches.

by examining data collected in this way. As with most brief formulas this technique is not all-inclusive. Different hemodynamic measurements for specific clinical situations are necessary. Specific examples are included in the case studies.

The routine collection of hemodynamic data from the right and left sides of the heart with appropriate sampling for blood oxygen saturations and CO measurements can be accomplished rapidly and safely in less than 30 minutes. CO by the thermodilution technique is routine. Fick (oxygen consumption method) CO is used for valvular lesions. Green dye is no longer available to measure suspected cardiac shunts. Arterial, vena caval, right atrial (RA), and pulmonary artery (PA) oxygen saturations are collected routinely. Multiple oxygen saturation samples are obtained throughout the right and left sides of the heart for intracardiac shunt identification.

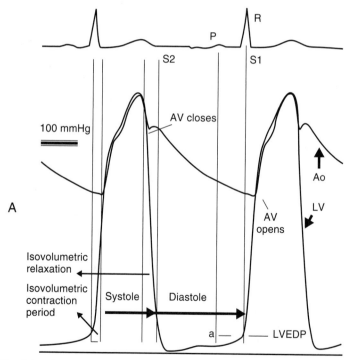

Fig. 3-2 **A,** Normal left ventricular *(LV)* and aortic *(Ao)* pressure with electrocardiogram. *P,* P wave; *R,* R wave; *S₁, S₂,* first and second heart sounds; *LVEDP,* LV end-diastolic pressure. Scale mark indicates 100 mm Hg.
Continued

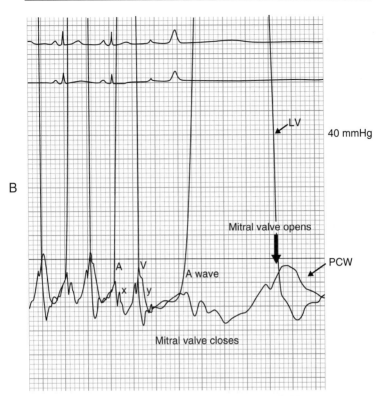

Fig. 3-2, cont'd   B, LV and pulmonary capillary wedge *(PCW)* pressures on 0 to 40 mm Hg scale. *A,* A wave; *V,* V wave corresponding to mitral valve opening and closing; *x,* x descent; *y,* y descent.

RIGHT- AND LEFT-SIDED HEART CATHETERIZATION

The protocol used during right-sided heart catheterization is summarized in Box 3-1. Right-sided heart catheterization is not required for all studies of the left side of the heart.

Indications

Right-sided heart catheterization is indicated for patients with a history of dyspnea, valvular heart disease, or intracardiac shunts. Patients with a history of pulmonary edema occurring on a previous hospital admission often have only dyspnea with no objective evidence of left ventricular (LV) dysfunction (e.g., chest film, echocardiography). Dyspnea caused by lung

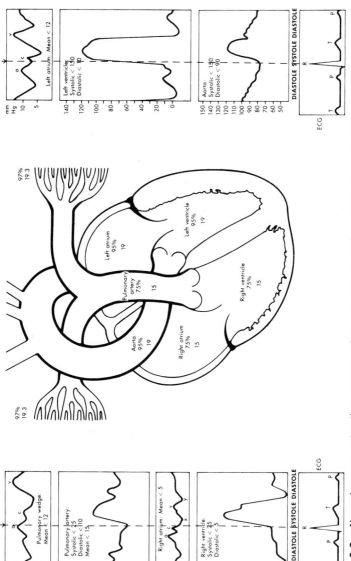

Fig. 3-3 Normal oxygen saturation, oxygen volume percentage, and pressure ranges in heart chambers and great vessels with pressure tracings in relation to electrocardiogram.

disease cannot be differentiated from that caused by pulmonary hypertension or LV dysfunction.

Complications of Right-Sided Heart Catheterization

The most common problem during right-sided heart catheterization is arrhythmia resulting from stimulation of the right ventricular (RV) outflow tract, which may result in atrioventricular block or, rarely, right bundle-branch block (Table 3-1). Significant but transient ventricular arrhythmias

---

Box 3-1

Right-Sided Heart Catheterization Protocol

Right Atrium (RA)
Advance catheter to inferior vena cava
Obtain oxygen saturation sample (1-ml heparinized* syringe). Advance catheter to RA
Turn recorder on (40 mm Hg scale); zero pressure
Record phasic pressure (25 mm/sec paper speed)
Check mean pressure (10 mm/sec paper speed), inspiration maneuver, phasic pressure; zero check pressure
Turn recorder off

Right Ventricle (RV)
Advance catheter to RV
Turn recorder on; record phasic pressure (25 mm/sec paper speed)
Zero check pressure
Turn recorder off

Pulmonary Capillary Wedge (PCW)
Advance catheter to PCW
Turn recorder on
Record phasic/mean/phasic pressure (25/10/25 mm/sec paper speed)

Pulmonary Artery (PA)
From PCW, let balloon down, pull catheter back for PA pressure
Record phasic/mean/phasic pressure (25/10/25 mm/sec paper speed)
Zero check pressure
Turn recorder off
Obtain oxygen saturation samples

---

*Only 1 to 2 drops of heparin should be aspirated and flushed out of 1-3-ml heparinized syringes.

Box 3-2

Left-Sided Heart Catheterization Protocol*

Matching Peripheral to Central Aortic Pressure

Pigtail catheter inserted through arterial sheath (sheath should be one French size larger than catheter)

Administer heparin (3000 to 5000 U per laboratory routine)

Advance catheter to aortic valve

Zero pigtail pressure (200 mm Hg scale)

Zero sheath pressure (200 mm Hg scale)

Turn recorder on; record femoral artery (sheath) and central aortic pressure (phasic/mean/phasic 25/10/25 mm/sec paper speed)

Zero both pressures

Turn recorder off

Aortic Valve Assessment

Advance pigtail to left ventricular chamber

Zero pressures; turn recorder on

Record left ventricular and femoral artery pressures (25 mm/sec speed, 200 scale) phasic/mean femoral artery/phasic pressure†

Turn recorder off

*Right-sided heart hemodynamic studies often precede left-sided heart studies. Simultaneous pressures of the left and right sides of the heart provide the most precise and accurate information.
†100 mm/sec paper speed if aortic valve gradient present.

Box 3-3

Combined Hemodynamic Measurements of the Left and Right Sides of the Heart

Begin studies after right-sided heart catheterization is completed with pulmonary capillary wedge (PCW) tracing ready and left ventricular (LV) protocol completed with pigtail catheter in left ventricle before LV pullback.

Aortic Valve Assessment

Follow left-sided heart protocol (see Box 3-2)

Mitral Valve Assessment

Zero PCW, femoral artery, and LV pressures

Turn recorder on; record LV versus PCW (50 mm/sec speed, 40 mm Hg scale) phasic/mean/phasic PCW pressure

Continued

Box 3-3

Combined Hemodynamic Measurements of the Left and Right Sides of the Heart—cont'd

Mitral Valve Assessment—cont'd
Zero check LV pressure
Let down balloon or pull back PCW to pulmonary artery (PA) (25 mm/sec speed, 40 mm Hg scale) and record phasic/mean/phasic PA pressure
Turn recorder off
Note: 100 mm/sec paper if mitral valve gradient present

Cardiac Output
Perform Fick oxygen collection (Waters oximetry hood)
Measure thermodilution outputs × 3
Obtain arterial and PA oxygen saturation samples (in duplicate)

Right-Sided Heart Pullback
Zero all pressures
Turn recorder on (25 mm/sec paper speed, 40 mm Hg scale)
Record PCW to PA phasic/mean/phasic pressure
Record PA to right ventricular (RV) pressure
Continue recording RV and add LV pressure (to establish presence of constrictive/restrictive physiology) (100 mm/sec paper speed, 40 mm Hg scale)
Zero check LV pressure
Record RV to right atrial (phasic/mean/phasic, 25/10/25 mm paper speed, 40 mm Hg scale zero check)
Turn recorder off
Note: Left ventriculography usually performed at this point

Postventriculography Hemodynamics
Zero check LV, aortic pressures
Turn recorder on
Record postventriculography LV end-diastolic pressure
(100 mm/sec paper speed, 40 mm Hg scale)
Perform LV pullback to aorta with femoral artery pressures displayed (25 mm/sec paper speed, 200 mm Hg scale)
Check mean aortic pressures
Zero pressures
Turn recorder off

occur in 30% to 60% of patients who undergo right-sided heart catheterization and are self-limited and do not require treatment. The arrhythmia is terminated when the catheter is readjusted. Sustained ventricular arrhythmias have been reported, especially in unstable patients or patients with electrolyte imbalance, acidosis, or concurrent myocardial ischemia. The prophylactic use of lidocaine is not necessary. In patients with left bundle-branch block, a temporary pacemaker may be needed if right bundle-branch block occurs during right-sided heart catheterization.

Use of Pulmonary Wedge Pressure. The pulmonary capillary wedge (PCW) pressure closely approximates left atrial (LA) pressure. PCW pressure overestimates LA pressure in patients with acute respiratory failure, chronic obstructive pulmonary disease with pulmonary hypertension, pulmonary venoconstriction, or LV failure with volume overload. Reported discrepancies between LA and PCW pressure may be caused in part by different types of catheters: balloon-tipped flotation catheters are soft with small lumens; LA pressure catheters (e.g., Brockenbrough or Mullins-type sheath) are stiff with large lumens. In most patients PCW pressure is sufficient to assess LV filling pressure. In patients with mitral valvular disease or mitral valve prostheses, a significant error may be introduced by using a balloon-tipped flotation catheter for

Table 3-1

Complications of Right-Sided Heart (Pulmonary Artery) Catheterization

	Major	Minor
Access	Pneumothorax	Hematoma
	Hemothorax	Thrombosis
	Tracheal perforation (subclavian route)	
	Sepsis	Cellulitis
Intracardiac	Right ventricular perforation	Ventricular arrhythmia
	Heart block (right bundle-branch block)	
	Pulmonary rupture	
	Pulmonary infarction	

PCW pressure assessment. Transseptal LA catheterization should be considered in these cases.

Rules for obtaining an accurate PCW pressure that agrees with LA pressure are as follows:

1. The operator should position the catheters correctly and verify the position through waveform, oximetry (oxygen saturation >95%), and fluoroscopy.

The position of catheters (end-hole wedge) is confirmed by oxygen saturation sample greater than 95% (obtaining this saturation not contaminated by low saturation PA blood is difficult when the balloon is inflated).

The operator should confirm that PCW pressure is not a damped PA pressure by using a precise *a* and *v* waveform timed against electrocardiogram (ECG) or LV pressure.

During fluoroscopy, when 2 ml of contrast material is injected into the catheter, a lack of contrast washout 15 seconds after injection indicates proper catheter position. A "fern" pattern of contrast seen on the fluoroscope may help when the hemodynamic tracing is in question in patients who are receiving mechanically assisted ventilation or in patients with rapid, deep inspiratory efforts.

2. A stiff, large-bore end-hole catheter should be used.
3. Connect the catheter to the pressure manifold with stiff, short pressure tubing.
4. The system should be thoroughly flushed before accepting wedge pressure.
5. For mitral valve area determinations the operator should correct for the time delay (i.e., phase shift the PCW pressure v wave to match the LV downstroke).

Left-Sided Heart Catheterization

The protocol for left-sided heart catheterization is summarized in Box 3-2. Indications for left-sided heart catheterization are summarized in Chapter 1 (see Table 1-2). A combined right-side and left-side heart protocol is the most precise and complete method of addressing most hemodynamic problems that are encountered in the catheterization laboratory (see Box 3-3).

COMPUTATIONS FOR HEMODYNAMIC MEASUREMENTS

When the hemodynamic data have been obtained, computations are made to clarify and enhance quantitation of cardiac function. In this section only the most common computations and standard formulas are provided. Computations most often used involve assessment of cardiac work, calculation of flow resistance, computation of valve areas, and shunt calculations. Specific derivations and applications of these formulas can be found elsewhere.

CO by Fick (O_2 consumption) method

$$CO = \frac{O_2 \text{ consumption (ml/min)}}{AVO_2 \text{ difference (ml } O_2/100 \text{ ml blood)} \times 10}$$

Oxygen consumption is measured from a metabolic "hood"; it can also be estimated as 3 ml O_2/kg or 125 ml/min/m². Arteriovenous oxygen (AVO_2) difference is calculated from arterial − mixed venous (PA) O_2 content, where O_2 content = saturation × 1.36 × hemoglobin.

For example, if the arterial saturation is 95%, then the O_2 content = 0.95 × 1.36 × 13.0 g = 16.7 ml, PA saturation is 65%, and O_2 consumption is 210 ml/min (70 kg × 3 ml/kg) or measured value, and CO would be determined as follows:

$$\frac{210}{(0.95 - 0.65) \times 1.36 \times 13.0 \times 10^*} = \frac{210}{53} = 3.96 \text{ L/min}$$

Cardiac index (CI) (L/min/m²)

$$CI = \frac{CO \text{ (L/min)}}{\text{Body surface area (BSA) (m}^2)}$$

Stroke volume (SV) (ml/beat)

$$SV = \frac{CO \text{ (ml/min)}}{\text{Heart rate (HR) (beats/min)}}$$

Stroke index (SI) (ml/beat/m²)

$$SI = \frac{SV \text{ (ml/beat)}}{BSA \text{ (m}^2)}$$

Stroke work (SW) (g · m)

SW = (mean LV systolic pressure − mean LV diastolic pressure)
    × stroke volume × 0.0144†

---

*Correction factor when using O_2 content in the Fick formula.
†0.0136 = conversion factor for mm Hg to cm H_2O.

Pulmonary arteriolar resistance (PAR) (units)

$$PAR = \frac{\text{Mean pulmonary arterial pressure} - \text{Mean LA pressure (or PCW pressure)}}{CO}$$

Total pulmonary resistance (TPR) (units)

$$TPR = \frac{\text{mean PA pressure}}{CO}$$

Systemic vascular resistance (SVR, Wood units)

$$SVR = \frac{\text{Mean systematic arterial pressure} - \text{mean right arterial pressure}}{CO}$$

Converting to resistance in metric units (dynes · sec · cm^{-5})

$$\text{SVR, PAR, TPR units} \times 80$$

COMPUTATIONS OF VALVE AREAS FROM PRESSURE GRADIENTS AND CARDIAC OUTPUT

A pressure gradient is the pressure difference across an area of valvular or vascular obstruction, such as a stenosis or an occlusion or narrowed valve (Fig. 3-4).

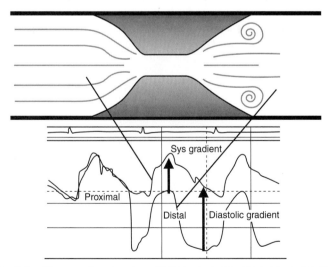

Fig. 3-4   Diagram of pressure gradient across a stenosis or narrowing. The pressure gradient is the difference between proximal and distal pressure. The pressure distal to the narrowing shows a systolic and a diastolic pressure gradient.

Variables That Affect Pressure Gradients

Physiologic Variables

1. Rate of blood flow (e.g., CO, coronary blood flow)
2. Resistance to flow
3. Proximal chamber pressure and compliance

Anatomic Variables

1. Shape and length of valve orifice
2. Tortuosities of the vessels (for arterial stenosis); folding of coronary artery by guidewire (i.e., pseudostenosis)
3. Multiple or serial lesions (for cardiac valves and arterial stenosis)

Artifactual Variables

1. Miscalibrated pressure transducers
2. Pressure leaks on catheter manifold or connecting tubing
3. Pressure tubing type, length, and connectors
4. Air in system
5. Catheter sizes (especially small diameters)
6. Fluid viscosity (viscous contrast material tends to damp pressure wave)
7. Position of catheter side holes (aortic stenosis with pigtail catheter [see Fig. 3-56])

Valve area calculation

$$\text{Area (cm}^2) = \frac{\text{Valve flow (ml/sec)}}{K \times C \times \sqrt{\text{MVG}}}$$

where *MVG* is mean valvular gradient (mm Hg), *K* (44.3) is a derived constant by Gorlin and Gorlin, *C* is an empirical constant that is 1 for semilunar valves and tricuspid valve and 0.85 for mitral valve, and *valve flow* is measured in milliliters per second during the diastolic or systolic flow period.

Mitral valve flow

$$\frac{\text{CO (ml/min)}}{\text{Diastolic filling period (sec/min)}}$$

where diastolic filling period (sec/min) = diastolic period (sec/beat) × HR.

Aortic valve flow

$$\frac{CO \ (ml/min)}{Systolic \ ejection \ period \ (sec/min)}$$

where systolic ejection period (sec/min) = systolic period (sec/beat) × HR.

EXAMPLES OF AORTIC AND MITRAL VALVE AREA CALCULATIONS

Notes for data used in the following calculations: A scale factor is calculated as millimeters of mercury per centimeter of paper deflection; however, 200 mm Hg full scale may not be exactly 10 cm on the recording paper. When CO is used, conversion should be to milliliters per minute, not liters per minute. When computing flow, the ejection period and filling period are converted to fractions of the period in seconds by measuring the paper distance and converting that to time (i.e., 4.1 cm for systolic ejection period = 4.1 cm × 1 sec/10 cm = 0.41 second).

   Data obtained at catheterization for aortic stenosis (Fig. 3-5)
   1. CO = 4 L/min = 4000 ml/min
   2. HR = 60 beats/min

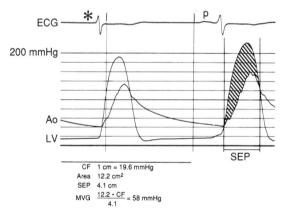

Fig. 3-5   Aortic valve area is determined from the planimetered area of the aortic valve gradient. The aortic valve gradient area *(shaded area)* is bounded by the systolic ejection period *(SEP)*. *Ao,* Aortic pressure; *LV,* left ventricular pressure (scale 0 to 200 mm Hg); *CF,* correction factor or scale factor; *MVG,* mean value gradient. See text for details.

3. Scale factor to convert recording deflection to pressure = 1 cm = 19.6 mm Hg (directly measured paper calibration lines of 200 mm Hg)
4. Tracing of LV-aortic pressures at 100 cm/sec paper speed (if femoral artery pressure is used shifting aortic upstroke to match LV upstroke *reduces* true gradient area)

Step 1: Planimeter 5 aortic-LV gradients and average (if atrial fibrillation, planimeter 10 beats).

$$Area = 12.20 \ cm^2$$

Step 2: Measure systolic ejection periods (SEP) and average.

$$SEP = 4.1 \ cm \ (next \ convert \ to \ time).$$
$$4.1 \times 1 \ sec/10 \ cm = 0.41 \ second$$

Step 3: Convert planimeter area to mean systolic pressure gradient.

$$Mean \ valve \ gradient = (area \times scale \ factor)/SEP$$

$$12.2 \ cm^2 \times \frac{19.6 \ mm \ Hg/1 \ cm}{4.1 \ cm} = \frac{239}{4.1} = 58 \ mm \ Hg$$

Note: For gradient only, SEP remains in centimeters because of scale factor.

Step 4: Compute aortic valve flow.

$$\frac{CO}{SEP \times HR} = \frac{4000}{0.41 \ sec/beat \times 60 \ beats/min} = \frac{4000}{24.6} = 162.6$$

Note: SEP now in sec/beat.

Step 5: Compute aortic valve area.

$$\frac{Aortic \ valve \ flow}{1.0 \times 44.3\sqrt{gradient}} = \frac{162.6}{44.3 \times \sqrt{58}} = \frac{162.6}{44.3 \times 7.6}$$

$$= \frac{162.6}{336.6} = 0.48 \ cm^2$$

Notes on the aortic valve gradient: The mean pressure gradient is measured by planimetry of the superimposed aortic (Ao) and LV pressure tracings. Peak-to-peak pressure gradients are easily seen and are often used as an estimate of the severity of stenosis. The peak-to-peak gradient is not equivalent to mean gradient for mild and moderate stenosis, but is often close to mean gradient for severe stenosis. The *delay* in pressure transmission and pressure wave reflection from the proximal aorta to the femoral artery artificially *increases* the mean gradient. Femoral pressure overshoot (amplification) reduces the true gradient. If the femoral arterial pressure is used, phase shifting of the femoral arterial pressure to the left ventricle upstroke may be important. In patients with low gradients (i.e., <35 mm Hg), more accurate valve areas were obtained with *unadjusted* LV-Ao pressure tracings. Optimally a second catheter can be positioned directly above the aortic valve to reduce transmission delay and femoral pressure amplification. A long (>30 cm) arterial sheath can be used. Transseptal cardiac catheterization can also be performed to obtain direct LV pressure (see Fig. 3-5).

Simplified formulas provide quick in-laboratory determinations of aortic valve area. Aortic valve area can be estimated closely as CO divided by the square root of the LV-aortic peak-to-peak pressure difference.

$$\text{Peak-to-peak gradient} = 65 \text{ mm Hg}$$
$$CO = 5 \text{ L/min}$$
$$\text{Quick valve area (Hakke formula)} = \frac{5 \text{ L/min}}{\sqrt{65}}$$
$$= \frac{5 \text{ L/min}}{8}$$
$$= 0.63 \text{ cm}^2$$

Note: The quick formulas for valve area differ from the Gorlin formula by 18 ± 13% in patients with bradycardia (<65 beats/min) or tachycardia (>100 beats/min).

The Gorlin equation at *low*-flow states *overestimates* the severity of valve stenosis. In low-flow states (CO <2.5 L/min), the Gorlin formula should be modified to employ the mean transvalvular gradient with new empirically derived constants.

USE OF VALVE RESISTANCE FOR AORTIC STENOSIS

Valve resistance, a measure of valve obstruction, has been shown to have clinical use. Although this index was first proposed around the same time that the Gorlin valve area formula was first reported, valve resistance has not been used because the units of dynes · second · cm^{-5} were not well related to clinical outcome.

Although they have obvious strengths, valve area measurements have practical and theoretical limitations. Area is a planar measurement without consideration of the funnel-like nature of the mitral inflow or the more tubelike configuration of the aortic outlet. Valve area is based on laminar flow of a nonviscous fluid. Turbulence and blood viscosity are not considered. The constant in the denominator of the Gorlin formula is the square root of gravity, 2 gH, and assumes that blood flow is gravity driven rather than pulsatile as in the arterial system.

Valve areas of less than 0.7 cm² are almost always associated with an important clinical syndrome, and areas of greater than 1.1 cm² are usually not associated with significant symptoms, but areas between these two measurements are in a gray zone. One of the most common clinical situations is found in a patient with a valve area of 0.9 to 1.0 cm², a low transvalve pressure gradient, low CO, and poor LV function. There is uncertainty regarding the outcome after valve replacement, as well as a high mortality rate if ventricular function does not improve after surgery.

Valve resistance provides an alternative method to assess valve obstruction. It is calculated using the same variables used for valve area measurement. In contrast to valve area, the mean pressure gradient is considered to be a linear variable rather than taken as a square root term (Fig. 3-6). The contribution of pressure gradient to the magnitude of valve resistance is greater. Resistance has also been shown to be more constant than valve area under conditions of changing CO.

Resistance necessarily has a close relationship to valve area. Fig. 3-7 shows resistance and area calculated in a group of patients before and after balloon aortic valve dilation. Resistance rises sharply above a valve area of 0.7 cm². The

VALVE RESISTANCE
$$dynes \cdot sec \cdot cm^{-5}$$

$$\left[\frac{\text{Mean Gradient}}{\left(\dfrac{\text{C.O.(L/min)}}{\text{SEP(sec/min)}} \right) \times 60} \right] \times 80$$

Fig. 3-6   Formula for valve resistance. *CO,* Cardiac output; *SEP,* systolic ejection period.

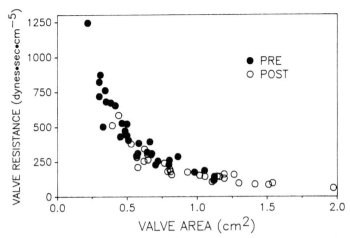

Fig. 3-7 Comparison of valve area by Gorlin formula versus valve resistance before *(pre)* and after *(post)* aortic valvuloplasty. Valve resistance less than 200 dynes · sec · cm^{-5} is associated with minimal obstruction; greater than 250 dynes · sec · cm^{-5} with significant obstruction. This measure complements and refines valve area decision making. (From Feldman T, Ford L, Chiu YC, et al: *J Heart Valve Dis* 1:55-64, 1992.)

shoulder of this curve is 0.7 to 1.1 cm^2, which is the common area of indeterminate significance of Gorlin aortic valve area. Some patients in this gray zone tend to have higher valve resistance than others. It has been shown in this setting that patients with resistance greater than 250 dynes · sec · cm^{-5} are more likely to have significant obstruction than patients with resistance less than 200 dynes · sec · cm^{-5}. There is also a gray zone in using this index, and some patients may have resistance less than 250 dynes · sec · cm^{-5} despite a planar valve area of 0.7 to 0.8 cm^2.

Resistance is a complementary index, not a replacement for valve area. Valve resistance is not expected to remain consistent. Some of the changes in valve area observed in a single patient under different conditions or at different times might be more acceptable when considered as changes in valve resistance and not in planar area. As with peripheral resistance, valve resistance is interpreted in the context of the clinical conditions under which it is measured. A peripheral resistance of 1000 dynes · sec · cm^{-5} has a different significance in a patient with presumed sepsis than it does in a patient with LV failure. Similarly, we can expect valve resistance to vary as CO changes.

Catheter Selection for Aortic Stenosis

Initial catheter selection is a matter of operator choice based on previous experience. The pigtail ventriculography catheter is a good initial choice in most cases. The operator crosses the aortic valve with a 0.038-inch, straight-tipped safety guidewire, extending the wire and straightening the pigtail with a slight angled bend. The operator should direct the wire into the area of highest turbulence as detected by jet impaction on the wire, and note the movement as visualized on the fluoroscopy monitor. Manipulation of the wire and catheter allows positioning of the wire in various directions needed to cross the valve. Advancing the pigtail over the wire and, in most cases, rapidly positioning the catheter for ventriculography and hemodynamic studies is a simple operation. When this method is successful it is a one-step procedure, and for this reason the pigtail catheter is a logical first choice. Other catheter choices for crossing the aortic valve include the left and, occasionally, right Amplatz catheter, right Judkins catheter, multipurpose catheter, and specially designed catheters that have been reported in the technical literature. When the operator uses alternative catheters, use of the left and right Judkins curves also permits coronary angiography to be obtained between catheter exchanges. All but the pigtail catheter are generally unsuitable for LV angiography. It should not require more than 15 to 20 minutes for the operator to cross the aortic valve, and if great difficulty is encountered, a transseptal approach should be considered early in the procedure.

Points to Remember for Crossing the Aortic Valve with Guidewires

1. Adequate heparinization (5000-U bolus) should be maintained. Frequent catheter flushing is performed.
2. A maximal time of 3 minutes per crossing attempt is required before wire withdrawal, wiping, and flushing of the catheter.
3. A 0.035-inch guidewire may be insufficiently stiff to support the catheter on crossing severely deformed, calcific aortic valves, and a 0.038-inch guidewire should

be substituted. Large catheters that accept this size of wire should be used.

4. Guidewire configurations that lead to the coronary ostia should be avoided to prevent dissection of the coronary arteries, which would complicate this otherwise benign maneuver.

5. Manipulation of the wire should be gentle to avoid damaging the valve, lifting atheromas, or causing a perforation of the cusps or aortic root.

Data from Catheterization Laboratory for Calculation of Mitral Valve Area. Fig. 3-8 is a hemodynamic tracing to calculate mitral valve area.

1. Cardiac output = 3.5 L/min = 3500 ml/min
2. Heart rate = 80 beats/min
3. Scale factor = 1 cm = 3.9 mm Hg (40 mm Hg full scale)
4. Tracing of LV-PCW pressure at 100 mm/sec paper speed = (10 cm/sec paper speed) (align PCW v wave with downstroke of LV pressure)

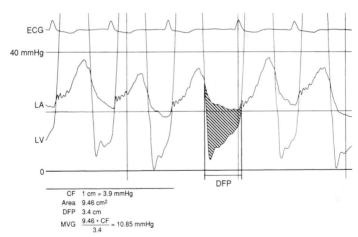

CF	1 cm = 3.9 mmHg
Area	9.46 cm²
DFP	3.4 cm
MVG	$\dfrac{9.46 \cdot CF}{3.4}$ = 10.85 mmHg

Fig. 3-8   Hemodynamic tracing used to calculate mitral valve area. The shaded area is the diastolic mitral valve gradient surrounded by the diastolic filling period *(DFP)*. *CF,* Correction factor or scale factor; *LA,* left atrial pressure; *LV,* left ventricular pressure (scale 0 to 40 mm Hg); *MVG,* mean value gradient. See text for details.

Step 1: Planimeter 5 LV-PCW areas (10 if in atrial fibrillation).

$$\text{Area} = 9.46 \text{ cm}^2$$

Step 2: Measure diastolic filling period (DFP).

DFP = 3.4 cm (then convert to time)
3.4 cm × 1 sec/10 cm = 0.34 second

Step 3: Convert planimetered area to mean diastolic pressure gradient.

$$
\begin{aligned}
\text{MVG} \ &= \ \frac{\text{area} \times \text{scale factor}}{\text{DFP}} \\
&= \ \frac{9.46 \text{ cm}^2 \times 3.9 \text{ mm Hg/1 cm}}{3.4 \text{ cm}} \\
&= \ \frac{36.9}{3.4} \\
&= \ 10.85 \text{ mm Hg}
\end{aligned}
$$

Step 4: Compute mitral valve flow.

For the mitral gradient, similar to aortic valve areas, DFP is in centimeters at this point owing to scale factor.

$$
\begin{aligned}
\frac{\text{CO (ml/min)}}{\text{DFP} \times \text{HR}} \ &= \ \frac{3500 \text{ ml/min}}{3.4 \text{ cm} \times (1 \text{ sec/10 cm}) \times 80 \text{ beats/min}} \\
&= \ \frac{3500}{0.34 \times 80} \\
&= \ \frac{3500}{27.2} \\
&= \ 128.7
\end{aligned}
$$

Step 5: Compute mitral valve area.

$$
\frac{\text{Mitral valve flow}}{0.85 \times 44.3 \sqrt{10.85}} \ = \ \frac{128.7}{0.85 \times 44.3 \times 3.3} \ = \ \frac{128.7}{124.3} \ = \ 1.0 \text{ cm}^2
$$

Notes on mitral valve gradient: Obtaining an accurate PCW pressure (discussed earlier in this chapter and in Chapter 2) is crucial. PCW pressure overestimates LA pressure (transseptal catheterization) in patients with prosthetic mitral valves. Overestimation is caused in part by large v waves increasing the phase delay, making correction and alignment of pressure tracings difficult.

Use of direct LA pressure from transseptal measurement is the most accurate method. Transseptal catheterization should be performed to confirm large pressure gradients, especially for suspected prosthetic mitral stenosis. However, if the PCW pressure/LV pressure tracings show no significant gradients, transseptal catheterization is unnecessary. A worksheet for valve area calculation is shown in Fig. 3-9.

Tricuspid Valve Gradients. Because small gradients (5 mm Hg) across the tricuspid valve may lead to significant clinical symptoms, precise measurement of hemodynamics through two large-lumen catheters may be required. Pressures through two catheters (or through the two lumens of a balloon-tipped catheter if correctly positioned) should be matched before placement in the right atrium (RA) and right ventricle (RV) to avoid technical error. The valve area formula should be used for mitral stenosis. Validation of the Gorlin equation and constant for the tricuspid or pulmonic valves has not been established.

Pulmonic Valve Stenosis. A pulmonary valvular stenosis gradient (Fig. 3-10) is obtained by catheter "pullback," continuously measuring pressure during catheter withdrawal across the stenotic valve. Two catheters, multiple-lumen balloon-tipped catheters, or double-lumen Cournand catheters are more precise, however, and can record simultaneous PA and RV pressures in the manner used for aortic valve stenosis. There is no validated formula for pulmonary valve area. Prognostic data are based on RV pressure and gradient alone.

MEASUREMENT OF CARDIAC OUTPUT

In the cardiac catheterization laboratory, CO is determined by one of two techniques: (1) measurement of oxygen consumption (Fick technique) or (2) indicator dilution technique (thermodilution using a PA catheter).

Fick Principle for Measurement of Cardiac Output

The Fick principle states that uptake or release of a substance by any organ is the product of the arteriovenous concentration difference of the substance and the blood flow to that organ. Pulmonary blood flow (which is equal to systemic blood flow in the absence of an intracardiac shunt) is determined by measuring the arteriovenous difference of oxygen across the lungs and the uptake of oxygen from room air by the lungs. CO

Determination of mitral valve gradient and area

Cardiac output (CO)   ml/min
Diastolic filling period per beat (dfp true)   sec/beat
Heart rate   beats/min
Diastolic filling period per minute (DFP) = HR × dfp   sec/min
Empiric constant (with true dfp)   0.85
Mitral diastolic mean gradient (by planimetry)   mm Hg

$$\text{Mitral valve flow} = \frac{CO}{DFP} = \boxed{} = \boxed{} \ ml/sec$$

$$\text{Mitral valve area} = \frac{\text{Mitral valve flow}}{0.85 \times 44.3 \times \sqrt{\text{mitral valve diastolic gradient}}} = \boxed{\frac{}{}} = \boxed{} \ cm^2$$

Determination of aortic valve gradient and area

Cardiac output (CO)   ml/min
Systolic ejection period per beat (sep)   sec/beat
Heart rate   beats/min
Systolic ejection period per minute (SEP) = HR × sep   sec/min
Empiric constant   1
Aortic systolic mean gradient (by planimetry)   mm Hg

$$\text{Aortic valve flow} = \frac{CO}{SEP} = \boxed{} = \boxed{} \ ml/sec$$

$$\text{Aortic valve area} = \frac{\text{Aortic valve flow}}{1 \times 44.3 \times \sqrt{\text{aortic valve systolic gradient}}} = \boxed{\frac{}{}} = \boxed{} \ cm^2$$

Fig. 3-9 Worksheet for determination of valve areas. (Modified from Grossman W: *Cardiac catheterization and angiography*, ed 3, Philadelphia, 1986, Lea & Febiger.)

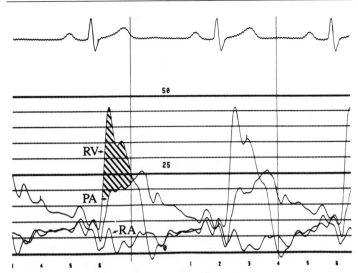

Fig. 3-10   Hemodynamic tracings from a patient with pulmonary stenosis. The shaded area is pulmonary stenosis gradient (scale 0 to 50 mm Hg; time lines are 1 second). *PA,* Pulmonary artery pressure; *RV,* right ventricular pressure; *RA,* right atrial pressure.

is calculated as oxygen consumption divided by the arteriovenous oxygen concentration difference. The arteriovenous oxygen consumption difference is calculated (in milliliters of oxygen) from the difference in LV oxygen content (1.36 × hemoglobin × LV O_2 saturation × 10) minus the PA (mixed venous) oxygen content (1.36 × hemoglobin × PA O_2 saturation × 10). In the cardiac catheterization laboratory, oxygen consumption is measured by the polarographic cell method.

Polarographic Cell Method (Metabolic Hood). The polarographic cell method uses a polarographic oxygen sensor cell to measure the oxygen content of expired air (Fig. 3-11). Room air is withdrawn at a constant rate through a plastic hood that is placed over the patient's head while the patient is in a supine position. The unit measures the contents of the hood (room air/expired air) through flexible tubing to the polarographic oxygen-sensing cell. The metabolic rate meter gives a readout of oxygen consumption in liters per minute.

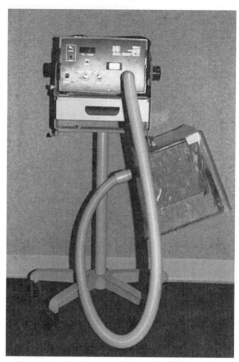

Fig. 3-11 Metabolic (Waters) hood for determination of oxygen consumption. See text for details.

FICK OXYGEN CONSUMPTION METHOD

The Fick technique is the most accurate method of assessing CO, particularly in patients with low CO. Simultaneous reliable measurements of the arteriovenous oxygen content difference and oxygen consumption are crucial for an accurate value. Determination of oxygen consumption requires that patients breathe comfortably at a steady state. If a steady state is not achieved because of anxiety, dyspnea, or any condition in which measurement of oxygen is spuriously elevated, an abnormally high CO is calculated. Conversely, shallow breathing (alveolar hypoventilation), commonly seen with oversedation, results in a falsely low oxygen consumption and low CO determination.

Supplemental oxygen is often administered to a patient during diagnostic cardiac catheterization. Mixing the supplemental oxygen with room air makes determination of the oxygen content of the inspired air difficult (if not impossible) to calculate. Supplemental oxygen therapy should be discontinued at least 10 to 15 minutes before determination of CO by the Fick technique. If oxygen cannot be discontinued safely, an alternative to the Fick technique should be used.

INDICATOR DILUTION CARDIAC OUTPUT PRINCIPLE

The indicator dilution technique is based on the principle that a single injection of a known amount of an indicator (e.g., cold saline for the thermodilution technique) injected into the central circulation mixes completely with blood and changes concentration as it flows to a more distal location. The change in the indicator concentration (or temperature) is plotted over time; the area under the curve is planimetered to calculate CO. The most common indicator dilution technique used in the cardiac catheterization laboratory is the thermodilution method. The indocyanine method for shunt studies is no longer used.

Thermodilution Indicator Method

The thermodilution indicator method requires a PA balloon flotation catheter (Swan-Ganz) with a thermistor at the tip. Iced or room-temperature saline is the indicator substance. Iced (4° C) or room temperature (20° C) saline is cold relative to blood at normal body temperature (37° C). The basic Swan-Ganz catheter is a triple-lumen design. The proximal port, located 30 cm from the tip, is used for RA pressure measurement and for rapid infusion of the saline during CO determination, the distal end hole is used for pressure measurement, and the lumen is used to inflate the balloon. A thermistor at the distal tip measures the blood temperature.

The balloon serves two purposes: (1) it is a positioning aid, and (2) it facilitates measurement of the PCW pressure. The inflated balloon helps to direct the catheter into the PA by "floating" with the flow of blood through the right heart chambers. When positioned in the PA, the catheter can be advanced to the distal pulmonary vasculature, "wedging" in a small branch. The balloon forms a seal that isolates the tip from PA flow. This separation ensures that the pressure measured beyond the balloon is the pulmonary capillary pressure, which is generally equal to the LA pressure. An additional feature of this catheter is a small thermistor near the end of the catheter. The thermistor is positioned in the PA when the proximal port is in the right atrium.

Measuring Cardiac Output

CO is determined by rapid injection 10 ml of saline (iced or at room temperature) through the proximal port of the PA catheter. An external thermistor measures the temperature of the injectate. Complete mixing of the injectate with blood causes a decrease in the blood temperature, which is sensed by the distal thermistor. The CO computer calculates the change in the indicator concentration (temperature over time) to determine the CO in liters per minute.

For saline injections coiled tubing systems that are immersed in an ice water bath are commercially available to facilitate cooling of the injectate. With this system the injectate is withdrawn from a room-temperature bag of intravenous fluid, through the coil, and into the injectate syringe. Special syringes are available that isolate the operator's hand from the injectate syringe. This isolation prevents warming of the injectate by the operator's hand.

Notes on Thermodilution Technique

To obtain consistent, reliable results, the physician and the members of the technical staff must employ good technique. The following steps contribute to thermodilution CO accuracy.

1. The catheter must be positioned properly in the PA. Excessive coiling of the catheter in the RA or RV can result in poor positioning of the dual thermistor in relation to the injectate port. This problem is sometimes encountered with a large, dilated right side of the heart. In these instances, a 0.025-inch guidewire should be used to give additional stiffness to the catheter. A wedged catheter does not register the appropriate temperature change.

2. Most thermodilution systems require that a computation constant (on the output computer) be used. The computer should be set to the proper computation constant depending on the system being used. Some computers provide a table that gives a constant corres-

ponding to the injectate volume, the injectate temperature, and size and type of catheter being used.

3. The precise amount of injectate must be injected. In adults 10 ml is the commonly used volume, and 5 ml is typical in children. In adults for whom fluid restriction is important, a smaller bolus of injectate may be desired. If so, the clinician must remember to change the computation constant on the output computer to reflect the change in injectate volume.

4. Warming the barrel of the injectate syringe in the palm of the hand should be avoided. This warming introduces error into the output calculation. Special syringe holders are available to alleviate this problem.

5. The start button must be coordinated. The technician must press the start button on the computer simultaneously with the delivery of the injectate. Injection before the release of the start button by the technician is a common error. When this happens, the computer does not recognize the full bolus of injectate being delivered.

6. The bolus should be delivered rapidly at a consistent flow rate.

7. The catheter should be securely connected to the computer. If the interface cable from the CO computer is nonsterile, care should be taken that the sterile field is not violated (special cable drapes are available).

8. If room temperature saline is used, there should be at least a 10° C difference between the injectate and body temperature. Most computers have built-in sensors that enable the technician to check these parameters before the start of the procedure.

9. Three to five CO values should be obtained. Erroneous values may be recorded but are ignored in the final averaging of results.

10. The thermodilution technique is inaccurate with tricuspid regurgitation or low CO. Both conditions interfere with the normal flow of injectate past the sensing thermistor.

ANGIOGRAPHIC CARDIAC OUTPUT

CO determined angiographically is computed as the stroke volume (end-diastolic volume minus the end-systolic volume) times the heart rate. Angiographic CO provides the best estimate of CO through a stenotic valve when any degree of regurgitation is present. Errors in stroke volume computation are increased with enlarged ventricles, especially when single-plane cineangiography is employed. Angiographic CO is not determined simultaneously with a transvalvular gradient; additional error may be introduced by delay in simultaneous measurements. A calibrated ventriculogram is also necessary.

DIFFERENCES AMONG CARDIAC OUTPUT TECHNIQUES

Discrepancies exist among Fick, thermodilution, and indocyanine green dye determinations of CO in patients with low CO or in patients with aortic or mitral regurgitation. In low-flow states or in valvular regurgitation, recirculation of the indicator (i.e., cold saline or green dye) may appear as a distortion on the curve downslope before reaching baseline. Failure to reach accurate baseline results in inaccurate CO determinations. In patients with mitral and aortic valve regurgitation and low CO, the dye dilution method varied by more than 20% from the Fick method.

Thermodilution is inaccurate in low CO states. Tricuspid regurgitation or intracardiac shunts further reduce the accuracy of thermodilution. In patients with low CO, Hillis and others found the Fick/thermodilution percentage difference averaged 10 ± 10%. In patients with aortic or mitral regurgitation, the Fick/thermodilution percentage difference was 7 ± 7%. Thermodilution is preferable to green dye because right-sided injection and right-sided sampling (of the cold indicator) yield a curve that is less subject to recirculation-induced distortion than right-sided injection and left-sided sampling of green dye.

INTRACARDIAC SHUNTS

A shunt is an abnormal communication between the left and right heart chambers. The direction of blood flowing through the shunt is left to right, right to left, or sometimes bi-directional. In the absence of shunting, the pulmonary blood flow (right side of the heart) is equal to the systemic blood flow. Table 3-2 lists intracardiac shunt locations. A left-to-right shunt increases the amount of blood to the right side of the heart and increases pulmonary blood flow, now the sum of the

Table 3-2

Cardiac Shunt Locations

Location	Earliest Step-Up Location (for Left-to-Right Shunts)
Atrial Septal Defects	
Primum (low)	RA, RV
Secundum (mid)	RA
Sinus venosus (high)	RA
Partial anomalous pulmonary venous return (pulmonary veins entering right atrium)	RA
Ventricular Septal Defects	
Membranous (high)	RV
Muscular (mid)	RV
Apical (low)	RV
Aorticopulmonary Window (Connection of Aorta to Pulmonary Artery)	PA
Patent Ductus Arteriosus (Normally Closed Ao-PA Connection at Birth)	PA

Ao, Aortic; *PA,* pulmonary artery; *RA,* right atrium; *RV,* right ventricle.

systemic blood flow plus shunt flow. With a right-to-left shunt, the amount of blood shunted from the right side of the heart to the left is added to that normally ejected into the systemic circulation, making systemic blood flow greater than pulmonary blood flow by the amount of the shunt (Fig. 3-12). Intracardiac shunts have been evaluated by four methods: (1) oximetry, (2) indocyanine green dye dilution curves (Fig. 3-13), (3) angiography, and (4) radioactive tracers. Table 3-3 compares methods of shunt detection.

Oximetry Procedure: Diagnostic Saturation Run

Oximetry is the method most commonly used to assess cardiac shunts. A diagnostic "saturation run" uses heparinized 1- to 3-ml syringes to obtain blood from the PAs and regions of the RV, RA, superior vena cava (SVC), and inferior vena cava (IVC) in a rapid, organized manner. A large-bore end-hole or side-hole catheter (multipurpose) is preferred for rapid sampling.

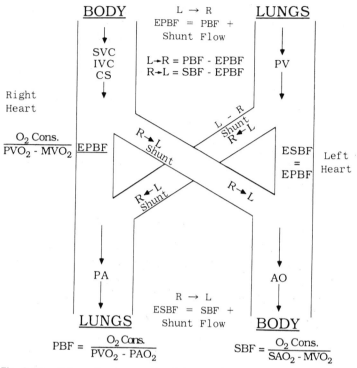

Fig. 3-12 Schematic diagram for right-to-left and left-to-right shunting across the heart. *L*, Left; *R*, right; *PBF*, pulmonary blood flow; *EPBF*, effective pulmonary blood flow; *SBF*, systemic blood flow; *ESBF*, effective systemic blood flow; *O₂ Cons.*, oxygen consumption; *PAO₂*, pulmonary artery oxygen saturation or content; *PVO₂*, pulmonary venous oxygen saturation or content; *MVO₂*, mixed venous oxygen saturation or content; *SAO₂*, systemic arterial oxygen saturation or content; *SVC*, superior vena cava; *IVC*, inferior vena cava; *CS*, coronary sinus; *Ao*, aorta; *PA*, pulmonary artery.

Samples can also be obtained from a standard balloon-tipped Swan-Ganz–type catheter. Saturation syringes should be heparinized with less than 0.5 ml. The labels and list of sample sites should also be prepared in advance (Box 3-4).

The saturation run begins after diagnostic hemodynamic data and CO have been obtained and before right-sided heart pullback. With the catheter positioned in the right or left PA, oxygen consumption (Fick method) is measured. After the oxygen consumption measurement is completed, one operator

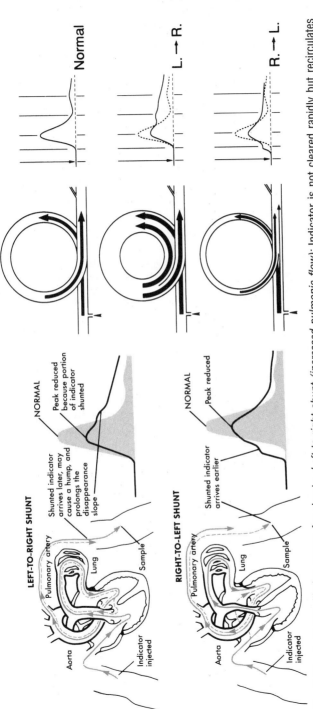

Fig. 3-13 Indicator dilution curves for shunts. *Left-to-right shunt (increased pulmonic flow):* Indicator is not cleared rapidly but recirculates through central circulation via defect. Based on magnitude of shunt, a constant fraction leaves the central pool with each circulation. Maximal deflection is reduced, and the disappearance is prolonged as a result of slow clearance. *Right-to-left shunt (decreased pulmonic flow):* A portion of the indicator passes directly to the arterial circulation via the defect without passing through the lungs and arrives at the arterial sampling site before the portion that did traverse the pulmonary circulation.

Table 3-3

Comparison of Methods to Detect, Localize, and Quantitate Intracardiac Left-to-Right Shunting

Detection Method	Able to Localize?	Able to Quantitate?	Minimal Qp/Qs Reliably Detected
Oximetry	Yes	Yes	1.5-1.9 Atrium
			1.3-1.5 Ventricle
			1.3 Great vessels
Indocyanine green			
Carter et al.*	No	Yes	1.35
Gamma variate	No	Yes	1.15
Hydrogen	No	No	1.01
Angiography	Yes	No	Unknown
Radionuclide	No	Yes	1.15
Echocardiography	Yes	Yes	Unknown

*Data from Boehrer JD, Lange RA, Willard JE, et al: *Am Heart J* 124:448-455, 1992.

manipulates the catheter under fluoroscopic and pressure control, while the assistant aspirates the blood samples at each location along the run. Each new sample is obtained after several milliliters of blood have been withdrawn and discarded within the catheter left from the previous site. If a sample cannot be obtained from a specific site because of ventricular ectopy, it may be necessary to reposition the catheter or skip the sample site until the rest of the run has been completed. The entire diagnostic run should take approximately 5 to 7 minutes.

Oxygen Step-Up. A left-to-right shunt is suggested at a chamber or vessel when a step-up, or increase, of oxygen content in that chamber or vessel exceeds that of a proximal compartment (beyond a normal variation in the oxygen content between the right heart chambers). A step-up in oxygen saturation at the PA by more than 7% (above the RA saturation) is indicative of a left-to-right shunt at the atrial level (Table 3-4). Similarly the desaturation of arterialized blood samples from the left heart chambers and aorta suggests a right-to-left shunt. In determining the site of the right-to-left shunt, sequential sampling can be made from the LA, LV, and aorta.

Box 3-4

Sample Sites for Oxygen Saturations During Diagnostic Saturation Run

Right Side of the Heart
Left pulmonary artery (PA)
Right PA
Main PA
PA_{PV} (above pulmonary valve)
Right ventricle, below pulmonary valve (RV_{PV})
RV (mid)
RV (apex)
RV_{TV} (tricuspid valve)
Right atrium at tricuspid valve (RA_{TV})
RA (mid)
Superior vena cava (SVC), high
SVC (low)
RA (high)
RA (low)
Inferior vena cava (IVC), high (just beneath heart, above hepatic vein)
IVC (low, above renal vein, but below hepatic vein)

Left Side of the Heart
Arterial saturation, aortic
(If possible cross atrial septal defect, pulmonary vein saturation)
Patent foramen ovale or left atrium

Mixed venous blood is assumed to be fully mixed PA blood. If there is a left-to-right shunt, mixed venous blood is measured one chamber proximal to the step-up. In the case of an atrial septal defect, the mixed venous oxygen content is computed from the weighted average of vena caval blood (i.e., as the sum of three times the SVC plus one IVC oxygen content and divided by four).

When pulmonary venous blood is not collected, PVO_2 (pulmonary vein) percentage saturation is assumed to be 95%.

Shunt Calculation. The Fick or left-sided indicator dilution methods of CO determination are employed to measure systemic flow (see Fig. 3-12). Using the Fick method, the following formulas apply:

Table 3-4

Oxygen Saturation Values for Shunt Detection

Level of Shunt	Significant Step-Up Difference* O_2 % Saturation
Atrial (SVC/IVC to right aorta)	≥7
Ventricular	≥5
Great vessel	≥5

SVC, Superior vena cava; IVC, inferior vena cava; PA, pulmonary artery pressure.
*Difference between distal and proximal chamber. For example, for ASD:

$$PA - \frac{3\ SVC + 1\ IVC}{4} \quad \text{(should be ≤7\% normally)}$$

Systemic flow (L/min)

$$= \frac{O_2 \text{ consumption (ml/min)}}{10 \times \text{arterial} - \text{mixed venous } O_2 \text{ difference (vol \%)}}$$

Pulmonary flow (L/min)

$$= \frac{O_2 \text{ consumption (ml/min)}}{10 \times \text{pulmonary vein} - \text{pulmonary artery } O_2 \text{ difference (vol \%)}}$$

Normally the effective pulmonary blood flow is equal to the systemic blood flow.

In a left-to-right shunt (see Fig. 3-12) the effective pulmonary blood flow is increased (by the amount of the shunt) as follows:

Effective pulmonary flow = systemic flow + shunt flow
(left-to-right)   (1)

In a right-to-left shunt, the effective pulmonary blood flow is decreased (by the amount of the shunt):

Effective pulmonary flow = systemic flow − shunt flow
(right-to-left)   (2)

The shunt volume is determined by use of Equations (1) and (2).

The ratio of pulmonary to systemic flow (called Qp/Qs, where Q is flow, p is pulmonary, and s is systemic) for a left-to-right shunt is called the shunt fraction. Flow ratios, Qp/Qs, greater than 1.5 often require closure.

Example for Left-to-Right Shunt Atrial Septal Defect Calculation

Data obtained at catheterization:

$$\text{Hemoglobin} = 13 \text{ g}$$
$$O_2 \text{ consumption} = 210 \text{ ml/min}$$

Location	Saturation (%)	Location	Saturation (%)
Arterial	92	PA	83
SVC	70	Pulmonary vein	95
Mid RA	85	IVC	68
Low RA	68		

Step 1: Compute O_2 content.

$$\text{Arterial } O_2 \text{ content} = 0.92 \times 1.36 \times 13.0 \times 10 = 163$$

$$\text{Mixed venous } O_2 \text{ content} = \frac{(.70 + .70 + .70 + .68)}{4} = 0.69$$
$$\times 1.36 \times 13.0 \times 10 = 122$$

$$\text{Pulmonary artery } O_2 \text{ content} = (0.83 \times 1.36 \times 13.0 \times 10) = 147$$

$$\text{Pulmonary vein } O_2 \text{ content} = (0.95 \times 1.36 \times 13.0 \times 10) = 168$$

Step 2: Compute systemic flow [Equation (1)].

$$\frac{210 \text{ ml/min}}{163 - 122} = \frac{210}{41}$$
$$Qs = 5.12$$

Step 3: Compute pulmonary flow [Equation (2)].

$$\frac{210}{168 - 147} = \frac{210}{21}$$
$$Qp = 10$$

Step 4: Compute Qp/Qs.

$$\frac{10}{5.1} = 1.96$$

Example for Simplified Qp/Qs Formula Using Saturations Only

$$\frac{Qp}{Qs} = \frac{SAO_2 - MVO_2}{PVO_2 - PAO_2} \quad \frac{Art - MV}{PV - PA}$$

Where *Art* is arterial; SAO_2, systemic artery oxygen saturation; PVO_2, pulmonary vein oxygen saturation; MVO_2, mixed venous oxygen saturation; and PAO_2, pulmonary artery oxygen saturation.

Using saturation data from example of left-to-right ASD:

$$\frac{Qp}{Qs} = \frac{92 - 69}{95 - 83} = \frac{23}{12}$$
$$= 1.92$$

Example for Right-to-Left Shunt
Data obtained at catheterization:

Hemoglobin = 15 g
O_2 consumption = 195 ml/min

Location	Saturation (%)	Location	Saturation (%)
Arterial	89	LA	88
SVC	81	PA	82
Mid RA	83	PV	96
Low RA	82	IVC	70

Step 1: Compute O_2 content.

Arterial O_2 content = $(0.89 \times 15 \times 1.36 \times 10)$ = 181 ml/L
$= 167$ ml/L

Pulmonary artery O_2 content = $(0.82 \times 15 \times 1.36 \times 10)$ = 167 ml/L

Pulmonary vein O_2 content = $(0.96 \times 15 \times 1.36 \times 10)$ = 195 ml/L

Step 2: Compute systemic flow [Equation (1)].

$$\frac{O_2 \text{ consumption}}{SAO_2 - PAO_2} = \frac{195}{181 - 167} = \frac{195}{14}$$
$$Qs = 13.9$$

Step 3: Compute pulmonary blood flow [Equation (2)].

$$\frac{O_2 \text{ consumption}}{PVO_2 - PAO_2} = \frac{195}{195 - 167} = \frac{195}{28}$$
$$Qp = 7.0$$

Step 4: Compute Qp/Qs.

$$\frac{7.0}{13.9} = 0.5 \text{ (right-to-left shunt)}$$

Limitations of the Oximetric Technique
1. Because of its low sensitivity, oximetry may fail to detect small (<1) shunts.
2. The application of the Fick principle to calculate blood flow presumes a steady state during the diagnostic run and measurement of oxygen consumption (i.e., timely

collection of saturation sample within a period when the oxygen consumption and CO are stable).

3. The oximetry method also assumes that complete mixing is achieved instantly and that the blood samples obtained are representative of blood in the respective compartment.

4. The rate of systemic blood flow is important in detecting a shunt by oximetry. A high systemic flow tends to equalize the arteriovenous oxygen difference across a given vascular bed. In the presence of elevated systemic blood flow the mixed venous oxygen saturation is higher than normal and intrachamber variability caused by streaming is blunted. By contrast, when the systemic blood flow is reduced and the mixed venous oxygen saturation is lower, a larger step-up must be detected before a significant left-to-right shunt is diagnosed.

Arteriovenous indocyanine green dilution curves were relied on in detecting shunting when the oximetry values showed a left-to-right shunt in excess of 26% of the pulmonary flow. A venovenous (right-side injection and right-side sampling) dye dilution curve was more sensitive in this situation (see Fig. 3-13).

Angiography

Angiography is a *nonquantitative* method used to localize either left-to-right or right-to-left shunts. The angiographic method may be useful when origin of the shunt cannot be entered. The shunt can be detected by injection of contrast medium into the closest proximal chamber. The left anterior oblique view with cranial angulation puts the interatrial and interventricular septae on edge, which provides an ideal view for detection of contrast medium passage across the atrial and ventricular septal defects (see Chapter 4 for angiographic views to visualize an intracardiac shunt).

Radioactive Tracers

Radioactive tracers for shunts are administered by vein in the nuclear medicine department and provide a useful estimate of shunt flow. Radioactivity seen in the brain or kidneys after right-sided injection means that the tracer has passed through an intracardiac shunt (right-to-left), and has escaped entrapment by the lungs.

EQUIPMENT USED FOR HEMODYNAMIC STUDY
Pressure Manifold Setup

The optimal set of transducers, tubing, and manifolds for any laboratory is that which is cost efficient, familiar, accurate, and simple to use. Several varieties of disposable and reusable manifolds exist (Fig. 3-14). A variety of transducers, positioned either on the manifold or at the side of the catheterization table, are suitable. For research studies, special transducer-tipped micromanometer pressure catheters and guidewires are used for the high-fidelity pressure recordings. High-fidelity recordings are not necessary for routine clinical hemodynamic studies; accurate measurements can be obtained with fluid-filled systems if appropriate precautions in the setup are taken. Some clear plastic manifolds have four ports, for a pressure and zero line at the first, saline flush solution at the second, contrast media at the third, and a closed waste line (to minimize contamination of personnel and laboratory) at the fourth stopcock.

All injections into the arterial system are performed with hand syringes or with an appropriately cleared power injection setup. For best waveform results, pressure tubing should be short and stiff. Ideally the transducer is as close to the catheter as possible.

For optimal pressure measurements the tubing length from the catheter to the transducer should be minimized. Longer tubing contributes to poorer quality tracings (more "fling" artifact). The zero level is set at midchest (measured antero-posterior diameter of the patient divided by two). When the transducer is raised above zero level, pressure is artificially lower. When the transducer is lower than zero, pressure is artificially higher. When abnormally low pressures are seen initially, the operator should recheck the zero for proper positioning (at midchest) and check for air bubbles or loose connections.

Physiologic Recorder

The physiologic monitor-recorder is the primary instrument used for the processing and recording of hemodynamic signals. The typical monitor in the cardiac catheterization laboratory is a multichannel unit that can process, display, and record electrocardiogram (ECG) signals, pressure tracings, and direct current (DC) inputs from external sources (e.g., thermo-

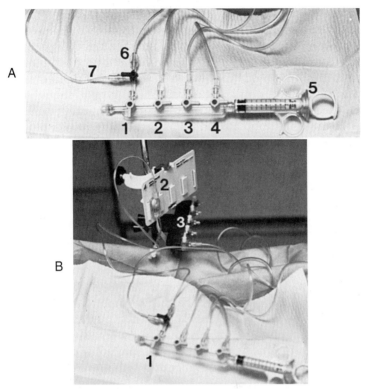

Fig. 3-14   A, Pressure manifold used for coronary angiography. *1,* The connection to the patient at the end of a plastic, movable, swivel connector. This also connects to *6* and *7,* which are the pressure and zero lines. *2,* Saline flush line; *3,* contrast line; *4,* waste line; *5,* control syringe. **B,** Close-up of the pressure manifold. *1* is connected to the transducer and zero lines; *2,* transducer on holder; *3,* off-table zero.

dilution). Most recorders have multichannel inputs (6 to 20 inputs). The number of channels determines how many individual signals are displayed and recorded simultaneously. For routine cardiac catheterization, one ECG signal and two to three pressure signals are normally recorded. In certain complex cases, such as electrophysiology studies and cases with complex congenital or valvular heart disease, it is common to use 4 to 18 channels. The physiologic recording channels must be set up and calibrated before each case.

Pressure Amplifiers. The pressure amplifier of the physiologic monitor connects with the pressure transducer and provides the pressure wave from the intravascular catheter. The transducer and amplifier convert the mechanical energy of a pulsatile column of fluid in the catheter to an electrical signal that is displayed on the monitor-recorder. The system should be checked at the start of each day to ensure that signal deflection is accurate and calibrated to a known pressure from a blood pressure cuff.

Calibration. The transducer-amplifier of the physiologic monitor system should be calibrated daily. A common technique uses a mercury manometer and applies a known pressure to the transducer. The gain setting on the amplifier is adjusted so that the amplitude of the signal matches the pressure that is being applied.

Electronic Calibration. Most recorders have an electronic calibration that allows the operator to input an electronic pressure standard. This feature provides a convenient means for simulating pressure signals to calibrate the display. A "cal" (calibration) signal at the end of each physiologic recording can be used to document the range on which the recording was made.

Display Settings for Recording Paper-Video Monitor. The operator has many choices when setting the display for physiologic monitoring. These include the following:
1. *Time lines*—This is the time interval at which a vertical line appears on the recording paper. The usual choices, in seconds, are 0.01, 0.04, 0.1, 0.2, 0.5, 1 and 5 (Figs. 3-15 and 3-16). The typical setting for a routine case is 1-second time lines (i.e., a line each second). For special studies or when a faster paper speed is used, a faster time line sequence should be used. It is important to know the time line interval used because certain calculations are made from the time line interval (e.g., heart rate, diastolic filling times). If the paper speed is known, the time line interval can be measured and calculated. A full-page inscription of time lines should be used to assist the timing of pressure wave changes (see Fig. 3-16).

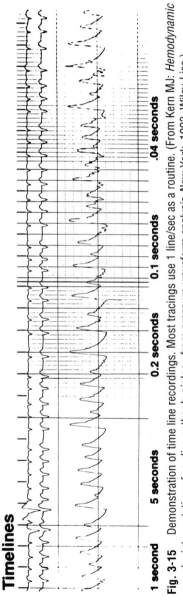

Fig. 3-15   Demonstration of time line recordings. Most tracings use 1 line/sec as a routine. (From Kern MJ: *Hemodynamic rounds: interpretation of cardiac pathophysiology from pressure waveform analysis*, New York, 1993, Wiley-Liss.)

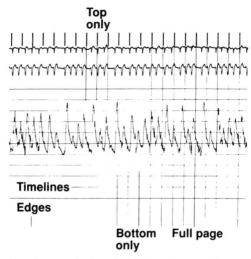

Fig. 3-16 Time lines can be inscribed differently across the recording paper. For accurate and easy timing of hemodynamic events (i.e., correlation with pressure waves), full-page time lines should be used *(far right side)*. (From Kern MJ, Aguirre F, Donohue T: *Cathet Cardiovasc Diagn* 27:147-154, 1992.)

2. *Paper speed.* The rate of paper speed can be changed by the operator. The paper speed choices for most recorders range from 5 to 500 mm/sec. The typical choice for most procedures is 25 mm/sec. In certain hemodynamic studies, 50 and 100 mm/sec are used. Slower paper speeds (10 and 5 mm/sec) are used to record the mean pressure or to conserve paper in long hemodynamic studies. In some recorders, different paper types (photographically faster) may be necessary if paper speed greater than 150 mm/sec is used.

3. *Sweep speed (video monitor).* This control gives the operator the choice of changing the sweep of the oscilloscope monitor. On some monitors, this feature is linked to the paper speed.

4. *Calibration lines.* This switch allows the operator to set the number and spacing of the horizontal calibration lines on the monitor and the paper. A usual configuration is 10 cm per full-scale spacing. Positioning of the calibration lines can be changed on some recorders, which can be a source of error (Fig. 3-17).

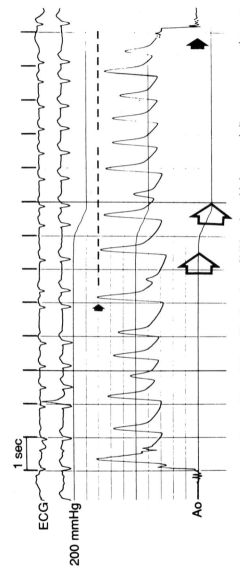

Fig. 3-17   Effect of changing position of the calibration lines. Shifting the grid downward *(two open arrows)* causes an erroneous increase in systolic aortic pressure from 160 to nearly 180 mm Hg. At low pressures this could be a critical problem. Note the confirmation of the error by the zero recheck at the far right arrow. *Ao,* Aortic pressure. (From Kern MJ, Aguirre F, Donohue T: *Cathet Cardiovasc Diagn* 27:147-154, 1992.)

HEMODYNAMIC RECORDING TECHNIQUES

Certain basic techniques are required to obtain high-quality hemodynamic recordings. The following are some suggestions that aid in providing consistent, reliable data:

1. At the start of each procedure, the patient's name, the date, and calibration inputs are placed on the recording paper.
2. The recording technician zeros the transducers-recorder properly. Transducers should be placed at the midchest level and opened to air before reference zeros are set. The midchest point can be measured with a ruler and marked for later reference.
3. The technician indicates what scale is being used during the recording. If simultaneous tracings are being recorded, good technique dictates that all channels be placed on the same scale factor. This may not always be possible but should be encouraged. (Some units print the scale on the paper automatically.)
4. The recording technician should anticipate changes in the recording technique as the catheter is moved to new positions. Pressure scales and recording paper speed are changed as needed.

Example: For monitoring of right atrial pressure in a patient with pulmonary hypertension, a full-scale 0 to 50 mm Hg may be appropriate. As the catheter passes through the tricuspid valve, the RV pressure may be greater than 50 mm Hg. The technician should observe this, anticipate the change, and quickly change the scale (e.g., 0 to 100 mm Hg full scale) accordingly. This is an instance when the recording paper should be marked accurately so that there is no question when the physician reviews the tracings as to what scale was used.

HEMODYNAMIC EXAMPLES AND ARTIFACTS
Normal Right Ventricular and Right Atrial Pressure Waves

The respiratory influences on RA pressure are shown in Fig. 3-18. Simultaneous RV and RA pressures (0 to 40 mm Hg scale) are shown in Fig. 3-19. The atrial filling wave a and ventricular filling wave v correspond to the right ventricular pressure tracing. Following the a wave is the X descent, and following the v wave is the normal Y descent. These features may be altered in the presence of disease or obscured in patients who

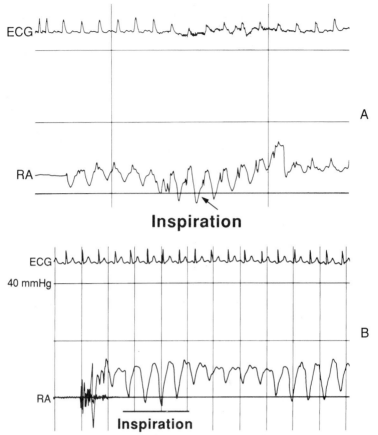

Fig. 3-18   A, Normal decrease in right atrial *(RA)* pressure during inspiration (scale 0 to 40 mm Hg). Note increase in Y descent *(arrow).* **B,** Abnormal response of right atrial pressure to inspiration in a patient with constrictive physiology or heart failure. Although Y descent is exaggerated, no corresponding fall in a or v wave height occurs.

have atrial arrhythmias. The notch (*closed arrow,* Fig. 3-19) on the top of the RV tracing is the "ringing" of a fluid-filled catheter. This rebound or ringing is also evident on the early diastolic part of the pressure wave (*open arrow,* bottom of same beat).

Fig. 3-20 shows the continuous pressure on pullback (*) across the interatrial septum from the left atrium to the right

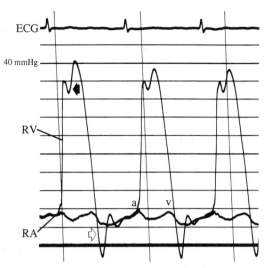

Fig. 3-19 Right atrial *(RA)* and right ventricular *(RV)* tracings in a normal patient. *Closed arrow,* Notch of ringing or overshoot on right ventricular pressure rise; *open arrow,* ringing and overshoot of decline in right ventricular pressure at early diastole; *a,* atrial wave; *v,* ventricular filling wave.

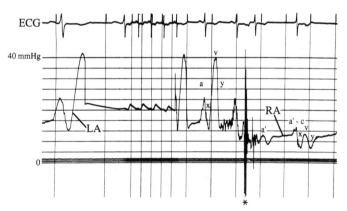

Fig. 3-20 Hemodynamic tracing of left atrium *(LA)* with catheter pullback to right atrium *(RA)* across the intraatrial septum. See text for details of waveform analysis.

atrium of a patient with aortic stenosis and shows the differences between LA and RA a and v waves. The v waves on the left atrium are prominent with their corresponding X and Y descents. In the right atrium the a and v waves are present but less striking. In general RA a waves are bigger than v waves. In the left atrium v waves are more prominent than a waves.

Right Atrial Pressure with Tricuspid Regurgitation

In contrast to the normal pattern (see Fig. 3-19), the RA pressure rises throughout RV systole when tricuspid valvular regurgitation pushes blood back into the right atrium (Fig. 3-21). In this patient the RA pressure during diastole matches the RV pressure, indicating no tricuspid stenosis. Tricuspid regurgitation is also evident in Fig. 3-21. RV and RA pressure are elevated (RV systolic, 70 mm Hg; RA mean pressure, 17 mm Hg). The RA pressure shows striking regurgitant waves during systole. A small gradient exists between the right atrium (higher tracing) and right ventricle (lower tracing) during diastole because of mild tricuspid stenosis (a narrow and limited opening of the tricuspid valve). In patients with tricuspid regurgitation, large pulsatile waves in the jugular, hepatic, and femoral venous system may be easily seen or palpated (Fig. 3-22).

Right Atrial Pressure in a Patient with Atrioventricular Dissociation

Normal a waves represent atrial contraction into the ventricle with no obstruction to inflow. In an atrioventricular block the atria are not contracting at the proper time in relation to the ventricles (Fig. 3-23). Immediately after the QRS, the ventricles contract and the tricuspid and mitral valves close. If the P wave (and atrial contraction) comes after the tricuspid valve is closed, a giant a or cannon wave can be seen. When atrioventricular synchrony (normal sequence) occurs on beats 6 and 7, the a waves return, proportional in size to the timing of the atrial contraction, emptying blood before ventricular systole (QRS). Similar findings may be seen when the dissociation is caused by a pacemaker. Giant a waves occur during pacing (Fig. 3-24).

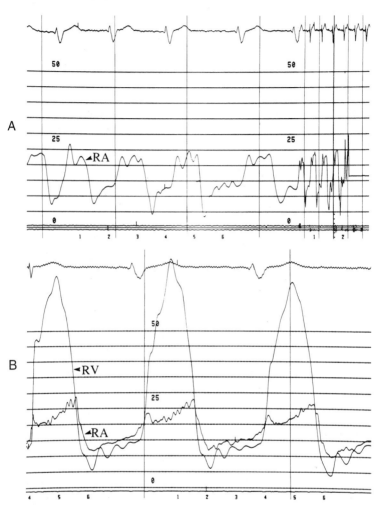

Fig. 3-21 **A,** Right atrial *(RA)* pressure in a patient with severe tricuspid regurgitation. **B,** When right atrial pressure is paired with simultaneous right ventricular *(RV)* pressure, tricuspid regurgitation can be seen associated with tricuspid stenosis as the separation (gradient) between the RA and RV pressures during diastole. See text for details.

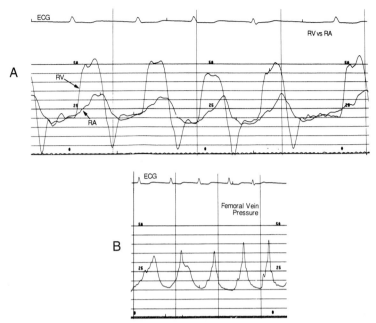

Fig. 3-22   A, Right ventricular *(RV)* and right atrial *(RA)* pressures (scale 0 to 50 mm Hg) showing severe tricuspid regurgitation. **B,** Note transmission of regurgitant wave to the femoral vein (sheath).

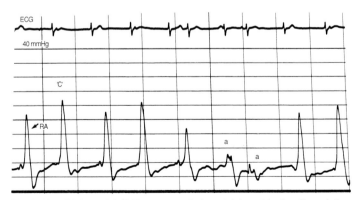

Fig. 3-23   Right atrial *(RA)* pressure during atrial-ventricular dissociation. *C,* Cannon wave; *a,* small a wave during synchrony of the atrial and ventricular activity. See text for details.

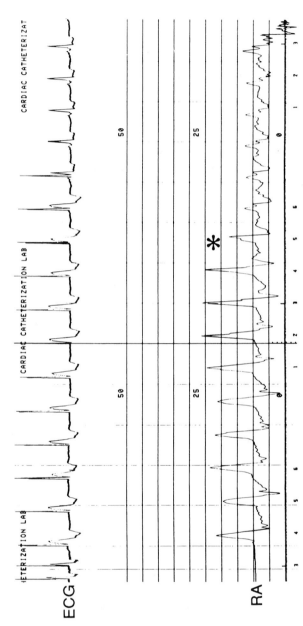

Fig. 3-24 Right atrial (*RA*) pressure during and after temporary right ventricular pacing. ECG shows large pacer spikes associated with giant a waves on right atrial pressure. Fusion beats begin at the asterisk, and the timing of an atrial contraction begins to precede ventricular activation, resulting in normal a waves.

Pulmonary Capillary Wedge Pressure and Left Atrial Pressure with Simultaneous Transseptal and Right-Sided Heart Catheterization

The PCW pressure is measured through a 7 F fluid-filled, balloon-tipped catheter; the LA pressure is measured through a Brockenbrough catheter (Fig. 3-25). The LA pressure rise precedes that of the PCW pressure for every waveform by approximately 100 to 150 ms. The good correspondence (generally) of these two pressures permits clinical use of PCW pressure for most standard hemodynamic cases (a, a′ and v, v′ are the LA and PCW pressures, respectively). Lists of pathologic changes of the atrial, systemic, and pulmonary pressure waveforms and some possible causes for the abnormalities are provided in Boxes 3-5 through 3-7.

Normal Femoral Arterial and Central Aortic Pressures

The femoral arterial (FA) pressure measured through the side arm of the femoral arterial sheath (8 F) is matched against pressure in the pigtail catheter (7 F) positioned above the aortic valve (Fig. 3-26). These pressures normally correspond closely. There is a slight overshoot of the more peripheral FA pressure (Fig. 3-26, *A*). Also, by observing the time of upstroke of the pressures, the operator can distinguish the central aortic pressure (first rising). The mean of the two pressures is identical (Fig. 3-26, *B*).

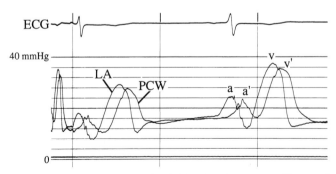

Fig. 3-25   Simultaneous left atrial *(LA)* and pulmonary capillary wedge *(PCW)* tracings. (The patient has aortic stenosis with high ventricular filling pressure.) See text for details.

Box 3-5

Pathologic Changes of the Atrial Pressure Waveforms

Elevated mean atrial pressure (right atrial [RA] >4 to 8 mm Hg, left atrial [LA] >8 to 12 mm Hg)

Insufficiency of the following chamber (i.e., ventricle)

Stenosis or insufficiency of the atrioventricular (AV) valve

Hypervolemia

Pericardial disease or effusion

Congestive heart failure or infarction

Low Mean Atrial Pressure

Hypovolemia

Zero line artifact

A (Atrial Contraction) Wave

Elevated a wave

Hypertrophy or decreased ventricular compliance (i.e., stiff heart)

Mitral or tricuspid insufficiency

Mitral or tricuspid stenosis

Decreased atrial pressure-volume compliance curve (i.e., stiffer chamber) (*case example:* see Fig. 3-25)

Missing a wave

Atrial arrest

Atrial fibrillation

Atrial flutter

False lowered a wave in patients with a large c-v wave

V (Diastolic Filling) Wave

Elevated v waves in

Increased flow (e.g., atrial or ventricular septal defect)

AV valve insufficiency (in the case of severe insufficiency, the high v wave is called ventricularization of the trial pulse curve) (mitral regurgitation; see Fig. 3-40)

Atrial fibrillation

Atrial fibrillation and AV-valvular insufficiency (in cases of atrial fibrillation, valvular insufficiency can be diagnosed on the basis of the atrial pulse curve only if the v wave is markedly elevated) (*case example:* large v wave, see Fig. 3-41)

X and Y Descents (Atrial Pressure Waves)

Missing in atrial fibrillation (*normal case example:* LA, RA, see Fig. 3-20)

Special abnormalities of the atrial pressure wave

Box 3-5

Pathologic Changes of the Atrial Pressure Waveforms—cont'd

X and Y Descents (Atrial Pressure Waves)—cont'd

Equalization of the RA and LA pressures in severe atrial septal defect or cardiac constriction

Inspiratory increase of the mean RA pressure in constrictive pericarditis

Multiple pressure wave deformities of the atrial pulse curve in patients with rhythm disturbances (e.g., pacemakers, multifocal atrial tachycardia)

Saw-tooth deformity of the atrial pressure in atrial flutter

Dissociation of atrial and ventricular chamber pressure waves and corresponding intracardiac ECG in Ebstein's abnormality (atrialization of right ventricle)

Fig. 3-27 shows simultaneous arterial pressure with LV pressure. Satisfactory assessment of most aortic valvular lesions can be achieved if the operator matches the pressures before crossing the aortic valve. The phase lag and normal overshoot of the arterial pressure compared with the LV pressure should be noted. The aortic and LV pressure tracings here and in Figure 3-28 are characteristic for most patients when an 8 F femoral arterial sheath and a 7 F pigtail catheter are used in the procedure.

The contribution of atrial filling to systemic pressure can be seen in Fig. 3-28. The normal sinus beats (1 and 2) with simultaneous aortic (FA) and LV pressure tracings show a systolic pressure of 175 mm Hg (scale 0 to 200 mm Hg) and aortic diastolic pressure of 70 mm Hg. Atrial contribution is lost because of a-v dissociation (*arrow,* Fig. 3-28), and a pacemaker rhythm takes over. The systolic pressure falls dramatically to 118 mm Hg and gradually returns as atrial activity becomes more connected to the QRS.

Normal Right-Sided Heart Pressures on Catheter Pullback

Normal pressures of the right side of the heart are shown during continuous pressure recording (using a balloon-tipped PA catheter) on catheter pullback from PA to RV and RA (0 to 40 mm Hg scale) (Fig. 3-29). Simultaneous LV and RV pressures are compared on the same scale and fast (50 mm/sec) paper speed. Premature ventricular contractions are common when the catheter contacts the RV outflow tract.

Box 3-6

Pathologic Changes of the Ventricular Pressure Waveforms

Systolic Pressure
Elevated
Pulmonary or arterial hypertension
Pulmonary stenosis, aortic stenosis, aortic insufficiency

Decreased
Hypovolemic state
Cardiac congestion, cardiac failure, tamponade, infarction

End-Diastolic Pressure
Elevated
Hypervolemia
Hypertrophy
Decreased compliance
Cardiac failure, tamponade
Aortic insufficiency

Decreased
Hypovolemia
Tricuspid stenosis, mitral stenosis

a Wave on Ventricular Pressure Trace
Decreased or missing in the following
Mitral stenosis, tricuspid stenosis
Mitral insufficiency, tricuspid insufficiency (if left or right ventricular compliance is increased)
Atrial fibrillation
Atrial flutter
Atrial arrest
Severe aortic insufficiency

Early Rapid Diastolic Pressure "Dip" with Mid-Diastolic "Plateau" (Flat Wave)
Artifact (bradycardia)
Constrictive pericarditis with elevated diastolic plateau
Restrictive cardiomyopathy

Box 3-7

Special Abnormalities of the Pressure Waves

Pulmonary Artery Pressure
Elevated
Primary or secondary pulmonary hypertension
Large left-to-right shunt
Peripheral pulmonary stenosis
Mitral stenosis, regurgitation, congestive heart failure

Decreased
Hypovolemia
Pulmonary stenosis (valvular, subvalvular, and peripheral)
Ebstein's anomaly
Hypoplastic right heart syndrome
Tricuspid stenosis and tricuspid atresia

Aortic Pressure
Elevated
Arterial hypertension

Decreased
Aortic stenosis
Low cardiac output
Shock

Wide Aortic Pulse Pressure
Arterial hypertension
Aortic insufficiency
Large left-to-right shunt (e.g., open ductus, aortopulmonary window, truncus arteriosus communis, perforated sinus Valsalva–aneurysm)

Narrow Aortic Pulse Pressure
Aortic stenosis
Heart failure
Cardiac tamponade
Shock

Arterial Pulsus Bisferiens (Spiked Pulse)
Aortic insufficiency
Obstructive hypertrophic cardiomyopathy

Continued

Box 3-7

Special Abnormalities of the Pressure Waves—cont'd

Pulsus Paradoxus (Abnormally Large Decrease in Arterial Pressure Systolic Peaks During Inspiration [>10 mm Hg])
Cardiac tamponade

Pulsus Parvus (Weak) and Tardus (Slow) (Delayed and Reduced Arterial Pressure)
Aortic stenosis

Pulsus Alternans (Alternating Strong and Weak Arterial Pressure)
Congestive heart failure
Cardiomyopathy

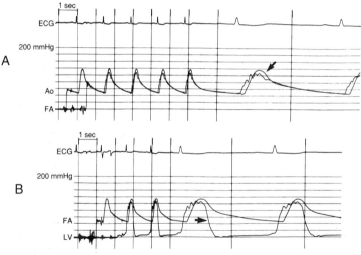

Fig. 3-26   A, Simultaneous hemodynamic tracings of femoral artery *(FA)* pressure, taken through the side arm of the 8 F sheath and central aortic *(Ao)* pressures. Ao pressure is obtained through the 7 F pigtail catheter. The overshoot of the FA pressure *(arrow)* and lag in the pressure upstroke are the normal characteristics for the femoral tracings. **B,** FA and left ventricular *(LV)* pressure *(arrow)*.

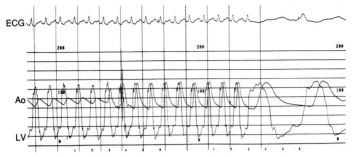

Fig. 3-27   Simultaneous aortic *(Ao)* pressure (from the femoral artery sheath) and left ventricular *(LV)* pressure from the pigtail catheter. Note the damped femoral artery tracing at the left side with the delayed upstroke. After the femoral artery sheath is flushed *(right side)*, systolic pressure matches LV pressure. For the clinical determination of Ao valve gradients, this technique is satisfactory in most patients.

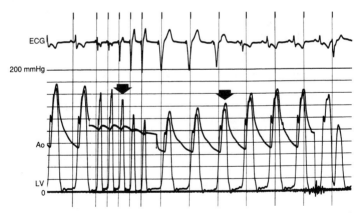

Fig. 3-28   Simultaneous hemodynamic tracings of aortic *(Ao)* and left ventricular *(LV)* pressures in a patient with a pacemaker. Loss of atrial contraction (paced beats) decreases ventricular filling with loss of systemic pressure. *Left arrow,* Initiation of ventricular pacing with loss of the atrial contribution to LV filling; *right arrow,* return of atrial synchrony and normal sinus rhythm. The systemic pressures are increased markedly during normal sinus rhythm.

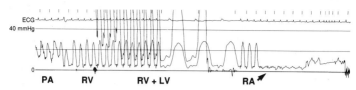

Fig. 3-29 Continuous hemodynamic tracing during catheter pullback from pulmonary artery *(PA)* to right atrium *(RA)*. Differences in left ventricular *(LV)* and right ventricular *(RV)* pressures are shown (0 to 40 mm Hg full scale).

Large v Waves on the Pulmonary Capillary Wedge Tracing

LV and PCW pressures generally match well in diastole (0 to 40 mm Hg scale) (Fig. 3-30). The PCW a wave (a′) follows the LV a wave by 150 ms (beat 1). The v wave is large. There is no important diastolic PCW-LV gradient. On beat 2, because of late atrial activity, loss of the LV a wave is shown by the different initial upstroke of the LV pressures. The PCW has large, late a and v waves. The v wave on a PCW pressure tracing is usually associated with significant mitral regurgitation. Large v waves are neither highly sensitive nor specific for mitral regurgitation, however. Large v waves may also be present with ventricular septal defect or with any condition in which the LA

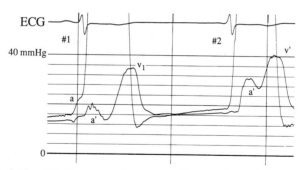

Fig. 3-30 Simultaneous pulmonary capillary wedge and left ventricular pressures in a patient who has loss of atrial activity *(beat 2)*. On beat 1 the a wave is evident on left ventricle *(a)* and pulmonary capillary wedge pressure *(a′)*. The a wave is lost in beat 2 with no atrial activity. The a′ wave is considerably higher because of its contraction against the closed mitral valve. See text for details.

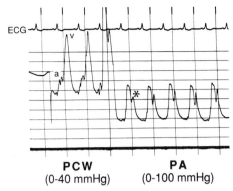

ECG

v

a

*

PCW
(0-40 mmHg)

PA
(0-100 mmHg)

Fig. 3-31   Giant v waves on the pulmonary capillary wedge *(PCW)* tracing can be transmitted to the pulmonary artery *(PA)* pressure, producing a notch (*) on the PA downslope.

volume (e.g., ventricular septal defect) or left atrial pressure relationship (the stiffness or compliance) is increased (e.g., rheumatic heart disease, postcardiac surgery, and infiltrative heart diseases). Mitral valve obstruction from any cause and congestive heart failure in the absence of mitral regurgitation are also associated with large v waves. Giant v waves, also seen in Fig. 3-30, may be large enough to be transmitted to the PA pressure, which causes a notch on the diastolic downslope (Fig. 3-31).

Aortic Stenosis

Simultaneous LV and Ao pressure tracings in a patient with minimal aortic stenosis (0 to 200 mm Hg scale) are shown in Fig. 3-32. The pressures were measured with a Millar high-fidelity catheter with two transducers on the tip of the catheter (see Chapter 6). Peak-to-peak Ao–LV pressure difference is only 10 mm Hg. The mean gradient (area between Ao and LV during systole) is 15 mm Hg. The rapid aortic upstroke shows the effect of the turbulent jet of the narrowed valve vibrating the catheter. There is no lag in the timing of the Ao pressure rise with respect to the LV. A higher LV pressure may also be seen after an extrasystolic beat, called *postextrasystolic accentuation* (Fig. 3-33).

The atrial contraction is important in patients with aortic stenosis (Fig. 3-34). Simultaneous Ao and LV pressure

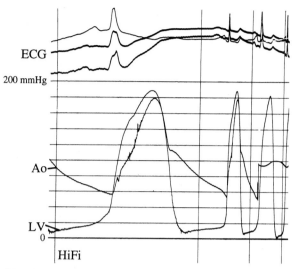

Fig. 3-32 Simultaneous aortic *(Ao)* and left ventricular *(LV)* pressures from dual micromanometer-tipped (high-fidelity *[HiFi]*) catheter in a patient with mild aortic stenosis. See text for details.

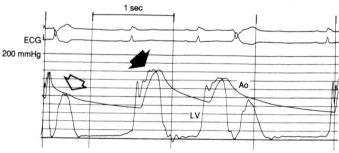

Fig. 3-33 Postextrasystolic accentuation of left ventricular *(LV)* and aortic *(Ao)* pressures *(closed arrow)* after a premature ventricular contraction *(open arrow)*. This patient does not have Ao stenosis. The premature ventricular contraction does not generate pressure sufficient to open the aortic valve and results in a dropped beat when the peripheral pulse rate is counted. (From Kern MJ, Donohue T, Bach R, et al: *Cathet Cardiovasc Diagn* 27:223-227, 1992.)

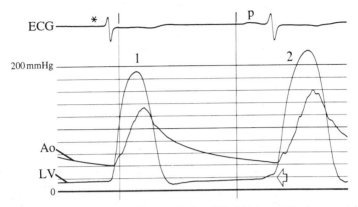

Fig. 3-34 Simultaneous left ventricular *(LV)* (obtained with transseptal technique) and aortic *(Ao)* pressures from fluid-filled catheter systems. Note the contribution of atrial contraction *(arrow)* to the change in LV and systemic pressures on beat 2. *p*, p wave; *, absence of p wave on this tracing. The wide pulse pressure also is indicative of Ao insufficiency. See text for details.

(transseptal approach, 0 to 200 mm Hg scale) shows that atrial activity is absent in the first beat, a junctional beat (*). Without the atrial contribution, Ao systolic pressure is 132 mm Hg, and LV systolic pressure is 190 mm Hg. In the following beat, number 3 atrial activity (P wave) precedes the QRS, and the Ao pressure increases to 160 mm Hg; LV pressure increases to 225 mm Hg, representing an approximately 25% increase in pressure augmentation. This effect is crucial in patients with poor LV function. Two additional features of this tracing are worthy of note; the a wave on the LV pressure tracing (*arrow,* Fig. 3-34) can be seen on the LV beat 2, and aortic regurgitation may be present when a wide pulse pressure (aortic systolic-diastolic pressure) greater than 50 to 60 mm Hg is observed. The aortic pressure has decreased to less than or equal to 50 mm Hg at the end of diastole. Bradycardia may also produce a wide pulse pressure.

Left Ventricular Gradient Below the Aortic Valve

Hypertrophic cardiomyopathy is a condition in which thick heart muscle, especially inside the LV chamber, contracts so hard that it obstructs flow out of the ventricle and by its own

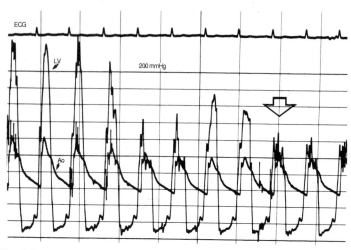

Fig. 3-35 Simultaneous left ventricular *(LV)* and aortic *(Ao)* pressures in a patient with obstructive hypertrophic cardiomyopathy during pullback of the catheter from the distal portion of the left ventricle. The pressure gradient between the aorta and left ventricle is lost. LV systolic pressure matches Ao pressure during catheter pullback before the catheter is pulled out of the left ventricle *(arrow)*. There is no true Ao valve gradient. This LV-Ao gradient is located in the mid-left ventricular wall beneath the Ao valve. The arrow indicates the matching of Ao and LV systolic pressures in the proximal chamber. See text for details.

contraction produces a pressure gradient with a normal aortic valve. Fig. 3-35 depicts simultaneous LV and Ao pressure showing large Ao-LV gradient (LV pressure, 220 mm Hg; Ao pressure, 120 mm Hg). On pullback of the LV catheter (multipurpose) from the distal LV to a position just beneath the aortic valve, the Ao-LV gradient disappears (see the LV pressure matching with Ao pressure, *arrow*, Fig. 3-35). Table 3-5 lists provocative maneuvers to increase an outflow tract gradient in patients with hypertrophic cardiomyopathies.

Aortic Regurgitation

Figs. 3-36 through 3-38 illustrate simultaneous Ao and LV pressures (0 to 200 mm Hg scale) in several patients with different degrees of aortic regurgitation. The characteristic hemodynamic feature of this condition is a wide pulse

Table 3-5

Provocative Tests for Hypertrophic Cardiomyopathy

Drug or Maneuver	Mechanism Increasing Ao-LV Gradient
Drugs	
Dobutamine	Increased myocardial contractility
Isoproterenol	Increased myocardial contractility, decreased blood pressure
Amyl nitrite	Decreased systemic arterial pressure (peripheral vasodilatation), reflex increasing sympathetic tone, decreased venous return, and increased myocardial contractility
Nitroglycerin	Decreased venous return, decreased cardiac output, and increased narrowing of LV outflow tract
Maneuvers	
Extrasystole	Postextrasystolic increase in myocardial contractility
Valsalva's maneuver	Decreased venous return, decreased LV volume, and increased narrowing of outflow tract

Ao, Aortic; *LV,* left ventricular.
Stroke volume and systemic arterial pulse pressure decrease in the postextrasystolic beat (Brockenbrough-Braunwald sign). This is in contrast to valvular aortic stenosis, in which the postextrasystolic beat is characterized by increased stroke volume and systolic gradient and by increased systemic arterial pressure.

pressure. The aortic (femoral) brisk pressure upstroke can be seen easily. Often there is marked overshoot of the femoral arterial pressure. In Fig. 3-37 the large and prominent a wave shows the effect of first-degree atrioventricular (AV) block (long PR interval, *arrow*) on the LV pressure. Figure 3-36 diagrams the physiology of the Ao-LV gradient in diastole. No atrial contribution of LV pressure is present.

Fig. 3-38 illustrates hemodynamically severe aortic regurgitation indicated by rapidly increasing LV diastolic pressure and wide Ao pressure with near-equilibration of Ao and LV pressure at end diastole. Note the aortic pressure overshoot.

Mitral Regurgitation

In Figs. 3-39 and 3-40 large v waves in the PCW tracing represent LV pressure transmitted backward through an

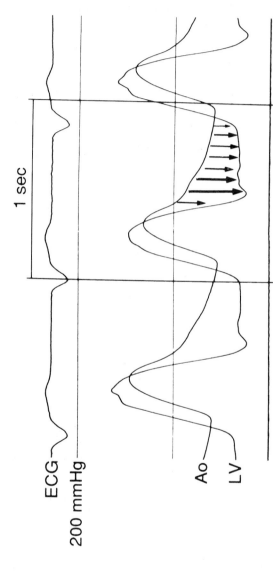

Fig. 3-36   Hemodynamic tracing in a patient with aortic insufficiency (and minimal aortic stenosis) showing the aortic (Ao)–left ventricular (LV) diastolic gradient (arrows) important for coronary perfusion. (Note loss of a wave because of paced rhythm.)

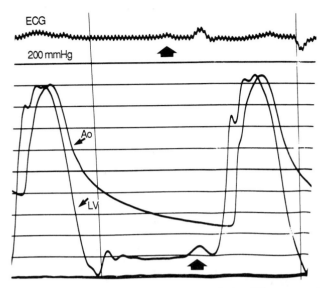

Fig. 3-37   Simultaneous aortic *(Ao)* and left ventricular *(LV)* pressures in a patient with aortic insufficiency. Note the absence of a systolic pressure gradient. The time delay in the Ao pressure upstroke indicates that femoral sheath pressure is used. The presence of a large and early a wave *(bottom arrow)* occurs with PR interval prolongation *(top arrow)*. See text for details.

incompetent mitral valve. The v wave occurs on the downstroke of the LV pressure. Fig. 3-40 shows large v waves (60 mm Hg) in a patient with mitral regurgitation. As noted in Fig. 3-30, however, v waves also reflect a change in the pressure-volume filling curve of the atrium.

Mitral Stenosis

In Fig. 3-41 simultaneous LV and PCW pressures show a mitral valve gradient throughout diastole. The a wave in the first beat is associated with a normal v wave. In the following beat, atrial activity is delayed and follows the QRS, contributing to large giant v wave (36 mm Hg). The augmented filling increases the mitral valve gradient. In some patients with mitral stenosis, balloon catheter valvuloplasty may be used to open a narrowed mitral orifice. Fig. 3-42 shows the mitral valve gradient before and after balloon catheter valvuloplasty. LA pressure is measured by the transseptal technique. Before

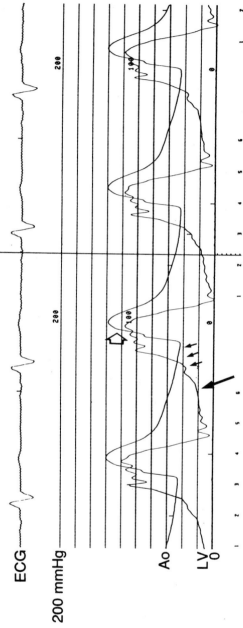

Fig. 3-38 Severe aortic regurgitation shown by rapidly increasing left ventricular (LV) diastolic pressure *(large black arrow)* and end-diastolic equilibration of aortic *(Ao)* and LV pressure *(three small arrows)*. Peripheral arterial pressure overshoot or amplification is caused by forceful LV ejection and compliant arterial system. (In this case, Ao pressure was matched with femoral artery sheath pressure.) (From Kern MJ, Aguirre FV: *Cathet Cardiovasc Diagn* 26:232–240, 1992.)

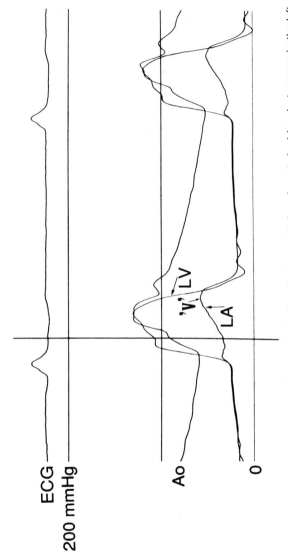

ECG

200 mmHg

'v'   LV

LA

Ao

0

Fig. 3-39   Hemodynamic tracings in a patient with mitral regurgitation characterized by giant v wave in the left atrial (*LA*) pressure. This v wave corresponds to marked increase in flow and volume into the left atrium. See text for details. *LV*, Left ventricular pressure; *Ao*, aortic pressure.

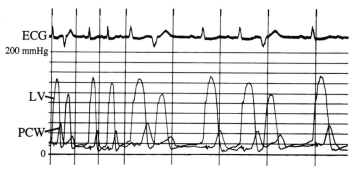

Fig. 3-40 Simultaneous left ventricular *(LV)* and pulmonary capillary wedge *(PCW)* pressures in a patient with mitral regurgitation. During ventricular ectopic activity (premature beats), large v waves (60 mm Hg) on the PCW pressure are seen. Giant v waves are hallmarks of severe mitral regurgitation. See text for details.

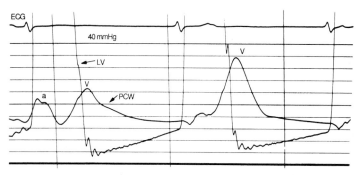

Fig. 3-41 Simultaneous pulmonary capillary wedge *(PCW)* and left ventricular *(LV)* pressures in a patient with mitral stenosis. The contribution of atrial contraction is evident on beat 1. Loss of atrial activity on beat 2 results in loss of the a wave and a giant v wave with an increased mitral valve gradient. See text for details.

valvuloplasty, the large gradient of 16 mm Hg resulted in a mitral valve area of 1 cm^2. After valvuloplasty, the gradient is considerably less (5 mm Hg). The valve area increased to 2.1 cm^2.

Mitral valve gradients are influenced by heart rate. When the rhythm is irregular (atrial fibrillation), calculations of gradients should be made from the average of 10 beats. Fig. 3-43

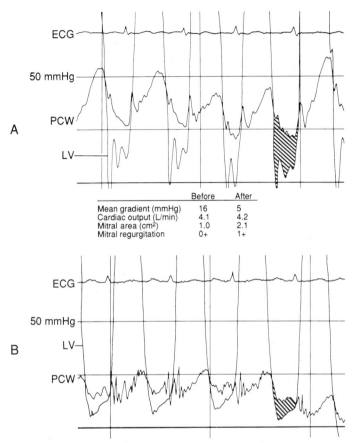

		Before	After
Mean gradient (mmHg)		16	5
Cardiac output (L/min)		4.1	4.2
Mitral area (cm²)		1.0	2.1
Mitral regurgitation		0+	1+

Fig. 3-42 Hemodynamic tracings in a patient with mitral stenosis **A,** before and **B,** after mitral valvuloplasty. The mean diastolic gradient of 16 mm Hg before valvuloplasty was reduced to 5 mm Hg after valvuloplasty, increasing the mitral valve area from 1 to 2.1 cm². *LV,* Left ventricular pressure; *PCW,* pulmonary capillary wedge pressure. See text for details.

illustrates the effect of RR cycle length on the mitral stenosis gradient.

Mixed Mitral Stenosis and Regurgitation

Fig. 3-44 illustrates simultaneous LV and PCW pressures (0 to 40 mm Hg scale) showing giant v waves with persistent PCW-LV gradient during diastole. Left ventriculography confirmed

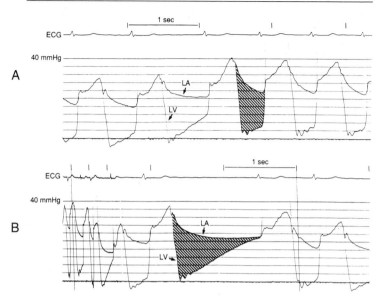

Fig. 3-43 Changing mitral stenosis gradient with heart rate (RR interval). **A,** Short RR interval is associated with gradient (shaded area) of 22 mm Hg. **B,** Long RR interval has a mean gradient of 29 mm Hg. When computing mean valve area in atrial fibrillation, average 10 beats. *LA,* Left atrial pressure; *LV,* left ventricular pressure. (From Kern MJ, Aguirre F: *Cathet Cardiovasc Diagn* 26:308-315, 1992.)

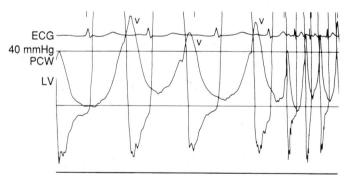

Fig. 3-44 Simultaneous left ventricular *(LV)* and pulmonary capillary wedge *(PCW)* pressures in a patient with severe mixed mitral regurgitation and mitral stenosis. The large v wave and the persistent diastolic gradient are characteristic of mixed mitral valvular disease. See text for details.

significant mitral regurgitation. The slope of the v waves in mitral regurgitation and stenosis is flatter than that in which large v waves are associated with isolated regurgitant flow (see Fig. 3-30).

Differences in Right Ventricular and Left Ventricular Pressures in Patients with Mitral Stenosis

Normal RV and LV pressures are separated by greater than 5 mm Hg in early and late diastole, and the RV pressure tracing is usually contained completely within the LV pressure tracing (Fig. 3-45). The diastolic ventricular pressures normally differ in slope and end-diastolic pressure. The a waves also differ in size because of the lower compliance (stiffer) left ventricle. Changes in the RV-LV pressure relationship are related to ventricular septal interaction and occur in pulmonary hypertension, bundle-branch block, myocardial infarction, RV volume overload, and, most commonly, pericardial constrictive physiology.

RV and LV pressures in a patient with left bundle-branch block are shown in Fig. 3-46. The timing of ventricular

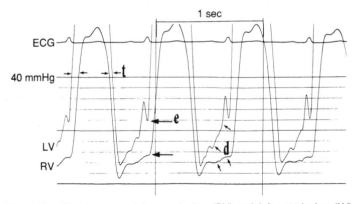

Fig. 3-45 Simultaneous right ventricular *(RV)* and left ventricular *(LV)* pressures in a patient with mild pulmonary hypertension. Note the different diastolic upslopes *(e)* and end-diastolic pressure *(d)*. The RV tracing is entirely within the LV tracing *(t)*, a normal pattern. (From Kern MJ: *Hemodynamic rounds: interpretation of cardiac pathophysiology from pressure waveform analysis,* New York, 1993, Wiley-Liss.)

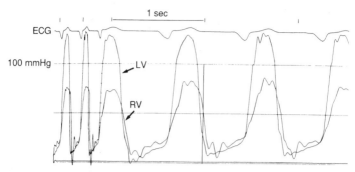

Fig. 3-46   Right ventricular *(RV)* and left ventricular *(LV)* pressures in a patient with left bundle-branch block and pulmonary hypertension. Note delay in RV pressure downslope falling outside LV pressure tracing. See text for details. (From Kern MJ: *Hemodynamic rounds: interpretation of cardiac pathophysiology from pressure waveform analysis,* New York, 1993, Wiley-Liss.)

activation is delayed in the bundle-branch block. RV pressure decline occurs outside the LV pressure. The clinical importance of this observation is unknown.

Constrictive Pericarditis

Constrictive pericarditis produces abnormal hemodynamics characterized by low arterial pressure, tachycardia, Kussmaul's sign (inspiratory increase in RA pressure), M or W configuration on RA pressure, and dip and plateau of early rapid diastolic filling with abrupt cessation caused by pericardial constraint (Fig. 3-47). In a comparison of constriction with tamponade physiology, the two are differentiated by the RA waveform (elevated and blunted in tamponade) and pulsus paradoxus (inspiratory decrease in arterial pressure in tamponade). Because these two entities are similar in their early stages, the RA pressures may also be similar. Two-dimensional echocardiography shows the amount of pericardial fluid and RA and RV chamber collapse of tamponade physiology. See Chapter 8 on pericardiocentesis for details of tamponade.

In Fig. 3-48 matching of elevated diastolic pressures with an early dip followed by a plateau during diastole (first beat) is the characteristic pattern. Often, the classic dip-and-plateau

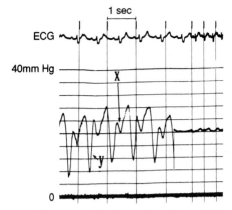

Fig. 3-47   Right atrial pressure showing pattern of constrictive physiology with large Y descent and smaller X descent. Mean right atrial pressure is 20 mm Hg.

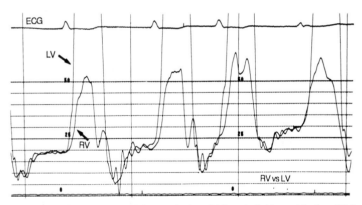

Fig. 3-48   Simultaneous left ventricular *(LV)* and right ventricular *(RV)* pressure tracing in a patient with constrictive pericarditis. Matching of diastolic pressures is one of the hallmarks of this condition. See text for details. Normal example of RV and LV pressures also is shown in Fig. 3-31. Note separation and increasing pressure in diastole.

configuration appears only during slow heart rates. Tachycardia and respiratory effort obscure the pattern, but matching of RV and LV pressures during diastole is consistent (Fig. 3-49). Dynamic respiratory variations differentiate constricture from a restrictive pathologic condition.

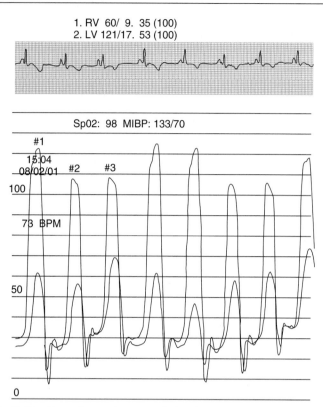

1. RV 60/ 9. 35 (100)
2. LV 121/17. 53 (100)

SpO2: 98 MIBP: 133/70

Fig. 3-49 Dynamic respiratory variation in constrictive and restrictive physiology. This example shows LV systolic pressure decrease when RV systolic pressure increases *(beat #3)* and is inconsistent with constrictive pericardial constraint.

Right Atrial Pressure in Patients with Constrictive Pericarditis

In Fig. 3-50 the characteristic pattern shows prominent Y descent with a classic M or W configuration of constrictive physiology. These waveforms are the altered X and Y troughs resulting from impaired ventricular filling. Myocardial restrictive heart disease or heart failure also shows this pattern occasionally. Fig. 3-51 shows pressure in patients with tamponade before and after pericardiocentesis.

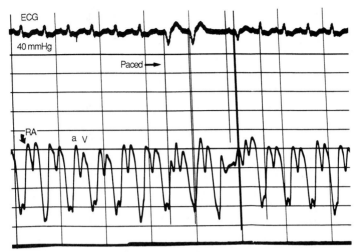

Fig. 3-50   Right atrial *(RA)* pressure in a patient with constrictive pericarditis showing abnormally elevated pressure with a classic M configuration. The elevated pressure with exaggerated Y descent is also seen in cardiomyopathy. See text for details.

Artifacts of Hemodynamic Tracings

Normal pressure curves from fluid-filled pressure systems are sharp without rounded contours. On the pressure tracings, narrow spikes or overshoot in the ventricular (right and left) pressure suggests underdamping (i.e., a too-sensitive pressure system). Wide, rounded waves indicate overdamping (i.e., not sensitive enough), usually produced by a problem in the fluid path to the transducer or a transducer that is not calibrated correctly.

Air Bubble. An air bubble in a LV pressure line produces a tracing with exaggerated systolic and diastolic overshoot (Fig. 3-52), suggesting underdamping. After the air bubble is flushed out, the sharp, crisp upstroke of the ventricular pressure shows a normal pressure rise. The short ring artifact of the pressure wave at peak LV pressure and during diastole should remain visible but occurs at a much higher frequency (i.e., shorter deflections). This pattern is an accurate waveform for a properly flushed fluid-filled catheter system.

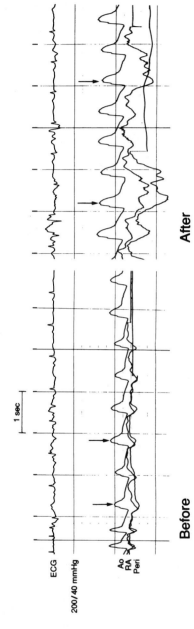

Fig. 3-51 Right atrial *(RA)*, pericardial *(Peri)*, and aortic *(Ao)* pressures in a patient with pericardial tamponade. Before pericardiocentesis, RA pressure has blunted X and Y descents. Arterial pressure shows pulsus paradoxus (inspiratory decrease >10 mm Hg of systolic pressure, *arrows*). After pericardiocentesis, pulsus paradoxus is absent, and RA waveform is more phasic. (From Kern MJ, Aguirre FV: *Cathet Cardiovasc Diagn* 26:152-158, 1992.)

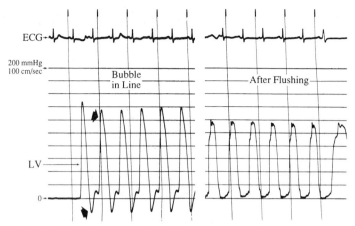

Fig. 3-52 Hemodynamic tracing showing the effect of an air bubble in a pressure line. Note the change in hemodynamic waveform after the bubble is flushed. The ringing artifact *(sharp points at arrows)* is eliminated, and fine detail of precise pressure is restored after flushing.

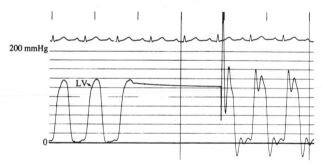

Fig. 3-53 *Left,* Left ventricular *(LV)* pressure tracing showing normally "damped" with viscous contrast media in the fluid path. *Right,* After flushing with saline, the tracing now is seen as underdamped with exaggerated ringing artifact.

Damping. Contrast media or a bubble in the pressure line can correct an underdamped tracing. Fig. 3-53 shows a suitable LV pressure with normal (or only slightly rounded) waveform. This tracing is a damped version of an underdamped signal that is apparent after flushing of the line (right side of tracing). Early diastolic and systolic portions of the pressure wave on

Table 3-6

Common Hemodynamic Recording Problems

Problem	Possible Cause	Solution
Overdamping*	Bubble or clot in line or transducer	Reflush system
	Small lumen of tubing system	Increase internal diameter of tubing
	Soft or compliant tubing	Use stiffer tubing
	Loose catheter connection	Tighten catheter
	Kink in catheter	Unkink catheter
Underdamping†	System tubing too stiff	Softer tubing
	System tubing too long	Shorten tubing
	Hyperdynamic state	Increase filter on amplifier
		Introduce small bubble or contrast media
	Catheter tip in turbulent jet	Reposition catheter
Loss of signal	Bad transducer	Change transducer
	Bad cable	Change cable
	Bad amplifier	Switch amplifier
	Catheter disconnected	Check connections
	Catheter obstructed/kinked	Flush/change catheter
Pressures do not return to zero	Same as above	Readjust zero line
		Recalibrate
		Check zero at midchest

Modified from Tilkian AG, Daily EK: *Cardiovascular procedures: diagnostic techniques and therapeutic procedures*, St Louis, 1986, Mosby.
*Overdamping system is not sensitive enough and yields flat or rounded tracings.
†Underdamping system is too sensitive and produces too much ringing or overshoot of tracings.

the right show striking overshoot underdamping. Table 3-6 lists common problems and solutions for hemodynamic waveforms.

Underdamping produces a "noisy" PCW pressure (Fig. 3-54). With instillation of contrast media into the catheter, underdamping is corrected, yielding a tracing with clearly interpretable waveforms (Fig. 3-55).

Catheter Malposition. A false aortic stenosis gradient is shown in Fig. 3-56. For measurement of LV and Ao pressures, all the

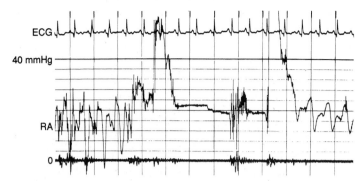

Fig. 3-54 Right atrial *(RA)* pressure tracing showing marked underdamped ringing artifact. Instillation of viscous contrast media damps the system, producing excellent waveforms.

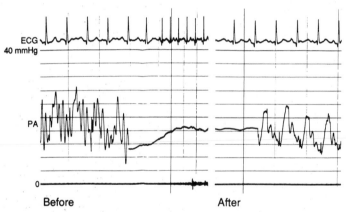

Before   After

Fig. 3-55 Pulmonary artery *(PA)* pressure after contrast medium has been instilled to produce some damping of the previously underdamped tracing, now showing excellent waveforms. See text for details.

side holes of the pigtail catheter must be under the aortic valve. In Fig. 3-56, *B*, the pigtail catheter is partly out of the left ventricle. The LV pressure is partly contaminated by Ao pressure, which reduces the LV-Ao gradient. This artifact also is evident by the abnormal diastolic waveform—a continued decline in diastolic pressure throughout the cycle. (LV diastolic pressure should be lowest in the first part of diastole with a

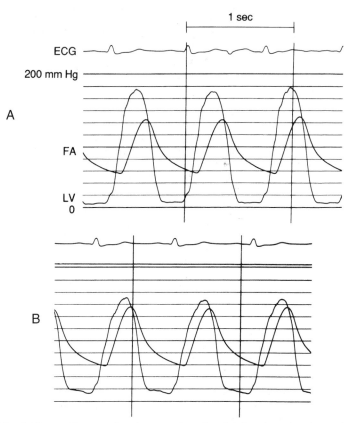

Fig. 3-56 A, True gradient is seen when the pigtail catheter is advanced fully across the aortic valve. *FA,* Femoral artery pressure; *LV,* left ventricular pressure. See text for details. **B,** Falsely low aortic stenosis gradient caused by pigtail catheter side holes in the aorta.

rising pressure across the diastolic period.) Fig. 3-56, *A,* shows the true gradient when the pigtail catheter is advanced slightly. This artifact is important and may lead to a conclusion of only minimal aortic valve disease if not appreciated (Figs. 3-57 and 3-58).

Catheter Movement. Inspiratory increases in RA mean pressure are Kussmaul's sign (Fig. 3-59) for constrictive pericarditis. However, on phasic examination of this waveform, the RA

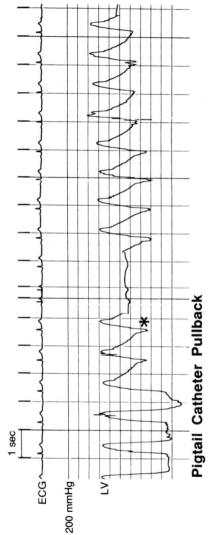

Pigtail Catheter Pullback

Fig. 3-57   A falsely wide aortic pulse pressure (*) with the use of a pigtail catheter is caused by incomplete withdrawal of all side holes outside the left ventricle (LV). On final catheter positioning (far right), aortic pressure is normal.

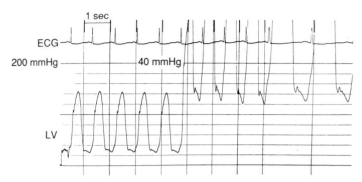

Fig. 3-58   Left ventricular *(LV)* diastolic pressure appears to fall during mid and late diastole. This pattern of impaired relaxation is seen in patients with hypertrophic cardiomyopathy. However, when one or more of the side holes of the pigtail catheter are in the aorta, the early diastolic pressure may be high and the LV filling pattern confused for abnormal relaxation.

pressure was elevated artifactually during inspiration by RV pressure as shown on the lower panel. The catheter inadvertently flipped into the right ventricle during inspiration. In a patient without clinical signs of constrictive or restrictive physiology, this artifact should be suspected; fluoroscopy or phasic pressure recording during inspiratory effort identifies this error.

Loose Connection.   Loss of pressure may be due to loose connection of tubing to catheter or tubing to manifold or to transducer (Fig. 3-60). An LV pressure that is lower than Ao pressure is due to this problem (unless Ao pressure is increased by another source, such as heterotopic transplant).

Damped Pulmonary Capillary Wedge Pressure.   The PCW pressure is satisfactory in most hemodynamic studies. In mitral valve disease, especially in patients who have had prosthetic mitral valves in place, however, the PCW pressure may not reflect LA pressure accurately. This difference is not a true artifact, but the difference in the two pressures may be clinically important. Fig. 3-61 shows simultaneous LA, PCW, and LV pressure tracings. The PCW pressure is delayed compared with directly measured LA pressure. Larger LA v waves without delay in downslope, in contrast to the PCW tracing,

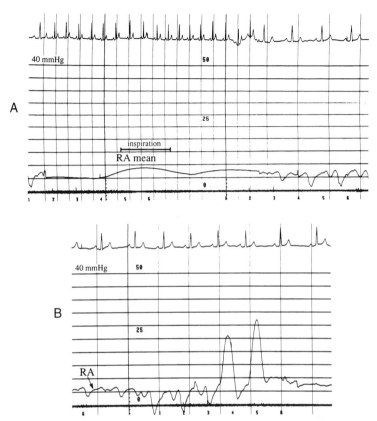

Fig. 3-59   A, Right atrial *(RA)* mean pressure increasing during inspiration. The artifact occurs when the catheter has moved accidentally into the right ventricular pressure. **B,** If not observed on phasic waveform, this artifact may be missed. See text for details.

show a major difference in the mitral valve gradient. The PCW-LV gradient may be much greater than the LA-LV gradient in some patients with mitral valve disease.

ELECTROCARDIOGRAPHY IN THE CARDIAC CATHETERIZATION LABORATORY

Basic electrocardiography may be unfamiliar to the new catheterization laboratory technician or nurse. This section reviews the fundamentals of electrocardiography as used in the cardiac catheterization laboratory for monitoring of patients.

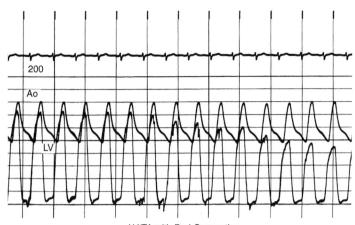

LV/FA with Bad Connection

Fig. 3-60 A loose connection on the left ventricular catheter to the pressure manifold causes loss of left ventricular pressure *(right side)*. Few real conditions produce an aortic *(Ao)* pressure higher than left ventricular *(LV)* pressure.

Cardiac Electrical System

Myocardial contraction is triggered by electrical activity. For every beat on the ECG, a corresponding pressure pulse usually occurs from myocardial contraction. The heart's electrical system has specialized tissue for the origination and transmission of electrical impulses. The normal sequence of electrical activation is shown in Figure F-1 and consists of the following: sinoatrial node → atrial tissue → AV node → bundle of His → bundle branches → Purkinje fibers → ventricular myocardium.

Electrocardiogram

The ECG is a graphic recording of electrical impulses that are generated by depolarization (contraction) and repolarization (relaxation) of the myocardium. The standard ECG includes six limb leads and six chest leads. The proper placement of electrodes for recording the 12-lead ECG is shown in Figures F-2 and F-3.

The ECG displays 12 leads that reflect different electrical views of the heart depolarization and repolarization. Typically, certain leads are associated with electrical activity from specific parts of the myocardium. Leads II, III, and aVF reflect electrical

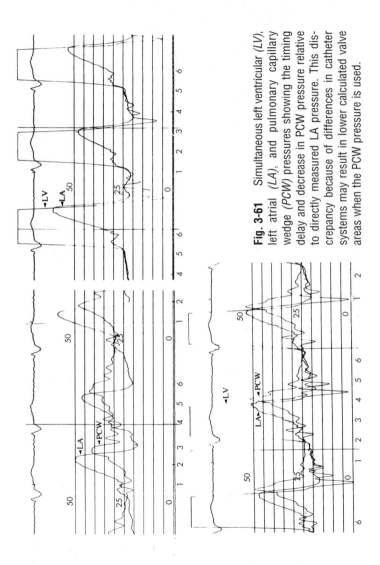

Fig. 3-61 Simultaneous left ventricular (*LV*), left atrial (*LA*), and pulmonary capillary wedge (*PCW*) pressures showing the timing delay and decrease in PCW pressure relative to directly measured LA pressure. This discrepancy because of differences in catheter systems may result in lower calculated valve areas when the PCW pressure is used.

activity in the inferior wall of the heart; leads I and aVL and chest leads V_5 and V_6, the lateral wall of the heart; chest leads V_1 and V_2, the septal region of the heart; and V_3 and V_4, the anterior wall of the heart. Electrical activity from the posterior wall of the heart is not directly recorded, and ischemia, injury, and necrosis are reflected by depolarization and repolarization abnormalities on the anterior surface of the heart (leads V_1 through V_3). In inferior-posterior myocardial infarction, ST segment, T wave changes, and Q waves are opposite in direction from an anterior myocardial infarction. During ischemia instead of ST depression, ST elevation occurs in leads V_1 to V_3. During acute injury, ST depression occurs; during infarction, a pathologic R wave rather than Q wave occurs in these leads.

COMPONENTS OF THE ELECTROCARDIOGRAM
(See Figs. F-4 and F-5)
P Wave

The sinus node normally is the pacemaker of the heart because the cells of the sinus node possess the greatest spontaneous automaticity (ability to initiate an impulse). As the electrical waves travel through the atrium, a P wave is produced on the surface ECG, which represents an electrical contraction (depolarization) of the atria. Mechanical contraction of the atria follows, which contributes to ventricular filling. From the atria the impulse travels through the AV node and through the His-Purkinje system and results in electrical activation of the ventricle. The P-R interval is the interval from the beginning of the P wave to the onset of the QRS and reflects conduction time from the sinoatrial node through the atria, AV node, and His-Purkinje system.

QRS Complex

After the P wave the next tracing on the ECG usually is the QRS complex, which represents ventricular depolarization. The electrical activation of the ventricle results in myocardial contraction (systole).

ST Segment and T Wave

The QRS is followed by the ST segment and T wave, which represent repolarization of the ventricles and correspond to myocardial relaxation (diastole). The period from the end of the QRS complex to the beginning of the T wave is called the ST segment. Depression or elevation of this segment from baseline may be produced by ischemia (depression) or acute injury (elevation).

Abnormal Rhythms

During sinus rhythm there is usually a regular rhythm with a normal sequence of activation. Premature beats are those that occur before the next expected beat. Premature ventricular contractions (PVCs) arise from abnormal electrical activity in the ventricles. The configuration of a PVC is usually a wide, bizarre QRS complex (see Fig. F-6, *A*). PVCs that occur from a single focus are referred to as *univocal* PVCs. PVCs that arise from different areas of the ventricles have different morphologies and are referred to as *multivocal* PVCs. Ventricular tachycardia is defined as the occurrence of three or more PVCs in a row (see Fig. F-6, *B*). A PVC may result in a reduced pressure pulse because of the abnormal activation sequence of the ventricle and the lack of coordination between atrial and ventricular contraction. During sustained ventricular tachycardia the blood pressure may drop dramatically. Ventricular fibrillation is the most disorganized and hemodynamically compromising arrhythmia that can occur (see Fig. F-6, *C*). During ventricular fibrillation, electrical activities are chaotic and uncoordinated so that no effective ventricular contraction takes place. As a result, no pulse or CO occurs, and clinical death results.

Typical Electrocardiographic Changes Seen in the Cardiac Catheterization Laboratory

Changes in the ST segment and T wave of the ECG may indicate a lack of blood flow to the myocardium through the coronary arteries. This lack of blood flow, referred to as ischemia, results in oxygen deprivation to the myocardium. If ischemia persists, tissue damage or death (necrosis) may occur. Dead tissue is referred to as infarcted. The ECG changes of ischemia and infarction are illustrated in Figures F-7 and F-8).

Ischemia can result in many different ECG changes. Ischemia affecting the entire depth of the myocardium (transmural) is detected as deep symmetric T wave inversion. T wave inversion can be seen in many conditions unrelated to ischemia (intracranial trauma, pulmonary embolism, myocardial contusion). Acute T wave changes occurring during anginal symptoms are specific for ischemia. Horizontal ST depression or downsloping ST segments are the hallmarks of subendocardial ischemia or infarction in many cases. Reversible depression favors ischemia, however. Nonspecific ST and T wave changes and normalization of T wave abnormalities over findings on a baseline ECG of a pain-free patient are also ECG findings consistent with ischemia.

The ECG findings of acute infarction occur in a stepwise temporal fashion. The earliest phase of infarction is associated with tall upright T waves that are referred to as hyperacute T waves. These T wave changes are usually followed shortly by the development of ST segment elevation in the region where myocardial damage is occurring. Conversely, reciprocal ST segment depression can be noted in the ECG leads recording from the opposing surface of the heart. In an acute inferior myocardial infarction, ST segment elevation is present in the inferior leads (II, III, and aVF), whereas ST segment depression is recorded simultaneously in the anterior leads (I, aVL, V, and V_2). Within hours of the onset of myocardial infarction, Q waves appear as a result of damage that occurs throughout all layers of the myocardium, resulting in a transmural or Q wave myocardial infarction. Myocardial necrosis results in an electrically silent segment that fails to contribute to the normal electrical forces of the heart during cardiac depolarization. An ECG lead recording over a segment of infarcted myocardium detects electrical forces moving away from the dead region, resulting in a negative Q wave. Infarctions that are confined to the subendocardial region do not result in Q wave formation and are termed *non–Q* wave or non-ST elevation myocardial infarctions.

Before a cardiac catheterization is performed, a baseline 12-lead ECG is obtained. The ECG can be used for comparison if symptoms develop during the procedure. During the catheterization one to three ECG leads are monitored continuously to evaluate for rhythm disturbances or ST segment and T wave changes that may indicate alterations in myocardial blood supply. During coronary angioplasty, balloon inflation temporarily interrupts the blood supply to the downstream myocardium. This interruption may result in reversible ischemia and transient ST segment and T wave changes. Persistent ST segment elevation or depression may indicate ongoing ischemia or acute myocardial injury. Other situations encountered in the cardiac catheterization laboratory that may result in ST segment or T wave changes include injection of contrast media into a coronary artery, occlusion of an artery with a diagnostic catheter (engaging the ostium of the left main or the right coronary artery), improper or incomplete deflation of an angioplasty balloon catheter, dissection of a coronary artery, coronary artery spasm, and blockage of a side branch by the balloon catheter or thrombus.

Rhythm disturbances are encountered commonly during cardiac catheterization. During right-sided heart catheterization, atrial arrhythmias and PVCs can result from catheter irritation. Catheter trauma to the right bundle branch can occur while attempting to float a catheter into the RV outflow tract. Although this situation often results in transient right bundle–branch block, complete heart block can be induced if preexisting left bundle–branch block is present. In this situation the operator must be prepared to pace the right ventricle until the right bundle recovers its function. PVCs and ventricular tachycardia can be induced by LV irritation from the ventriculography catheter or during contrast media injection. Bradycardia, sinus arrest, ventricular tachycardia, and ventricular fibrillation can result from contrast media injection of the coronary arteries (especially the right coronary artery). Catheter-induced coronary spasm can result in ventricular fibrillation caused by impaired coronary blood flow. The treatment of catheter-induced arrhythmias is straightforward; removing the catheter from the LV cavity or the coronary artery ostium is often enough to terminate the arrhythmia. Ventricular tachycardia or fibrillation that persists requires immediate resuscitation. If arrhythmias persist, the operator must investigate other underlying causes, including ischemia or electrolyte abnormalities. Prophylactic use of antiarrhythmic drugs to suppress arrhythmias during cardiac catheterization is not recommended. Coronary spasm during cardiac catheterization may be reversed by intracoronary infusion of nitroglycerin. Bradycardia and sinus node dysfunction can typically be reversed with vigorous coughing or the administration of atropine (see Chapter 4). Knowledge of and experience with the defibrillator in the cardiac catheterization laboratory are crucial (see Chapter 8).

Suggested Readings

Baim DS, Grossman W, editors: *Grossman's cardiac catheterization, angiography, and intervention,* Philadelphia, 2000, Lippincott Williams & Wilkins.

Brogan WC III, Lange RA, Hillis LD: Accuracy of various methods of measuring the transvalvular pressure gradient in aortic stenosis, *Am Heart J* 123:948-953, 1992.

Brown L, Kahl F, Link K, et al: Anatomic landmarks for use when measuring intracardiac pressure with fluid-filled catheters, *Am J Cardiol* 86:121-124, 2000.

Feldman T, Ford L, Chiu YC, Carroll J: Changes in valvular resistance, power dissipation and myocardial reserve with aortic valvuloplasty, *J Heart Valve Dis* 1:55-64, 1992.

Fuchs RM, Heuser RR, Yin FC, Brinker JA: Limitations of pulmonary wedge V waves in diagnosing mitral regurgitation, *Am J Cardiol* 49:849-854, 1982.

Gorlin R, Gorlin SG: Hydraulic formula for calculation of stenotic mitral valve, other cardiac valves, and central circulatory shunts, *Am Heart J* 41:1-29, 1951.

Hakki AH, Iskandrian AS, Bemis CE, et al: A simplified valve formula for the calculation of stenotic cardiac valve areas, *Circulation* 63:1050-1055, 1981.

Haskell RJ, French WJ: Accuracy of left atrial and pulmonary artery wedge pressure in pure mitral regurgitation in predicting left ventricular end-diastolic pressure, *Am J Cardiol* 61:136-141, 1988.

Hillis LD, Firth BG, Winniford MD: Analysis of factors affecting the variability of Fick versus indicator dilution measurements of cardiac output, *Am J Cardiol* 56:764-768, 1985.

Hillis LD, Winniford MD: The simplified formula for the calculation of aortic valve area: potential inaccuracies in patients with bradycardia or tachycardia, *Cathet Cardiovasc Diagn* 13:301-303, 1987.

Kern MJ: *Hemodynamic rounds series II,* New York, 1998, Wiley Liss.

Lange RA, Moore EM Jr, Cigarroa RG, Hillis LD: Use of pulmonary capillary wedge pressure to assess severity of mitral stenosis: is true left atrial pressure needed in this condition? *J Am Coll Cardiol* 13:825-829, 1989.

Mueller H, Chatterjee K, Davis K, et al: Present use of bedside right heart catheterization in patients with cardiac disease, *J Am Coll Cardiol* 32:840-864, 1998.

Schoenfeld MH, Palacios IF, Hutter AM Jr, et al: Underestimation of prosthetic mitral valve areas: role of transseptal catheterization in avoiding unnecessary repeat mitral valve surgery, *J Am Coll Cardiol* 5:1387-1392, 1985.

4

Angiographic Data

Saad Bitar and Morton J. Kern

Angiograms are the most important product of cardiac catheterization and often the most important tests that patients with cardiac disease can undergo. The risks of angiography are minimal, but operators must take special care in the performance of coronary and ventricular angiography. The expert angiographer must be concerned, competent, and experienced.

Optimal angiographic data collection is a process of linked steps. Failure of any link breaks the chain and may cause loss of all or part of the data. The chain begins with the nurse's positioning the patient on the table, then involves performance of the angiography, the recording and storing of the digital image, and finally the display of the image for review. Box 4-1 summarizes the major causes of poor angiograms.

The radiographic images are the visual representation of the vascular network connected to internal structures (organs) and, at times, predict the function of the circulation. Experienced operators obtain good-quality images without increasing the ordinary procedural radiation exposure to either the patient or the catheterization laboratory personnel.

CARDIAC ANGIOGRAPHY

CORONARY ARTERIOGRAPHY

The goal of coronary angiography is to visualize the coronary arteries, branches, collaterals, and anomalies with enough detail to make a precise diagnosis of and plan the treatment strategy for coronary artery disease. With percutaneous coronary interventions (PCI) (e.g., stents), the coronary angiographer is expected to document not only the presence of disease, but also its precise location relative to major and

217

Box 4-1

Causes for Poor Angiograms

Patient Factors
Size
Movement
Hardware (pacemaker, Harrison rods, multiple surgery with clips, silicone prosthesis)
Anatomic conditions (scoliosis, scarred lungs, large heart [fluid])

Angiographer Factors
Poor catheter seating (wrong catheter shape, size, anomalous origin, subselective cannulation)
Poor contrast opacification (weak injection, volume too small, diluted contrast material)

Equipment Factors
X-ray generator problems (high heat, quantum mottle, too high kilovoltage, too short pulse width, too long pulse width)
X-ray tube problems (anode pitting, wrong focal spot, beam geometry, proximity to image intensifier, poor collimation)

Image intensifier problems
Optical chain to TV (mirror malalignment, f-stop aperture control, overframing, focal length)
Cineangiographic camera (film gate malfunction, film travel misalignment, restricted travel)
Cineangiographic film or processing (poor sensitivity, latitude, poor exposure, poor development)
Cineangiographic projector (poor optical components)
Digital imaging program malfunction

---

minor side branches, thrombi, and areas of calcification in detail. For PCI, visualization of vessel bifurcations, origin of side branches, the portion of the vessel proximal to a significant lesion, and specific lesion characteristics (e.g., length, eccentricity, and calcium) is crucial. In the case of a total vessel occlusion, the distal vessel should be visualized as clearly as possible by the operator's injecting the coronary arteries that supply collaterals with a contrast medium, and taking cineangiograms with panning long enough to visualize late collateral vessel filling and to determine the length of the occluded segment because that helps determine revascularization strategy.

The routine coronary angiographic views should include visualization of the origin and course of the major vessels and their branches in at least two different planes. Coronary anatomy varies widely, and appropriately modified views must be individualized.

Techniques

Hand Injections for Coronary Arteriography. Contrast medium, a viscous, iodinated solution used to opacify the coronary arteries, can be injected by hand through a multivalve manifold. The tip of the syringe is kept pointed down (handle raised up) so that any small bubbles float up and are not injected into the circulatory system (Fig. 4-1). Flow rates are usually 2 to 4 ml/sec with volumes of 2 to 6 ml in the right coronary artery (RCA) and 7 to 10 ml in the left coronary artery (LCA). Hand injection of the coronary arteries offers advantages in ease of administration of intracoronary drugs and varying degrees of opacification for either severely diseased or high-flow coronary arteries. The use of disposable manifolds, syringes, and tubing is cost effective and safe.

Power Injections for Coronary Arteriography. Power injection of the coronary arteries has been used in thousands of cases in many laboratories and is as safe as hand injection. A power injector at a fixed setting might require several injections to find the optimal contrast delivery flow rate. Power injectors now incorporate hand controls, permitting precise operator touch–sensitive variable volume injectors (Acist; Bracco Diagnostics), and a computer touch screen for precise contrast delivery settings (Fig. 4-2). Typical settings for power injections are as follows:

RCA: 6 ml at 3 ml/sec; maximal psi 450
LCA: 10 ml at 4 ml/sec; maximal psi 450

Filming Frame Rates. The filming frame rates are usually 30 frames/sec. If the heart rate is greater than 95 beats/min, the rate of 60 frames/sec is used. Digital imaging uses similar frame rates, but 15 frames/sec may be standard in some laboratories.

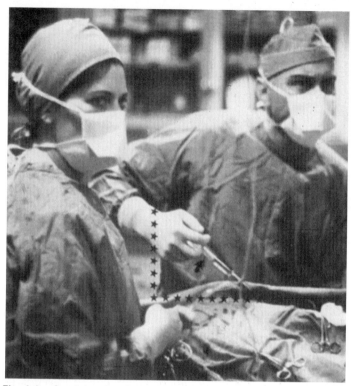

Fig. 4-1 Gensini performing coronary arteriography. Note the raised angle (30 degrees) of the injection syringe to keep out air bubbles. (From Gensini GG: *Coronary arteriography*, Mount Kisco, N.Y., 1975, Futura.)

Panning Techniques. Most laboratories use x-ray image screen sizes of 7 inches or less in diameter, which precludes having the entire coronary artery course visualized without panning over the heart to include late filling portions of the arterial segments. In addition, in most views some degree of panning is necessary to identify regions that are not seen from the initial setup position. Some branches may unexpectedly appear later from collateral filling or other unusual anatomic sources.

Angiographic View Setup Keys. One key to accurate, optimal coronary cineangiography, obtaining the most information for the least amount of movement, is the initial setup of the

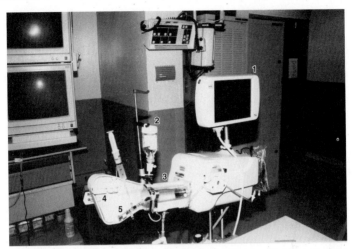

Fig. 4-2   Power injector (Bracco Diagnostics, Princeton N.J.). *1*, Operator touch screen to select injection of coronary arteries or ventriculography; *2*, large contrast bottle permits multiple patient studies because only the hand control and patient injection tubing are sterile and changed for each patient; *3*, injection syringe with piston; *4*, patient injection tubing; *5*, several valves and bubble detectors used to prevent contamination and inadvertent air injection.

catheter on the fluoroscope. Figure 4-3 shows the catheter–left main artery setup keys for left anterior oblique (LAO) views in the straight, cranial, and caudally angled projections. When the patient is positioned correctly and the setup key followed, only minimal panning is necessary to obtain the information. In the LAO view the operator pans down the left anterior descending (LAD) artery then rightward to identify collaterals going to the right coronary artery (RCA) or, if the circumflex artery is occluded, leftward to include collaterals going to the distal circumflex artery. For the RCA in the LAO position the operator pans downward and to the left toward the LAD artery to include late filling collaterals from the right to the LAD artery. These motions are diagrammed in Figure 4-3.

In the right anterior oblique (RAO) projections for the LCA and RCA, the operator pans downward to the apex to identify late filling, left-to-left or right-to-left collaterals. The initial setup keys for catheter tip position on the fluoroscope are summarized in Box 4-2 help the operator include all crucial information for coronary arteriography.

Imaging Views

To obtain optimal information from coronary cineangiography, the operator must use various views unveiling overlapped vessel segments. These views or projections highlight specific and distinct segments of the coronary anatomy and permit discrete visualization of underlying pathologic conditions. Understanding of the usefulness of various radiographic views (and nomenclature) is essential.

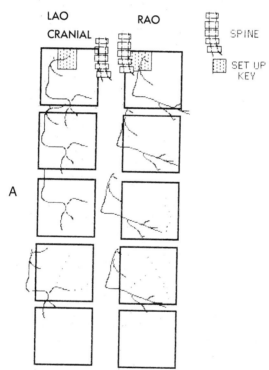

Fig. 4-3   Setup keys for panning during coronary arteriography. **A,** Right coronary artery *(RCA).* **B,** Left coronary artery *(LCA).* C, Lateral views. *LAO,* Left anterior oblique view; *RAO,* right anterior oblique view.   *Continued*

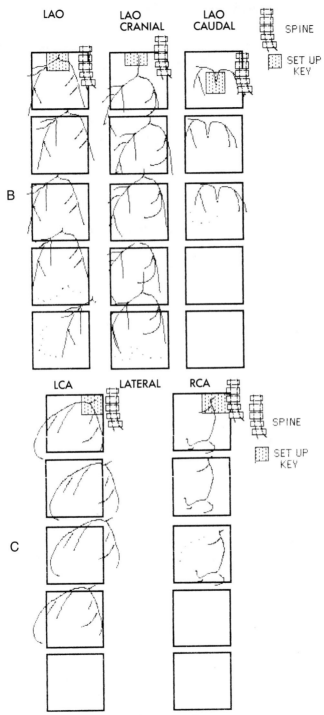

Fig. 4-3, cont'd For legend see opposite page.

Box 4-2

Setup Key Locations for Angiographic Views

Artery	View	Angulation	Setup Region on Screen* (No.)	Comment
LAD	LAO	Cranial	2	Set up on screen
	LAO	Caudal	5	Top, mid line
	RAO	Cranial	1	Top, left upper coronary
	RAO	Caudal	4	Middle, left side
RCA	LAO	Cranial/caudal	1, 2	Left upper coronary
	RAO	Cranial/caudal	1, 4	Left upper coronary
LAD or RCA	AP	Cranial	2	

AP, Anteroposterior; *LAD,* left anterior descending; *LAO,* left anterior oblique; *RAO,* right anterior oblique; *RCA,* right coronary artery.
*Fluroscreen grid.

1	2	3
4	5	6
7	8	9

Nomenclature for Angiographic Views. For all catheterization laboratories the x-ray source is *under* the table, and the image intensifier is directly above the patient (Fig. 4-4, Table 4-1, and Box 4-3). The source and image intensifier are moving in opposite directions in an imaginary circle around the patient positioned in the center. The body surface of the patient that faces the observer determines the specific view. This relationship holds true whether the patient is supine, standing, or rotated (Fig. 4-4).

Anteroposterior (AP) position. The image intensifier is directly over the patient with the beam traveling perpendicularly back to front (i.e., from posterior to anterior) to the patient lying flat on the x-ray table.

RAO position. The image intensifier is on the right side of the patient. *A,* anterior; *O,* oblique.

LAO position. The image intensifier is on the left side of the patient.

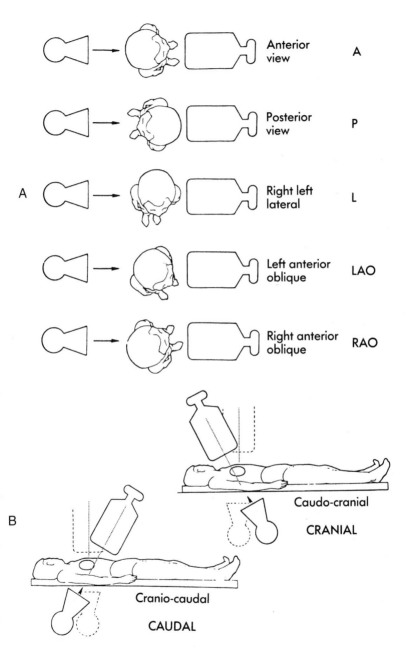

Fig. 4-4   For legend see page 226.   *Continued*

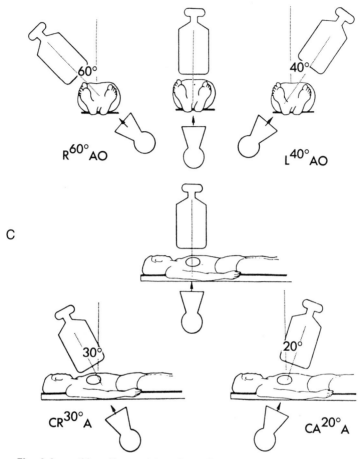

C

Fig. 4-4, cont'd Nomenclature for radiographic projections. The small black arrowheads show the direction of the x-ray beam. **A,** Anterior, posterior, lateral, and oblique. **B,** If the intensifier is tilted toward the feet of the patient, a caudal view is produced. If the intensifier is tilted toward the head of the patient, a cranial view is produced. **C,** Cranial *(CR)* and caudal *(CA)* oblique views. (Redrawn from Paulin S: *Cathet Cardiovasc Diagn* 7:341-344, 1981.)

Note: Think of the oblique view as turning the left or right shoulder forward (anterior) to the camera (image intensifier).

Cranial/caudal position. This nomenclature refers to image intensifier angles in relation to the patient's long axis.

Cranial. The image intensifier is tilted toward the *head* of the patient.

Table 4-1

Recommended "Key" Angiographic Views for Specific Coronary Artery Segments

Coronary Segment	Origin and Bifurcation	Course Through Body
Left main	AP	AP
	LAO cranial	LAO cranial
	LAO caudal*	
Proximal LAD	LAO cranial	LAO cranial
	RAO caudal	RAO caudal
Mid LAD	LAO cranial	
	RAO cranial	
	Lateral	
Distal LAD	AP	
	RAO cranial	
	Lateral	
Diagonal	LAO cranial	RAO cranial, caudal, or straight
Proximal circumflex	RAO cranial	
	RAO caudal	LAO caudal
	LAO caudal	
Intermediate	RAO caudal	RAO caudal
	LAO caudal	Lateral
Obtuse marginal	RAO caudal	RAO caudal
	LAO caudal	
	RAO cranial (distal marginals)	
Proximal RCA	LAO	
	Lateral	
Mid RCA	LAO	LAO
	Lateral	Lateral
	RAO	RAO
Distal RCA	LAO cranial	LAO cranial
	Lateral	Lateral
PDA	LAO cranial	RAO
Posterolateral	LAO cranial	RAO
	RAO cranial	RAO cranial

AP, Anteroposterior; *LAD,* left anterior descending artery; *LAO,* left anterior oblique; *PDA,* posterior descending artery (from RCA); *RAO,* right anterior oblique; *RCA,* right coronary artery.
*Horizontal hearts.

Box 4-3

Routine Coronary Angiographic Views

Left Coronary Artery

Straight AP or 5 degrees to 10 degrees RAO
30 degrees to 45 degrees LAO and 20 degrees to 30 degrees cranial
30 degrees to 40 degrees RAO and 20 degrees to 30 degrees caudal
5 degrees to 30 degrees RAO and 20 degrees to 45 degrees cranial
50 degrees to 60 degrees LAO and 10 degrees to 20 degrees caudal (spider view)
Lateral (optional)

For Concentration on Vessel Segment

Left main
LAD-circumflex bifurcation
circumflex + marginal branches
LAD + diagonals
LAD-circumflex bifurcation, circumflex, marginal branches
Bypass conduits to LAD

Right Coronary Artery

30 degrees to 45 degrees LAO and 15 degrees to 20 degrees cranial
30 degrees to 45 degrees RAO
Lateral (optional)

For Concentration on Vessel Segment

Proximal, mid, PDA
Proximal, mid, PDA

AP, Anteroposterior; *LAD,* left anterior descending artery; *LAO,* left anterior oblique; *PDA,* posterior descending artery (from right coronary artery); *RAO,* right anterior oblique.

Note: The lateral view is a useful addition to these views for both coronary arteries. In addition, the four most common views for the left coronary artery when performed LAO cranial, RAO caudal, RAO cranial, and LAO caudal form a box around the patient. Look first at the LAD (cranial views) and then at the circumflex (caudal views). This box should be on every study with rare exceptions.

Caudal. The image intensifier is tilted toward the *feet* of the patient.

Cranial and caudal views are used to "open" overlapped coronary segments that are *foreshortened* or obscured in regular views.

Note: Cranial views are best for the <u>LAD</u> artery; caudal views are best for the <u>circumflex</u> arteries.

The rationale for these routine angiographic views is as follows.

Left Coronary Artery.

1. The AP caudal or shallow RAO view displays the left main coronary artery (LMCA) in its entire perpendicular length (Figs. 4-5 to 4-7). In this view the proximal segments of the LAD and left circumflex arteries are displayed, but the branches are overlapped. After the left main segment, slight RAO or LAO angulation may be necessary to clear the density of the vertebrae and the catheter shaft in the thoracic descending aorta from covering the artery.

2. The LAO-cranial view also shows the LMCA (slightly foreshortened), LAD, and its diagonal branches. Septal (coursing to the left) and diagonal branches (to the right) are separated clearly. The circumflex artery and marginal branches are foreshortened and overlapped, although the posterolateral and posterior descending branches of left-dominant circulation are displayed clearly. Deep inspiration, which moves the density of the diaphragm down and out of the field, is helpful. The LAO angle (>30 degrees) should be set so that the LAD artery course is parallel to the spine and stays in the "lucent wedge" bordered by the spine on the medial edge and the curve of the diaphragm. Cranial angulation tilts the LMCA down and permits a view of the LAD/circumflex bifurcation. LAO-cranial angulation that is too steep or inspiration that is too shallow produces considerable overlapping with the diaphragm and liver, degrading the image.

3. The RAO-caudal view shows the LMCA bifurcation, perpendicular to that of the LAO-cranial angle. The

Text continued on page 239

A-P PROJECTION

The A-P projection allows a good visualization of the left main coronary artery.

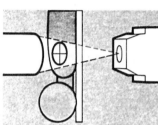

1. Left main coronary
2. Proximal part of LAD
3. Mid part of LAD
4. Distal part of LAD
5. Proximal circumflex artery
6. Distal circumflex artery
7. Left obtuse marginal artery
8. First diagonal artery
9. First septal perforating artery
10. Septal arteries
11. Auricular branch of the circumflex artery
12. Obtuse marginal artery n° 2.

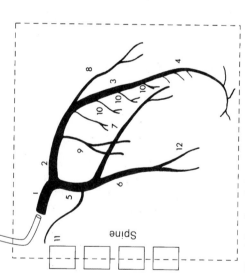

Fig. 4-5 A to E, Left coronary artery. **F to I,** Right coronary artery. *AP,* Anteroposterior; *LAD,* left anterior descending artery; *LAO,* left anterior oblique; *RAO,* right anterior oblique. (From Bertrand ME, editor: *Coronary arteriography,* Lille, France, 1979, French Society of Cardiology.)

Continued

RIGHT ANTERIOR OBLIQUE PROJECTION AT 30° (R.A.O. 30°)

The R.A.O. projection at 30° permits the entire circumflex system to be studied, as well as the first centimeters of the anterior interventricular artery.

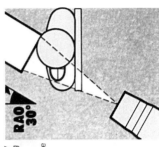

Continued

1. Left main coronary
2. Proximal part of LAD
3. Mid. part of LAD
4. Distal part of LAD
5. Proximal circumflex artery
6. Distal circumflex artery
7. Obtuse marginal artery
8. First diagonal artery
9. Second diagonal artery
10. First septal perforating artery
11. Septal arteries
12. Auricular branch of the circumflex artery

Fig. 4-5, cont'd   B, Left coronary artery.

LEFT ANTERIOR OBLIQUE PROJECTION AT 55/60° (L.A.O. 55/60°)

The LAO projection at 55°/60° mainly studies the diagonal arteries and the mid and distal parts of the LAD. On the other hand, the circumflex system is not well defined.

1. Left main coronary
2. Proximal part of LAD
3. Middle part of LAD
4. Distal part of LAD
5. Proximal circumflex artery
6. Distal circumflex artery
7. Left obtuse marginal artery
8. First diagonal artery
9. Second diagonal artery
10. First septal perforating artery
11 and 12. Septal arteries

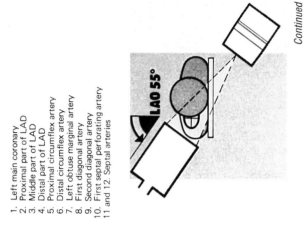

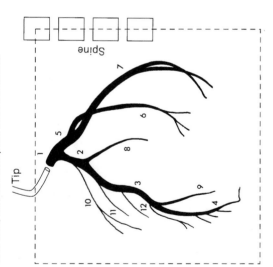

C

Continued

LEFT ANTERIOR OBLIQUE PROJECTION AT 55/60° COMBINED WITH A CRANIAL ANGULATION OF 20°

The cranial angulation of 20° combined with the LAO projection at 55°/60° is especially useful to study the left main coronary artery.

1. Left main coronary artery
2. Middle part of the LAD
3. Proximal circumflex artery
4. Obtuse marginal artery
5. First diagonal artery
6. Septal perforating artery

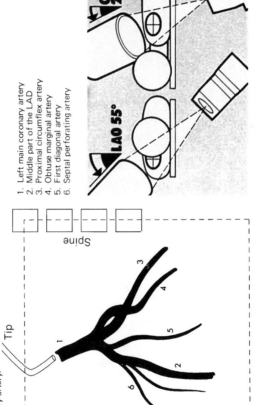

Fig. 4-5, cont'd   C and **D,** Left coronary artery.

Continued

LEFT LATERAL PROJECTION

The left lateral projection allows the study of the different segments of the anterior interventricular artery, the first diagonal artery, and the left marginal artery.

1. Left main coronary artery
2. Proximal part of LAD
3. Middle part of LAD
4. Distal part of LAD
5. Proximal circumflex artery
6. Distal circumflex artery
7. Obtuse marginal artery
8. First diagonal artery
9. Second diagonal artery
10. Septal arteries
11. Obtuse marginal artery no 2.

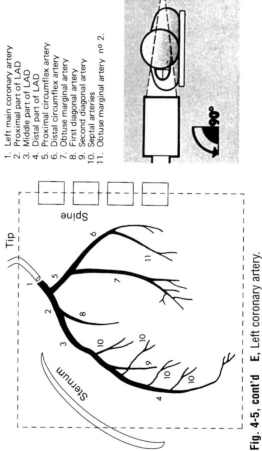

Fig. 4-5, cont'd **E,** Left coronary artery.

Continued

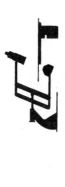

LEFT ANTERIOR OBLIQUE PROJECTION AT 45° COMBINED WITH A CAUDAL ANGULATION OF 15°

This projection allows the whole study of the R.C.A. and, especially, clearly defines the region of the crux of the heart.

1. First (horizontal) segment of the right coronary artery
2. Second (vertical) segment of the right coronary artery
3. Third (horizontal) segment of the right coronary artery
4. Posterior interventricular

5. Retroventricular artery
6. Conus branch
7. Artery of the sinus node
8. Right ventricular artery
9. Right marginal artery
10. Artery of the A-V node
11. Diaphragmatic artery

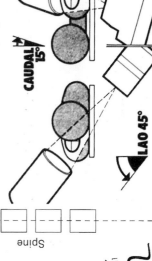

Continued

Fig. 4-5, cont'd   F, Right coronary artery.

RIGHT ANTERIOR OBLIQUE PROJECTION AT 45°

The RAO projection at 45° permits the survey of the second (vertical) segment of the right coronary artery, the posterior interventricular artery and the collateral branches (right ventricular and right marginal arteries). On the other hand, the first segment and the third segment as well as the retroventricular artery are not clearly defined. This projection also allows the visualization of the retrograde reopacification of the distal part of LAD proximally occluded.

1. First (horizontal) segment of the right coronary artery
2. Second (vertical) segment of the right coronary artery
3. Third (horizontal) segment of the right coronary artery
4. Posterior descending artery
5. Retroventricular artery
6. Conus branch
7. Artery of the sinus node
8. Right ventricular artery
9. Right marginal artery
10. Artery of the A-V node
11. Inferior septal arteries

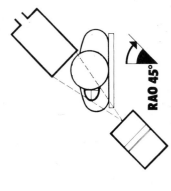

RAO 45°

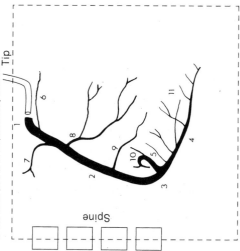

Spine

Tip

G

Continued

RIGHT ANTERIOR OBLIQUE PROJECTION AT 120° COMBINED WITH A CRANIAL ANGULATION OF 10°

This projection is very useful for studying the third horizontal segment, the crux of the heart, and the retroventricular artery and its branches.

1. First (horizontal) segment of the right coronary artery
2. Second (vertical) segment of the right coronary artery
3. Third (horizontal) segment of the right coronary artery
4. Posterior interventricular artery
5. Retroventricular artery
6. Diaphragmatic artery

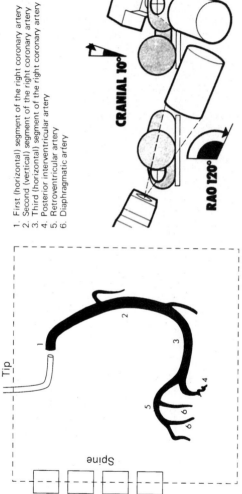

Fig. 4-5, cont'd   G and **H,** Right coronary artery.

Continued

LEFT LATERAL PROJECTION

This projection permits the study of the second (vertical) segment of the right coronary artery and the collateral branches (conus branch, right ventricular artery, right marginal artery).

1. First (horizontal) segment of the right coronary artery
2. Second (vertical) segment of the right coronary artery
3. Third (horizontal) segment of the right coronary artery
4. Posterior interventricular artery
5. Retroventricular artery
6. Conus branch
7. Artery of the sinus node
8. Right ventricular artery
9. Right marginal artery
10. Artery of the A-V node
11. Diaphragmatic artery
12. Inferior septal arteries

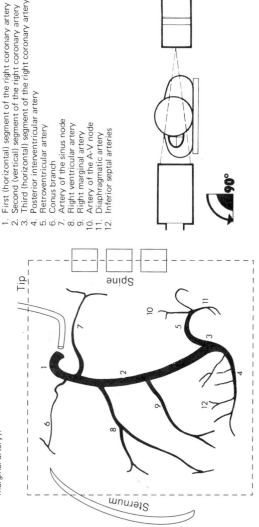

Fig. 4-5, cont'd I, Right coronary artery.

origin and course of the circumflex/obtuse marginal branches, ramus intermedius branch, and proximal LAD segment are seen clearly. This view is one of the two best for visualization of the circumflex artery. The LAD artery beyond the proximal segment is obscured by overlapped diagonals; however, the apical segment of the LAD artery is displayed clearly.

4. The RAO-cranial view is used to see the origins of the diagonals along the mid and distal LAD artery. Diagonal branch bifurcations are well visualized. The diagonal branches are projected upward. The proximal LAD and

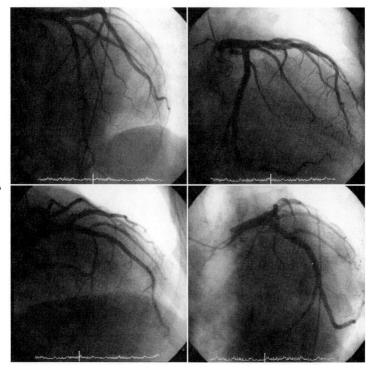

Fig. 4-6   A, Angiography of left coronary artery. *Top left,* Left anterior oblique cranial; *top right,* right anterior oblique (RAO) caudal; *bottom left,* RAO cranial; note origin of diagonal branches; *bottom right,* left anterior descending (LAO) caudal. Note origin of circumflex artery *(circumflex)* from left main coronary artery *(LM).*   *Continued*

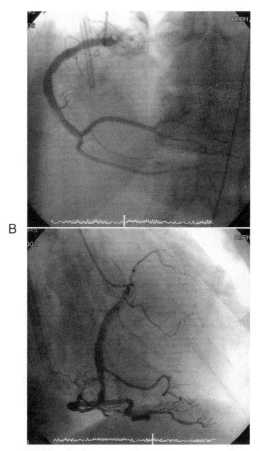

Fig. 4-6, cont'd B, Angiography of right coronary artery. *Top,* LAO, cranial; *bottom,* RAO.

circumflex usually are overlapped. Marginal branches may overlap, and the circumflex artery is foreshortened, but posterolateral branches are well visualized.

5. The LAO-caudal view ("spider" view) shows the LMCA (foreshortened) and bifurcation of the LMCA into the circumflex and LAD artery. Proximal and mid portions of the circumflex artery are usually seen clearly with the origins of obtuse marginal branches. Poor image quality may be caused by overlapping of the diaphragm and spine. Good separation of the vessel is more difficult in

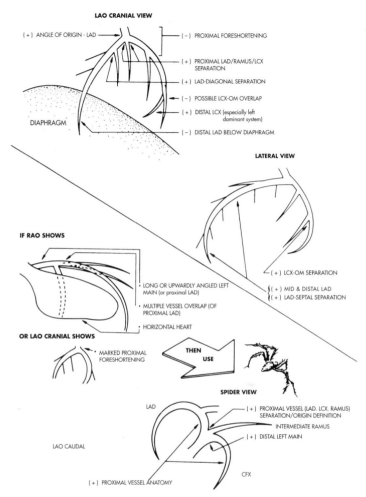

Fig. 4-7   Diagrammatic views of left coronary arteries showing special positioning to observe branch segments. *LAD,* Left anterior descending coronary artery; *LCX-OM,* left circumflex–obtuse marginal branch; *LAO,* left anterior oblique; *RAO,* right anterior oblique. See text for details. (From Boucher RA, et al: *Cathet Cardiovasc Diagn* 14:269-285, 1988.)

Continued

ADDENDUM:

EFFECTS OF ANGULATION ON DEFINING CORONARY ANATOMY

[(+) denotes aspect of vessel definition advantaged by selected view;
(–) denotes disadvantage of view]

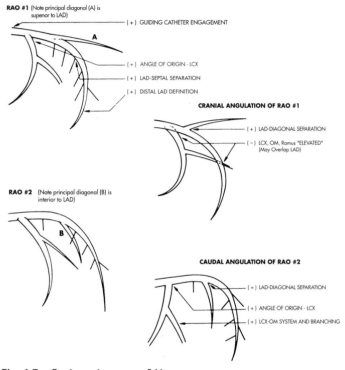

RAO #1 (Note principal diagonal (A) is
superior to LAD)

(+) GUIDING CATHETER ENGAGEMENT

(+) ANGLE OF ORIGIN - LCX

(+) LAD-SEPTAL SEPARATION

(+) DISTAL LAD DEFINITION

CRANIAL ANGULATION OF RAO #1

(+) LAD-DIAGONAL SEPARATION

(–) LCX, OM, Ramus "ELEVATED"
(May Overlap LAD)

RAO #2 (Note principal diagonal (B) is
interior to LAD)

CAUDAL ANGULATION OF RAO #2

(+) LAD-DIAGONAL SEPARATION

(+) ANGLE OF ORIGIN - LCX

(+) LCX-OM SYSTEM AND BRANCHING

Fig. 4-7 For legend see page 241.

vertically displaced hearts, such as in patients with chronic obstructive pulmonary disease, and more angulation is required to obtain an unobstructed view. The LAD artery is considerably foreshortened in this view.

6. A *lateral* view (image intensifier rotated 90 degrees, parallel with the floor) is the best view to show the mid and distal LAD artery. The LAD and circumflex arteries are well separated. Diagonals are usually overlapped. The (ramus) intermedius branch course is well

visualized. This view best shows insertions of bypass grafts into the mid LAD artery. Occasionally, slight caudal or cranial angulation is needed to visualize the segment of interest.

Right Coronary Artery.

1. The LAO-cranial view shows the origin of the RCA, the entire length of the mid RCA, and the posterior descending artery (PDA) bifurcation (crux) (see Figs. 4-5 to 4-7). Cranial angulation tilts the PDA down to see vessel contour and to reduce foreshortening. Deep inspiration is necessary to clear the diaphragm. The PDA and posterolateral branches are slightly foreshortened in this view.

2. The RAO view (no cranial or caudal angulation is generally needed) shows the mid RCA and the length of the PDA and posterolateral branches. Septal branches coursing upward from the PDA, supplying occluded LAD artery via collaterals, may be clearly identified. The posterolateral branches are overlapped and may need the addition of the cranial view.

3. The AP cranial view shows the origin of the RCA. The mid segment is foreshortened. This is the best view, however, to display the posterior descending and posterolateral branches of a dominant RCA system and the size of a collateralized LAD artery.

4. The lateral view also shows the RCA origin (especially in patients with more anteriorly oriented orifices) and mid RCA. The PDA and posterolateral branches are foreshortened.

Technical note: Because of individual variations in anatomy, small (1- to 2-ml) test injections during patient inspiration helps the operator obtain the appropriate oblique and axial (cranial-caudal) angulations and set up for panning.

Saphenous Vein Graft Angiographic Views. Coronary artery saphenous vein grafts are visualized in at least two views (LAO and RAO). It is important to show the aortic anastomosis, the body of the graft, and the distal anastomosis. The distal runoff and continued flow or collateral channels are also crucial. The graft-vessel anastomosis is seen best in the view that depicts the native vessel best. The graft views can be summarized as follows:

1. *RCA graft*—LAO cranial, RAO, and AP cranial
2. *LAD graft* (or internal mammary artery)—lateral, RAO cranial, LAO cranial, and AP (the lateral view is especially useful to visualize the anastomosis to the LAD)
3. *Circumflex (and obtuse marginal branches) grafts*—LAO caudal and RAO caudal
4. *Diagonal graft*—LAO cranial and RAO cranial

General strategy: The operator should perform the standard views while assessing the vessel key views for specific coronary artery segments (see Table 4-1) to determine the need for contingency views or an alteration or addition of special views.

Assessment of Coronary Stenoses.

Assessment of the Degree of Narrowing. The evaluation of the degree of a stenosis relates to the percentage reduction in the diameter of the vessel. This percentage is calculated in the projection where the greatest narrowing can be observed. Exact evaluation is almost impossible, and the lesions are roughly classified. The stenotic segment lumen is compared with a nearby lumen that does not appear to be obstructed but that may have diffuse atherosclerotic disease. The nearby lumen appears angiographically normal but may still be diseased (Figs. 4-8 and 4-9). This explains why postmortem examinations describe much more plaque than is seen on angiography. The percent diameter is estimated from the angiographically normal adjacent segment. Proximal segments may be larger than distal segments, which explains the large disparity between several observer estimates of stenosis severity. *Area stenosis* is greater than *diameter stenosis* and assumes the lumen is circular, whereas the lumen is usually eccentric. Six categories of vessel assessment can be distinguished in this way:

0	Normal coronary artery
1	Irregularities of the vessel
2	Narrowing of less than 50%
3	Stenosis between 50% and 75%
4	Stenosis between 75% and 95%
5	Total occlusion

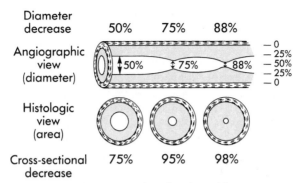

Fig. 4-8 Diagrammatic representation of angiographic versus postmortem analysis of coronary artery stenosis. (From Roberts WC: *Cardiovasc Med* 2:29-38, 1977.)

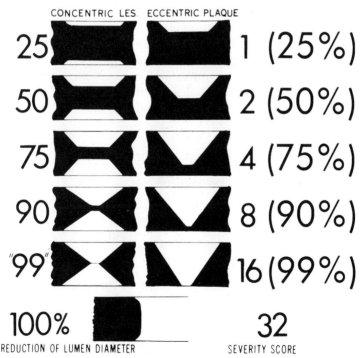

Fig. 4-9 Angiographic appearance of concentric and eccentric plaques with 25%, 50%, 75%, 90%, and 99% obstruction and complete occlusion (100%). *Les,* Lesion. (From Gensini GG: *Coronary arteriography,* Mount Kisco, N.Y., 1975, Futura.)

For nonquantitative reports the length of a stenosis is simply mentioned (e.g., LAD proximal segment stenosis diameter 25%, long or short). Other features of the coronary lesion may not be appreciated by angiography and require intravascular ultrasound imaging (Fig. 4-10).

Technical note: There is a ± 20% variation between readings of two or more experienced angiographers, especially for lesions 40% to 70% narrowed. Stenosis anatomy should not be confused with abnormal physiology (flow) and ischemia.

Classification of Distal Angiographic Contrast Runoff. The distal runoff is classified into four stages (also known as TIMI grade):

1. Normal distal runoff (TIMI 3)
2. Good distal runoff (TIMI 2)
3. Poor distal runoff (TIMI 1)
4. Absence of distal runoff (TIMI 0)

Contrast runoff is performed quantitatively by using cine frame counts from the first frame of the filled catheter tip to the frame in which contrast material is seen filling a predetermined distal arterial endpoint. Typically, a normal contrast frame count reflecting normal flow is 24 ± 10 frames.

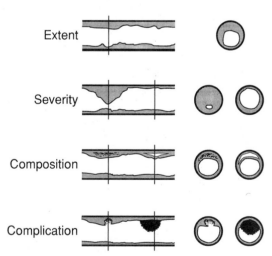

Fig. 4-10 Angiographic features that may not be appreciated on cine imaging and need intravascular ultrasound imaging.

Collateral Circulation. The reopacification of a totally or subtotally (99%) occluded vessel from antegrade or retrograde filling is defined as collateral filling. The collateral circulation is graded angiographically as follows:

Grade	Collateral Appearance
0	No collateral circulation
1	Very weak (ghostlike) reopacification
2	Reopacified segment, less dense than the feeding vessel and filling slowly
3	Reopacified segment as dense as the feeding vessel and filling rapidly

It is useful but difficult to establish the size of the recipient vessel exactly. The operator determines whether the collateral circulation is ipsilateral (e.g., same-side filling, proximal RCA to distal RCA collateral supply) or contralateral (e.g., opposite-side filling, LAD artery to distal RCA collateral supply). The operator identifies exactly which region is affected by collateral supply and stenoses in the artery feeding the collateral artery. The operator notes whether the opacification is forward (anterograde) or backward (retrograde). This evaluation is important for making decisions about which vessels might be protected or lost during coronary angioplasty.

PROBLEMS AND SOLUTIONS IN THE INTERPRETATION OF CORONARY ANGIOGRAMS
Vessel Overlap

Because coronary angioplasty requires a clear view of the target vessel that may be overlapped, multiple angles are required to reveal locations of lesions not previously considered important. Steeper angles or even AP cranial or caudal views are often helpful. For lesions whose significance remains uncertain, intravascular ultrasound imaging or physiologic measurements (fractional flow reserve, coronary flow reserve) should be considered.

Poor Artery Opacification

Poor contrast opacification of the vessel may lead to a false impression of an angiographically significant lesion or lucency that could be considered a clot. Inadequate mixing of contrast material and blood could be seen as a luminal irregularity. A satisfactory bolus injection of contrast material must be delivered if adequate opacification is to be achieved and the angiogram interpreted correctly. Contrast delivery can be enhanced by use of a larger catheter, injection during Valsalva maneuver phase III, or use of a power injector.

Total Coronary Occlusion

Total occlusion of a vessel may be erroneously suspected if the catheter injection site is subselective or if an anomalous origin or course of a vessel is not recognized. A short LMCA may lead to selective opacification of only the LAD artery and a presumption of a circumflex occlusion or anomalous origin of the circumflex artery. To address this case, an aortic cusp "flush" injection of contrast material may reveal the second vessel. Subselective injections into each vessel separately may be necessary if the LMCA is too short to opacify both vessels simultaneously. Similarly, subselective injection into a large RCA conus branch may not adequately visualize the main RCA. When target vessels are not well seen, the operator should consider anomalous origins of the coronary artery and review the aortogram and left ventriculography (see section on anomalous coronary arteries later in the chapter).

Coronary Spasm

Spontaneous or catheter-induced coronary artery spasm may appear as a fixed stenotic lesion. Catheter spasm has been observed in right and left coronary arteries (and the LMCA) and must be considered and excluded (by use of intracoronary nitroglycerin) before the narrowing is considered an organic lesion. Nitroglycerin reverses coronary spasm and should be administered when a question of catheter-induced spasm exists. Catheter-induced spasm may occur not only at the tip of the catheter touching the artery, but also more distally. Repositioning of the catheter and administration of nitroglycerin (100 to 200 µg through the catheter) clarify if the presumed lesion is structural or spastic. A change to a smaller diameter (4 F or 5 F) catheter or catheters that do not seat deeply may help.

Special Problems

Left Main Coronary Artery Stenosis. A commonly encountered and potentially critical problem is safe coronary angiography of patients who have LMCA stenosis. The approach to the patient with LMCA stenosis is one of the few situations in which the operator and team may directly affect the life and death of the patient.

LMCA stenosis is commonly associated with two clinical presentations:

1. Patients who show evidence of significant low workload ischemia or hypotension during exercise treadmill testing. Unstable angina may be caused by LMCA stenosis in about 10% of patients.
2. Patients with atypical angina. The clinical history and resting or stress ECG may not be helpful, and often patients with resting or atypical chest pain syndromes do not have previous exercise test data.

Technical notes for the angiography of the LMCA stenosis:

1. Either the Judkins femoral or the radial artery technique can be used safely. Access should be based on the operator's best working method.
2. Coronary arteriography before left ventriculography is recommended to obtain the most important information first, should a complication occur.
3. Careful slow advancement and seating of the Judkins left coronary catheter prevent this preshaped catheter from jumping into the ostia. This maneuver is important for an ostial narrowing. Continuous observation of pressure damping is also important.
4. If the catheter can be positioned beneath the ostia, a "cusp" flush of contrast material in the aortic sinus in an AP or shallow RAO projection may identify an ostial LMCA stenosis.
5. After catheter engagement the operator should look for aortic pressure wave deformation (damping). If pressure damping occurs, a limited contrast flush (1 to 2 ml) and rapid catheter withdrawal ("hit and run") during cineangiography should be performed to obtain a first look (Fig. 4-11). Rarely, aortic pressure damping occurs without LMCA narrowing because the coronary catheter is seated deeply and subselectively into the LAD artery. Gradual withdrawal and repositioning of the catheter may eliminate pressure damping. The absence of reflux of contrast media into the aortic root on coronary injection is associated with an ostial LMCA stenosis.

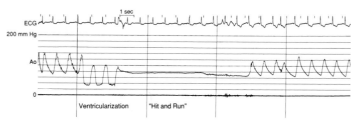

Fig. 4-11   Damping of aortic *(Ao)* pressure in the left main coronary artery with ventricularization in which immediate angiography was performed with removal of the catheter in a "hit-and-run" maneuver, rapidly restoring flow and perfusion after contrast media injection.

6. The number of coronary injections should be limited. Distal coronary artery anatomy suitable for bypass grafting is assessed from the few views (usually two or three) that are available. Additional injections should be kept to a minimum. Two projections, an LAO (cranial angulation) (Fig. 4-12, *A*) and a steeper RAO with caudal angulation (Fig. 4-12, *B*), are usually sufficient. An LAO-caudal projection for an ostial narrowing is sometimes better. Frequent catheter engagement of the LMCA segment and contrast jet stimulation of the lesion may precipitate coronary spasm or occlusion. In less critical LMCA stenosis with 40% to 60% narrowing, more views may be necessary. In some cases intravascular ultrasound imaging or physiologic measurements may be needed to assess lesion severity.

7. Nonionic or low-osmolar contrast agents should be used. Standard ionic contrast agents (e.g., meglumine diatrizoate) have been associated with lethal complications of hypotension, bradycardia, and reduced coronary perfusion. For the most part, hypotension and bradycardia have been eliminated with nonionic low-osmolar contrast agents.

8. After the left coronary views are completed, right coronary angiography is performed. If the RCA is occluded with a critical LMCA stenosis, intraaortic balloon pulsation, intensive care unit admission, and early coronary artery bypass graft surgery should be considered.

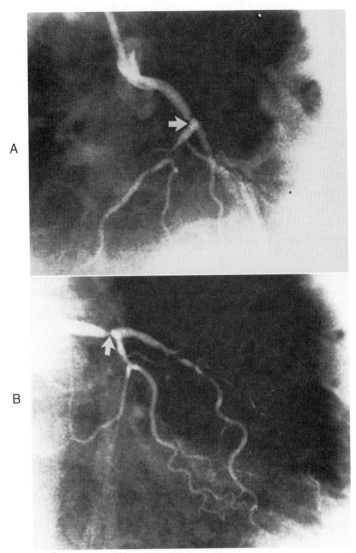

Fig. 4-12   Cineangiographic frame showing left main coronary stenosis *(arrow)*. **A,** Left anterior oblique projection. **B,** Right anterior oblique projection. See text for details.

Left Ventriculography in Patients with Left Main Coronary Artery Stenosis. In patients with LMCA stenosis, noninvasive techniques (two-dimensional and Doppler echocardiography, radionuclide angiography) to determine left ventricular (LV) function and mitral regurgitation may replace LV angiography. Safe contrast ventriculography can be performed with the use of low-volume (<30 ml) nonionic or low-osmolar contrast medium, facilitating a rapid "one-test (angiogram and left ventriculogram)" surgical decision. Digital subtraction ventriculography with a low-volume injection is often acceptable. Nonionic or low-osmolar contrast agents are preferred over standard ionic contrast media for these patients. Caution during LV catheter manipulation, including the pigtail catheter (especially in patients with LMCA stenosis and unstable angina), must be used to prevent a benign, transient arrhythmia from becoming a catastrophe. Left ventriculography should be considered only for patients who have a low risk/benefit ratio.

Important points for postcatheterization care of the patient with LMCA stenosis are as follows:

1. Prevention of hypotension is paramount. If an LMCA stenosis pressure gradient of 40 mm Hg, aortic diastolic blood pressure of 80 mm Hg, and LV end-diastolic pressure of 10 mm Hg is assumed, the coronary perfusion pressure can be approximated as $80 - (40 + 10) = 30$ mm Hg. If diastolic blood pressure decreases to 60 mm Hg, the perfusion pressure can decrease to 10 mm Hg, exacerbating myocardial ischemia and hypotension leading to a downward spiral of LV dysfunction and death.

2. Vasovagal reactions, especially during sheath removal, should be avoided if possible, and treated aggressively if they occur.

3. Adequate volumes of intravenous (IV) fluids (at least 1000 ml of normal saline in 4 hours) should be administered.

4. The patient's urine output should be monitored and adequate volume maintained.

5. Any signs of ischemia in the postcatheterization period must be attended to at once.

6. The patient's admission status should be changed from routine elective to urgent, requiring monitoring (e.g., in an intensive care unit).

7. The cardiothoracic surgeon should be notified. If a problem should develop, immediate communication between the cardiologist and surgeon makes a crucial difference in timing for urgent intervention. Insertion of an intraaortic balloon pump should be considered in patients with unstable angina or hemodynamic instability. Early consultation with the cardiothoracic surgeon helps determine timing of coronary artery bypass graft surgery.

Angiography of Common Coronary Anomalies. Misdiagnosis of an unsuspected anomalous origin of the coronary arteries is a potential problem for a busy angiographer. Because the natural history of a patient with an anomalous origin of a coronary artery may depend on the initial course of the anomalous vessel, it is the angiographer's responsibility to define accurately the origin and course of the vessel. It is an error to assume that a vessel is occluded when it has not been visualized because of an anomalous origin. Even experienced angiographers have difficulty delineating the true course of the anomalous vessel.

For the most critical anomaly, the left main anomalous origin from the right cusp, a simple "dot and eye" method for determining the proximal course of the anomalous artery from RAO ventriculogram, RAO aortogram, or selective RAO injection is proposed (Table 4-2). The RAO view best separates the normally positioned aorta and pulmonary artery (PA). Placement of right-sided catheters or injection of contrast material into the PA is unnecessary and often misleading.

Anomalous Origin of the Left Main Coronary Artery from the Right Sinus of Valsalva. When the LMCA arises from the right sinus of Valsalva or the proximal RCA, it may follow one of four pathways:

1. *Septal course.* The LMCA runs an intramuscular course through the septum along the floor of the right ventricular (RV) outflow tract (Fig. 4-13). It then surfaces in the midseptum, at which point it branches into the LAD artery and left circumflex artery. Because the artery divides in the midseptum, the initial portion of the circumflex artery courses toward the aorta (the normal

Table 4-2

Radiographic Appearance of Anomalous Origin of the Left Main Coronary Artery from the Right Sinus of Valsalva

Course of Anomalous Left Main Coronary	RAO AORTOGRAPHY OR VENTRICULOGRAPHY		LAD Length	Septal Branches Arising from LMCA
	Dot	Eye		
Septal	–	+ (upper CFX) (lower LMCA)	Short	Yes
Anterior	–	+ (upper LMCA) (lower CFX)	Short	No
Retroaortic	+ (posterior)	–	Normal	No
Interarterial	+ (anterior)	–	Normal	No

+, Present; –, absent. *Posterior* and *anterior* are in reference to the aorta root. *CFX*, Circumflex coronary artery; *LAD*, left anterior descending coronary artery; *LMCA*, left main coronary artery.

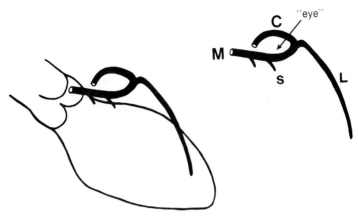

Fig. 4-13 Diagram of septal course of anomalous left coronary artery. *M,* Left main; *S,* septals; *C,* circumflex; *L,* left anterior descending artery.

position of the proximal LAD), and the LAD artery is relatively short (i.e., only mid and distal LAD are present). During RAO ventriculography, aortography, or coronary arteriography the LCMA and the circumflex coronary artery form an ellipse (similar to the shape of an eye) to the left of the aorta. The LMCA forms the inferior portion and the circumflex artery forms the superior portion. Septal perforating arteries are evident branching from the LMCA.

Note: This variant is considered benign and is not associated with myocardial ischemia.

2. *Anterior free wall course.* The LMCA crosses the anterior free wall of the right ventricle, then divides at the midseptum into the LAD and circumflex arteries (Fig. 4-14). Because the artery divides at the midseptum, the initial portion of the circumflex artery courses toward the aorta (the normal position of the proximal LAD), and the LAD artery is relatively short (i.e., only mid and distal LAD are present). During RAO ventriculography, aortography, or coronary arteriography, the LMCA and the circumflex artery form an ellipse ("eye") to the left of the aorta with the LMCA forming the superior portion and the circumflex forming the inferior portion.

Note: This variant has not been associated with myocardial ischemia.

3. *Retroaortic course.* The LMCA passes posteriorly around the aortic root to its normal position on the anterior surface of the heart (Fig. 4-15). It divides into the LAD and circumflex arteries at the normal point and gives rise to LAD and circumflex coronary arteries of normal length and course. During RAO ventriculography, aortography, or coronary angiography, the LMCA is seen "on end," *posterior* to the aorta, and appears as a radiopaque *dot.* This retroaortic dot signifies a posteriorly coursing anomalous vessel. (It is also seen with anomalous origin of circumflex from right sinus.)

Note: This variant is considered benign, and evidence of myocardial ischemia has been reported in only a few individuals.

4. *Interarterial course.* The LMCA courses between the aorta and PA to its normal position on the anterior surface of the heart (Fig. 4-16). It divides into the LAD and circumflex arteries at the normal point and gives rise to LAD and circumflex coronary arteries of normal length and course. During RAO ventriculography, aortography, or coronary arteriography, the LMCA is seen "on end," *anterior* to the aorta, and appears as a radiopaque dot to the left of the aortic root.

The interarterial course of the LMCA originating from the right sinus of Valsalva has been associated with exertional angina, syncope, and sudden death at a young age. Its identi-

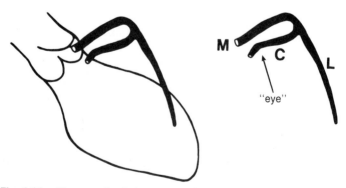

Fig. 4-14 Diagram of anterior course of anomalous left coronary artery. *M,* Left main; *C,* circumflex; *L,* left anterior descending artery.

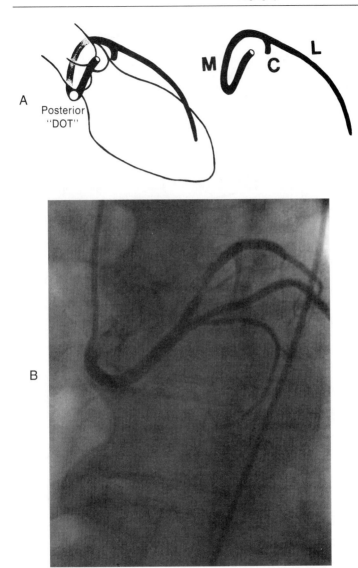

Fig. 4-15   A, Diagram of retroaortic course of anomalous left coronary artery. *M,* Left main; *C,* circumflex; *L,* left anterior descending artery. **B,** Intraseptal course of left main coronary artery from right sinus. The left main coronary artery, when it originates within the right sinus of Valsalva or from the proximal right coronary artery, may take an inferior and intraseptal course, a superior course anterior to the pulmonary artery, or a serpentine course between the great arteries (which carries a risk of sudden death).

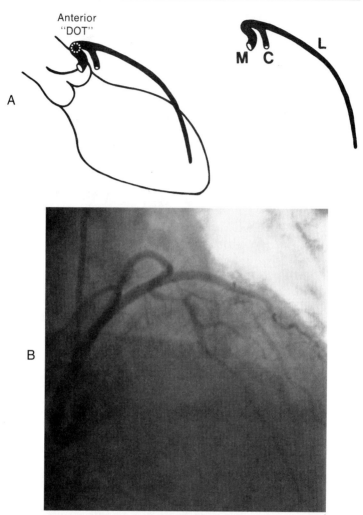

Fig. 4-16 **A,** Intraarterial course of left main coronary artery from right sinus. **B,** Anterior course after intraarterial path of anomalous left main coronary artery. *M,* left main; *C,* circumflex; *L,* left anterior descending artery.

fication is imperative. The mechanism causing myocardial ischemia is unclear, but it may be associated with slitlike orifice and ostial narrowing during activity rather than dynamic compression of the obliquely arising LMCA at the ostium as it courses between the aortic root and the root of the pulmonary trunk. When this anomaly is identified, coronary revascularization or translocation is indicated in patients with myocardial ischemia. The need for revascularization in older patients with this anomaly is less clear. A decision for revascularization should be based on the severity of concomitant obstructive coronary disease and inducible myocardial ischemia. The four types of anomalous courses of the LMCA are summarized in Table 4-2.

Anomalous Origin of the Circumflex Coronary Artery. The most common coronary anomaly is the circumflex artery arising from the proximal RCA. This feature is often suggested during left coronary angiography when the operator sees a long LMCA segment with a small or trivial circumflex branch. The circumflex artery may also be thought to be occluded. When the circumflex coronary artery arises from the right coronary cusp or the proximal RCA, it invariably follows a retroaortic course and passes posteriorly around the aortic root to its normal position (Figs. 4-17 and 4-18). During RAO ventriculography, aortography, or coronary angiography, the circumflex artery is seen "on end," appearing as a radiopaque dot posterior to the aorta. This variant is benign.

Anomalous Origin of the Right Coronary Artery from the Left Sinus of Valsalva. When the RCA arises from the left coronary cusp or the proximal LMCA, it generally follows only

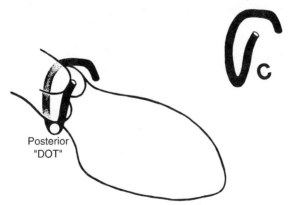

Posterior "DOT"

Fig. 4-17 Diagram of retroaortic course of circumflex (C) from the left coronary cusp.

A

B

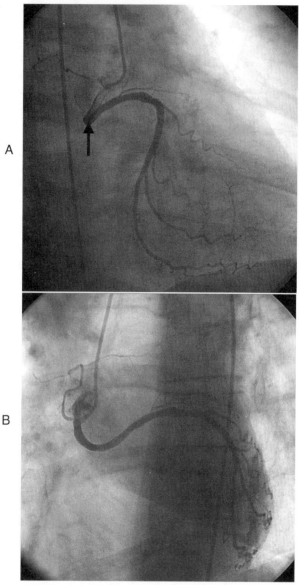

Fig. 4-18   A, The anomalous circumflex artery usually originates from the right sinus of Valsalva with a separate ostium or from the proximal right coronary artery. The typical course of this benign anomaly is retroaortic as it travels to the lateral surface of the left ventricle. Right anterior oblique view showing "dot" of anomalous retroaortic course of circumflex. **B,** Left anterior oblique view of anomalous circumflex.

one path, although other courses are theoretically possible (Fig. 4-19). The RCA courses between the aorta and PA to its normal position. During RAO ventriculography, aortography, or coronary arteriography, the RCA is seen "on end," anterior to the aorta, and appears as a radiopaque dot. This coronary anomaly has been associated with symptoms of myocardial ischemia, particularly when the RCA is dominant. Coronary revascularization should be considered when this anomaly is associated with symptoms of myocardial ischemia.

Anomalous Right Coronary Artery Above the Sinus of Valsalva or from Anterior Aortic Wall. The RCA may arise from an anterior location or high above the sinus of Valsalva. Aortic root flush injection helps locate the ostium for proper, subselective catheter selection (e.g., Amplatz left 2 or multipurpose). This variant is benign.

Anomalous Origin of the Left Anterior Descending Coronary Artery from the Right Sinus of Valsalva. When the LAD artery arises from the right aortic cusp or the proximal RCA, it generally follows one of two pathways, although other courses are possible.

1. *Anterior free wall course.* The LAD coronary artery crosses the anterior free wall of the RV, then at the midseptum turns toward the apex. During RAO ventriculography, aortography, or coronary arteriography the LAD artery is

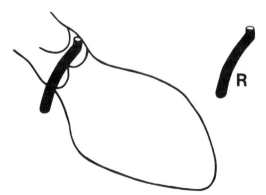

Fig. 4-19 Diagram of anterior course of right coronary artery *(R)* from the left coronary cusp.

seen as passing to the left and upward before turning toward the apex. This coronary anomaly is benign.

2. *Septal course.* The LAD coronary artery runs an intramuscular course through the septum, along the floor of the RV outflow tract. It then surfaces in the midseptum and turns toward the apex. During RAO ventriculography, aortography, or coronary arteriography the LAD artery is seen as passing to the left and downward before turning toward the apex. This anomaly is benign.

Left Anterior Descending and Circumflex Coronary Arteries from Separate Ostia in the Left Aortic Sinus. When the LAD and circumflex coronary arteries arise from separate ostia in the left coronary cusp, the normal proximal course is followed. Also, a conus branch has a separate ostium arising from the right coronary cusp.

VENTRICULOGRAPHY

The left ventriculogram is an integral part of every coronary arteriographic study. The motion of the walls of the heart can be observed and quantitated (Fig. 4-20). Abnormal wall motion indicates the presence of coronary ischemia, infarction, aneurysm, or hypertrophy (Fig. 4-21). Left ventriculography also provides quantitative information, such as the volume of the ventricle during systole and diastole, the ejection fraction, the rate of ejection, the quality of contractility, the presence of hypertrophic myopathy, and valvular regurgitation. Ventricular function predicts the long-term outcome of patients with coronary artery disease.

Ventriculography may be performed before or after coronary arteriography. Coronary arteriography is routinely performed first because ventricular function can be obtained through noninvasive methods in case of complications that terminate the study prematurely. In patients with LMCA stenosis, left ventriculography has often been omitted when postprocedural hypotension with ionic contrast media is anticipated. Low-volume, nonionic, or low–osmolar contrast ventriculograms can be performed with little or no hypotension for these patients. The same concerns apply to patients with critical aortic stenosis in whom hypotension after left ventriculography may cause heart failure from LV ischemic dysfunction.

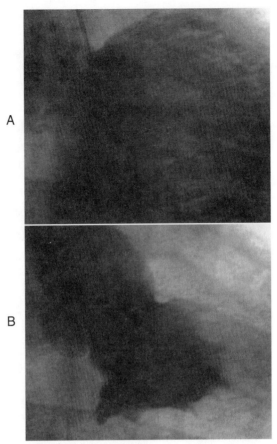

Fig. 4-20   A, Left ventriculographic frame in diastole 30-degree right anterior oblique projection. **B,** Left ventriculographic frame in systole.

Indications for Ventriculography

Indications for left ventriculography are as follows:

1. Identification of LV function for patients with coronary artery disease, myopathy, or valvular heart disease
2. Identification of ventricular septal defect
3. Quantitation of the degree of mitral regurgitation
4. Quantitation of the mass of myocardium for regression of hypertrophy or other similar research studies

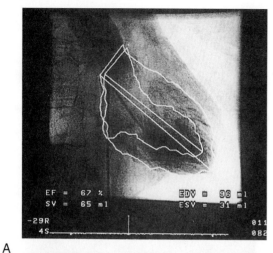

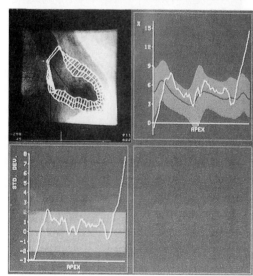

Fig. 4-21 Left ventriculographic wall motion analysis. **A,** Normal left ventricular (LV) wall motion shows concentric inward motion of all LV wall segments. Bottom panel shows chords and deviation from midline.

Continued

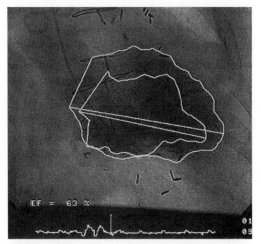

B

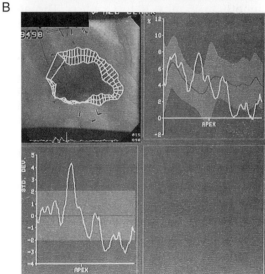

Fig. 4-21, cont'd   B, Inferior wall motion abnormality on left ventriculo-gram. Note failure of left ventricle to move inward on inferior wall. Bottom panel shows abnormal chords above mean values. The centerline method of regional wall motion analysis uses end-diastolic and end-systolic LV endocardial contours. Lower panels show how a centerline is constructed by the computer midway between the two contours. Motion is measured along 100 chords constructed perpendicular to the centerline. Motion at each chord is normalized by the end-diastolic perimeter to yield a shortening fraction. Motion along each chord is plotted for the patient *(dark line)*. The mean motion in the normal ventriculogram group *(thin line)* and 1 standard deviation (SD) above and below the mean *(dotted line)* are shown for comparison. Wall motion also is plotted as the difference in units of SDs from the normal mean *(right panel)*. The normal ventriculogram group mean is represented by the horizontal zero line.

Indications for right ventriculography are as follows:
1. Documentation of tricuspid regurgitation
2. Assessment of RV dysplasia for arrhythmias
3. Assessment of pulmonary stenosis.
4. Assessment of abnormalities of pulmonary outflow tract
5. Assessment of right-to-left ventricular shunts

Technical Notes for Ventriculography

Contrast Volume. Adequate visualization and opacification of the ventricle chambers are accomplished by delivery of a large bolus (30 to 45 ml) of x-ray contrast medium over a short period (1 to 3 seconds), always with a powered injection technique. Typical power injector settings for an average adult are total volume 30 to 45 ml at 10 to 15 ml/sec. The rate of rise to maximal pressure is also a variable that can be set for smoother contrast delivery, typically a 0.5-second rise time. With the catheter in the far apical position, a lower rate and volume can be used (e.g., 10 ml/sec for 30 to 35 ml). With operator-controlled injection (Acist), excellent ventriculograms can be obtained with 20-30 ml of contrast medium. The injection is stopped when the ventricle is satisfactorily opacified.

Catheter Position. The optimal catheter position for left ventriculography is one that avoids contact with the papillary muscles or positioning too close to the mitral valve, so that mitral regurgitation is not produced artificially. For most catheters a midcavity position seems best because contrast material fills most of the LV chamber and apex, and injection does not interfere with mitral valve function. In this position most pigtail catheter side holes are well below the aortic valve, which improves chamber opacification. Angled (145 degrees) catheters and helical tip designs (Halo catheter) may provide better quality ventriculography by the reduction of ectopy and mitral regurgitation.

The pigtail loop of the catheter may be coiled upward or downward in front of the mitral valve in the RAO plane as long as it does not interfere with mitral valve apparatus and reduce ectopy. Twisting of the pigtail loop with each beat indicates interference with the mitral valve apparatus.

When the position of the catheter is in question, a test injection of 5 to 8 ml of contrast material confirms proper catheter position (i.e., not entrapped in the valve structures or trabeculae). For right ventriculography a 7 F or 8 F Berman balloon-tipped catheter (with side holes proximal to balloon) produces excellent opacification. The angiographic projection of right ventriculography is not standardized. An AP cranial or lateral projection is commonly used.

Ventricular Ectopy. Ventricular ectopy during powerful contrast material injection is common and generally does not require lidocaine. A stable rhythm should be maintained before contrast material injection by careful catheter positioning between the papillary muscles and the inferior LV wall. Ventricular ectopy is commonly produced by use of end hole (e.g., multipurpose) catheters. A pigtail shape is safer.

Setup of Pressure Injectors. Pressure injectors are always used to deliver a preset contrast volume over a brief period. Higher injection pressures are needed for smaller diameter catheters (e.g., PSI set at 900 for 6 F and 1200 PSI for 4 F pigtail). Settings for injections are:
1. Flow rate (10 to 15 ml/sec)
2. Total volume (20 to 50 ml)
3. Pressure limit (900 to 1200 PSI)
4. Rise time (0.2 to 0.5 second)

All air and bubbles should be expelled from the transparent pressure injection syringe and tubing before any injection. This is a mandatory step of the setup. Physicians and nurses should be especially careful to avoid air injection. There is no excuse for injection of air during contrast ventriculography.

Left Ventriculography in Patients with Left Ventricular Dysfunction.
Patients with LV dysfunction and an elevated LV end-diastolic pressure (i.e., >25 mm Hg) may require a reduction in the LV end-diastolic pressure before ventriculography. Use of sublingual, IV, or intraventricular nitroglycerin (100- to 200-μg boluses) is a safe and rapid method of producing the desired results. As a rule, LV systolic pressure should be less than 180 mm Hg before contrast medium injection. Extreme caution should be used for compromised patients not responding to conventional medical treatment for heart failure (i.e., LV end-diastolic pressure >35 mm Hg). Nonionic or low-osmolar

contrast medium is recommended for patients with LV dysfunction to avoid adverse hemodynamic effects.

Operator Technique. During contrast material injection the physician performing the ventriculogram should be holding the catheter and the sheath, observing the physiologic monitor, and looking for problems (on the fluoroscope). Myocardial contrast staining, ventricular tachycardia, or other adverse events may occur. Rapid catheter withdrawal may be required. The distance the catheter must be pulled includes 10 to 15 cm to take out the slack around the aorta before the end of the catheter moves out of the ventricle. Use of small-diameter (e.g., 4 F to 5 F) catheters requires high pressures and does not allow flow rates greater than 13 ml/sec. Injector connections to the manifold or direct connection to the catheter must be secured so that inadvertent catheter-injector tubing separation does not spray the operator, patient, and laboratory with contrast material.

Instructions given to the patient by the operator before the injection avoid unexpected discomfort and ease the performance of the procedure. Informing the patient that the warm sensation caused by contrast vasodilation as pictures of the pumping chamber are taken lasts for 30 to 60 seconds and passes without incident is usually satisfactory.

Ventriculography Views. Standard left ventriculographic views are (1) a 30-degree RAO that visualizes the high lateral, anterior, apical, and inferior LV walls and (2) a 45- to 60-degree LAO, 20-degree cranial angulation that best identifies the lateral and septal LV walls. The LAO with cranial angulation provides a view of the interventricular septum, projected on edge and tilted downward to give the best view of ventricular septal defects and septal wall motion. Biplane ventriculography may be available in some catheterization laboratories. It involves increased radiation and more time spent positioning equipment. These considerations are offset by providing more information with less contrast media, which is often important, especially in children and patients with renal failure. If no biplane system is available, patients with coronary disease affecting the lateral wall should have a second left ventriculogram in 60-degree LAO, 20-degree cranial view.

Almost every such patient can tolerate an additional 30 to 40 ml of contrast material.

Film rates should be 30 to 60 frames/sec depending on heart rate (30 frames/sec for rates of <95 beats/min). A 9-inch image intensifier is routine. Image intensifier collimator "shutters" can be used to limit radiation scatter. Recommended views for valvular regurgitation are shown in Table 4-3. The angiographic quantitation of valvular regurgitation is shown in Table 4-4.

Complications of Ventriculography.

1. Cardiac arrhythmias, especially ventricular tachycardia and ventricular fibrillation, require immediate cardioversion.
2. Intramyocardial "staining," injection of contrast material into the myocardium, is generally transient and of no clinical importance unless it is deep or perforating (emergency pericardiocentesis may be required). Arrhythmias and staining are more common with the use of end hole catheters than with any other pigtail catheters.
3. Embolism from thrombi or air may occur. These events are minimized with careful catheter preparation, flushing, and systemic heparinization.

Table 4-3

Recommended Sites of Injection and Angiographic Projections in the Evaluation of Valvular Regurgitation and Shunts

	Filming Projections	Site of Injection
Type of Valvular Regurgitation		
Aortic	LAO, RAO	Aortic root
Mitral	RAO, cranial LAO (lateral)	Left ventricle
Tricuspid	RAO (shallow, lateral)	Right ventricle
Pulmonic	RAO, LAO, AP	Main PA
Type of Cardiac Shunt		
ASD	LAO, cranial	PA
VSD	LAO, cranial	Left ventricle
PDA	AP, cranial	Aorta

AP, Anteroposterior; *ASD,* atrial septal defect; *LAO,* left anterior oblique; *PA,* pulmonary artery; *PDA,* patent ductus arteriosus; *RAO,* right anterior oblique; *VSD,* ventricular septal defect.

Table 4-4

Angiographic Quantitation of Valvular Regurgitation

Mitral Regurgitation		Aortic Regurgitation	
+	Mild LA opacification; clears rapidly, often jetlike	+	Small regurgitant jet only; LV ejects contrast each systole
++	Moderate LA opacification, < LV	++	Regurgitant jet faintly opacifies LV cavity; not cleared each systole
+++	Diffuse contrast regurgitant; LA opacification = LV; LA significantly enlarged*	+++	Persistent LV opacification = aortic root density; LV enlargement*
++++	LA opacification > LV, persistent; systolic pulmonary vein opacification may occur; often marked LV enlargement*	++++	Persistent LV opacification > aortic root concentration; often marked LV enlargement*

LA, Left atrium; *LV*, left ventricle; *+*, 1; *++*, 2+; *+++*, 3+; *++++*, 4+.
*Chronic regurgitation.

4. Contrast-related complications noted previously, including allergic-type vasomotor collapse, may occur during this procedure. Transient hypotension (<15 to 30 seconds) is common with the use of ionic contrast media.

Regional Left Ventricular Wall Motion. The normal pattern of LV contraction has been defined as a uniform, almost concentric, inward motion of all points along the ventricular inner surface during systole. Uniform wall motion depends on the cooperative and sequential contraction of the heart muscle, producing maximal effective work at minimal energy costs. This coordinated contraction is called synergy. Uncoordinated contractions in the pattern of wall motion contraction (from ischemia, infarction, or myopathy) are termed asynergy. Abnormal LV wall motion is particularly obvious in patients with severe coronary artery disease or cardiomyopathy. There are three distinct types of asynergy (Fig. 4-22):

1. *Hypokinesia*—a diminished, but not absent, motion of one part of the LV wall (also called weak or poor contraction).

2. *Akinesia*—total lack of motion of a portion of the LV wall (i.e., no contraction).
3. *Dyskinesia*—paradoxical systolic motion or expansion of one part of the LV wall (i.e., an abnormal outward bulging during systole).

Several methods exist to analyze LV wall motion. A point system from the Coronary Artery Surgery Study (CASS) based on the regional severity of abnormal wall motion is used to produce a wall motion score that reflects overall LV function. The RAO and LAO left ventriculograms are divided into five segments. Points are assigned as follows:

1 = normal contraction
2 = moderate hypokinesis
3 = severe hypokinesis
4 = akinesis
5 = aneurysm-dyskinesis

A normal score is 5. Higher scores indicate more severe wall motion abnormalities.

For determination of quantitative regional wall motion abnormalities, three methods are used (also see Appendix F):

1. *Long-axis method.* Determination of the major long axis and division of the long axis into equal segments with perpendicular lines.
2. *Center point method.* Midpoint of the major axis and division of the lines radiating out from the center point.
3. *Centerline method.* A centerline is established between the end-diastolic and end-systolic borders, 100 perpendicular chords are drawn, and shortening of these chords determines wall motion abnormalities. Results are corrected with use of a normal motion value for each chord length. This is the preferred method for wall motion analysis (see Fig. 4-21).

Some of the methods of determining regional wall motion abnormality use computer planimetry that is available on most advanced x-ray systems.

Left Ventricular Volume Determination. LV volumes can be calculated from single-plane or biplane angiographic images (see Appendix F), but these methods generally overestimate true ventricular volume for two reasons: (1) a portion of the LV

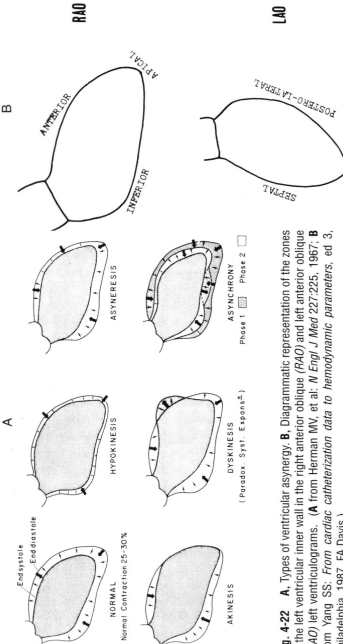

Fig. 4-22 A, Types of ventricular asynergy. **B**, Diagrammatic representation of the zones of the left ventricular inner wall in the right anterior oblique (*RAO*) and left anterior oblique (*LAO*) left ventriculograms. (**A** from Herman MV, et al: *N Engl J Med* 227:225, 1967; **B** from Yang SS: *From cardiac catheterization data to hemodynamic parameters*, ed 3, Philadelphia, 1987, FA Davis.)

chamber is occupied by papillary muscles and trabeculae and is incorporated into the ventricular area measurement, and (2) in the ventricular volume calculation, assuming the left ventricle is an ellipse when it is actually an irregular ovoid shape with variable margins overestimates volume.

The volume of the LV is computed by a formula previously calibrated against an image of known volume, such as a cast of a ventricle from an animal or postmortem specimen. The ventricular volume regression equation is determined specifically for the laboratory equipment in use. LV area is computed by the area-length method or Simpson's rule formula. The ventricular area is converted into a volume, assuming that the ventricle has an ellipsoid shape rotated around its long axis. Image distortion and magnification should be taken into consideration. Methods for determination of ventricular volume by biplane ventriculography are described in Appendix F. Adult values differ from values in children.

Measurements of Left Ventricular Contractility

Ejection fraction (EF, %) is calculated as:

$$EF = \frac{EDV - ESV}{EDV} \times 100$$

$$SV = EDV - ESV$$

where *EDV* is end-diastolic volume, *ESV* is end-systolic volume, and *SV* is stroke volume.

Velocity of circumferential fiber shortening (VCF, cm/sec) is calculated as:

$$\frac{\dfrac{D_{ed} - D_{es}}{D_{ed}}}{LVET}$$

where D_{ed} is diameter end diastole, D_{es} is diameter end systole, and *LVET* is LV ejection time (ms).

Measurement of Mitral Regurgitation

The severity of mitral regurgitation is semiquantitative based on the degree of contrast opacification of the left atrium during left ventriculography (Figs. 4-23 and 4-24 and see Table 4-4). Mitral regurgitation can also be quantitated by calculation of a regurgitant fraction.

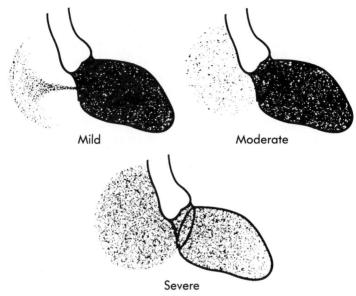

Fig. 4-23 Angiographic evaluation of mitral regurgitation. (From Pujadas G: *Coronary angiography in the medical and surgical treatment of ischemic heart disease,* New York, 1980, McGraw-Hill.)

The regurgitant fraction (RF) for patients with valvular regurgitation is calculated as follows:

$$RF = \frac{\text{regurgitant flow}}{\text{total flow}}$$

$$= \frac{\text{CO from angiogram} - \text{CO from Fick/thermodilution}}{\text{CO from angiogram}}$$

where CO is cardiac output. Semiquantitation of severity of regurgitation is determined as follows:

RF < 40%	Mild
RF = 40% to 60%	Moderate
RF > 60%	Severe

OTHER CARDIOVASCULAR ANGIOGRAPHIC STUDIES: ASCENDING AORTOGRAPHY

Indications for aortography include the following:
1. Aortic aneurysm or aortic dissection
2. Aortic insufficiency
3. Nonselective coronary or bypass graft arteriography

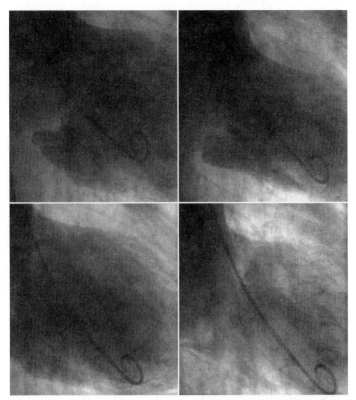

Fig. 4-24   Left ventriculogram in patient with mitral regurgitation. *Top left,* Early opacification of the left atrium (LA). *Top right and bottom left,* Denser opacification of LA. *Bottom right,* LA is more densely opacified than left ventricle after several beats. This is severe (4+) MR.

    4. Supravalvular aortic stenosis
    5. Brachiocephalic or arch vessel disease
    6. Coarctation of the aorta
    7. Aortic-to-PA or aortic-to-right-side heart (e.g., sinus of Valsalva fistula) communication
    8. Aortic or periaortic neoplastic disease
    9. Arterial thromboembolic disease
  10. Arterial inflammatory disease
Contraindications for aortography are as follows:
    1. Contrast media reaction
    2. Injection into false lumen of aortic dissection

3. End hole catheter malposition
4. Inability of the patient to tolerate additional radiographic contrast media

Although cut film is an established radiologic method, in cardiac catheterization laboratories, cineangiography is acceptable for patients with suspected dissection of the aorta.

Radiographic Projections for Aortography

Left Anterior Oblique or Lateral Projection. The LAO view is excellent for identifying dissection of the ascending aorta extending up to the neck vessels, optimally delineating the aortic arch; opening the aortic curvature; and providing clear views of the innominate, common carotid, and left subclavian arteries. The coronary arteries at the root of the aorta are displayed in a semilateral projection.

Right Anterior Oblique Projection. The descending thoracic aorta and the ascending aorta may be superimposed across the arch in the AP or LAO projection. The RAO view is more helpful in delineating the effect of dissection on the lower thoracic aorta and intercostal arteries and the origin of bypass grafts to the left coronary system.

There are no advantages to cranial or caudal tilts for viewing the aorta. In nonselective coronary arteriography in which aortic root angiography may help to identify a vein graft takeoff, the cranial and caudal angulation may provide some increased detail.

Angiographic Technique

Injection Rates. Aortography can be performed by use of a minimum flow rate of 15 to 25 ml/sec for total volumes of 40 to 60 ml. High-flow (≥ 5 F) catheters are required with standard power injectors. Film rates of 15 to 30 frames/sec are satisfactory.

Catheter Selection and Position. Use of catheters without end holes reduces the risk of extending or inducing a dissection during contrast medium injection. The catheter should be positioned just above the aortic valve but not close enough to interfere with valve opening or closing. For descending aortic dissection the catheter is positioned above the suspected proximal tear. Extreme caution should be used with guidewires during catheter placement.

Catheter position should be checked with a contrast test before full-volume injection. Figures 4-25 to 4-27 show

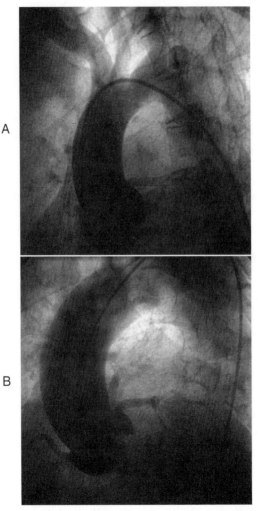

Fig. 4-25   **A,** Normal aortogram in left anterior oblique projection. **B,** Dilated ascending aorta.

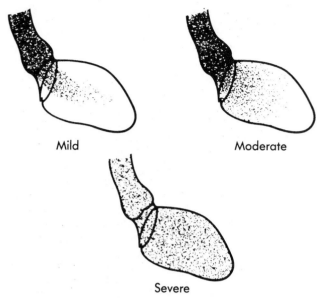

Mild   Moderate

Severe

Fig. 4-26 Angiographic evaluation of aortic regurgitation, right anterior oblique view. When the left anterior oblique view is used, overestimation of aortic regurgitation occurs. (From Pujadas G: *Coronary angiography in the medical and surgical treatment of ischemic heart disease,* New York, 1980, McGraw-Hill.)

examples of aortography and aortic regurgitation. Aortic regurgitation is estimated semiquantitatively as +1, +2, +3, or +4, depending on the opacification of the ventricle after the third cycle following contrast injection. Care should be taken to avoid entrapping the catheter in a false lumen of a suspected aortic dissection.

ABDOMINAL AORTOGRAPHY

Indications for abdominal aortography include the following:
1. Nonselective evaluation of renal arteries and mesenteric vessels
2. Abdominal aneurysm or dissection
3. Abdominal aortic atherosclerotic disease
4. Vascular assessment before intraaortic balloon pulsation insertion
5. Initial evaluation of claudication

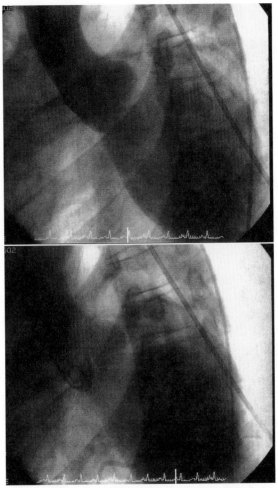

Fig. 4-27 *Top,* Cineframe showing aortic regurgitation from left anterior descending aortogram. Note equal opacification of left ventricle and aorta. *Bottom,* Left ventricle is still opacified after several beats. This is severe aortic regurgitation.

6. Evaluation of cause of difficult catheter movement for coronary angiography

The contraindications for abdominal aortography are the same as for thoracic aortography. Figure 4-28 shows typical findings in abdominal aortography in a patient with peripheral vascular disease.

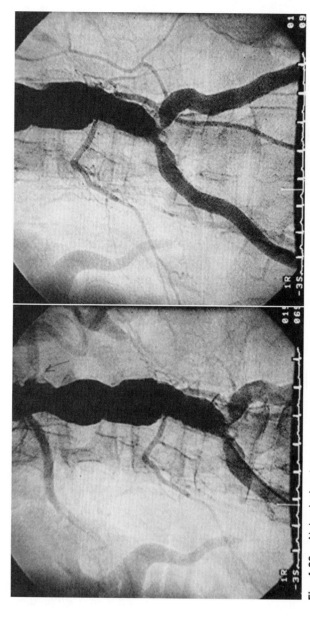

Fig. 4-28 Abdominal aortogram, anteroposterior projection. Aortography of the lower abdominal aorta shows bilateral iliac stenosis at its origin from the most distal part of the abdominal aorta.

PULMONARY ANGIOGRAPHY

Pulmonary angiography, the visualization of vascular abnormalities of the lung vessels (e.g., intraluminal defects representing pulmonary emboli, shunts, stenosis, arteriovenous [AV] malformation, and anomalous connections), should be preceded by the measurement of pressures of the right side of the heart. Indications for pulmonary angiography include the following:

1. Pulmonary embolism
2. Peripheral pulmonic stenosis or pulmonary AV fistula
3. Anomalous pulmonary venous drainage
4. Follow-through for left atrial opacification (suspected atrial myxoma, large thrombi)

Contraindications and precautions for pulmonary angiography are as follows:

1. Allergy to contrast agent
2. Pulmonary hypertension with PA systolic pressure (>60 mm Hg); extreme caution should be used (e.g., with primary pulmonary hypertension)
3. Acute RV volume overload (after injection of contrast medium, increased volume may produce RV failure, low cardiac output state, shock, or death)

Angiographic Technique

1. *Venous entry.* Femoral or brachial vein (percutaneous technique) is used, not cephalic vein. Before proceeding, the operator should consider whether percutaneous femoral vein approach may dislodge an iliofemoral clot. A brief contrast flush of the inferior vena cava is performed first. Noninvasive Doppler studies may also indicate thrombus. If thrombus is present, the brachial or internal jugular vein approach is used.
2. *Systemic arterial pressure monitoring.* Patients are often critically ill. Placement of a small arterial catheter in the femoral or radial artery to monitor pressure does not complicate the procedure.
3. *Selection of angiographic catheters.*
   a. Large-diameter 7 F or 8 F balloon-tipped flotation (Berman) catheters are easy to position. Ventriculographic pigtail catheters or Grollman catheters recoil less than balloon-tipped catheters.

b. *Caution:* A pacing catheter may be needed for patients with left bundle-branch block. Right bundle-branch block induced by passage of stiff catheters through the right side of the heart would result in asystole or complete heart block in these patients.

4. *Right heart hemodynamic measurements.* Right atrial (RA), RV, and PA pressures should be measured before angiography is performed. CO is also measured before angiography.

5. *Angiographic views.* The catheter is positioned in the proximal portion of right PA (or where lung scan defect is evident) (see Fig. 4-31). Injection rate depends on hemodynamics:

a. If resting PA pressures are normal, a rate of 30 to 40 ml at 20 ml/sec is used. Main PA injection is performed (30 frames/sec) in AP projection, panning to site of presumed ventilation or perfusion (i.e., lung scan) defect.

b. If pulmonary hypertension (PA systolic >60 mm Hg) or RV failure (RV diastolic or RA mean pressure >10 mm Hg) are present, contrast volume and flow rate are reduced for selective PA branch injection of 15 to 20 ml at 10 ml/sec.

c. Selective PA branch injections by hand syringe (10 ml) may visualize a filling defect of pulmonary emboli.

d. For subselective injection the catheter is positioned proximal to the lobar artery in question. Figure 4-29 diagrams the anatomy of the pulmonary arterial tree. The operator should not inject if the catheter is in the pulmonary capillary wedge position. The pressure tracing should not be damped (an end hole catheter should not be used to avoid accidental pulmonary capillary wedge injection).

e. Angiographic views should be oblique (RAO or LAO) ipsilateral to the artery imaged. The best view to visualize PA bifurcation and detect stenosis is 15- to 20-degree LAO with 35- to 40-degree cranial angulation.

6. *Filming rates.* A cineangiography rate of 30 frames/sec is adequate. (Because pulmonary arteries are not moving quickly, a slower rate is acceptable.) The filming run

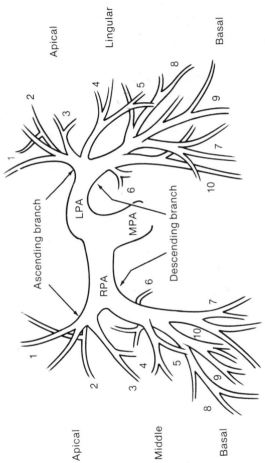

Fig. 4-29 Normal pulmonary arterial tree (anteroposterior projection). *MPA,* Main pulmonary artery; *RPA,* right pulmonary artery; *LPA,* left pulmonary artery. (From Tilkian AG, Daily EK: *Cardiovascular procedures: diagnostic techniques and therapeutic procedures,* St Louis, 1986, Mosby.)

should be long enough to visualize the levophase of left atrial filling. Subtraction images are also helpful if the patient is able to hold his or her breath.

Complications of Pulmonary Angiography

Problems and complications of right-sided heart catheterization (see Chapter 3) include cardiac perforation and arrhythmia. Angiography-related complications include bronchospasm, anaphylaxis, hypotension, and cardiogenic shock.

Interpretation of the Data

Hemodynamics. With acute pulmonary embolism a previously normal right ventricle fails at 40 to 60 mm Hg peak systolic pressure. The hemodynamic consequences of pulmonary embolization may be summarized as follows:

Obstruction of the Pulmonary Vasculature		Mean RA Pressure
Moderate	<25%	<10 mm Hg
Severe	25-50%	10 mm Hg
Massive	>50%	>10 mm Hg

Hypoxia increases cardiac output. Only with massive pulmonary embolism and RV failure will CO decrease. Systemic hypotension is a late-occurring premorbid event with pulmonary embolism.

Angiographic Findings. Criteria for an angiogram positive for pulmonary embolism include the following:
1. Intraluminal filling defects—not explicable by superimposed adjacent structures (Fig. 4-30)
2. Abrupt arterial cutoffs—when embolus completely occludes an artery

Associated suggestive but not definitive findings (both findings are common in patients with severe lung disease) of pulmonary embolism are as follows:
1. Oligemia—underperfused areas of lung
2. Asymmetry of flow—delayed filling by both sides is common with chronic obstructive pulmonary disease

PERIPHERAL VASCULAR ANGIOGRAPHY

When the techniques of coronary angiography have been mastered, peripheral vascular angiography is not difficult.

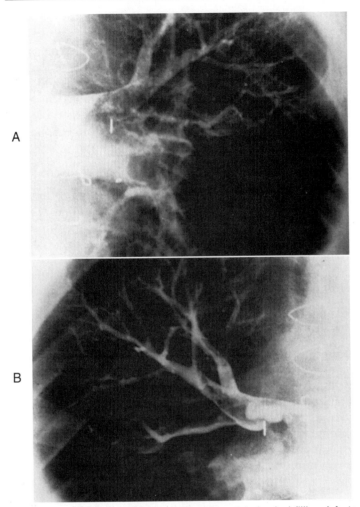

Fig. 4-30 Pulmonary arteriogram shows large intraluminal filling defects of pulmonary embolus within pulmonary arteries. **A,** Left upper lobe. **B,** Right middle and upper lobes.

Digital subtraction angiography is the method of choice for identifying peripheral vascular disease. Cineangiography can provide satisfactory information, however, if the filming time, frame rates, and contrast doses are properly established. Cineangiography is also helpful to detect the speed of vessel opacification and collateral filling.

Renal Arteriography

Selective renal arteriography is used to evaluate the renal artery origins and vasculature. Selective renal arterial injections provide the most detail and are obtained easily with a Judkins right 4 cm catheter. Note: For screening aortography, the renal artery origins usually arise at the L1 vertebra (just below the T12 ribs). The 30-degree ipsilateral oblique projection provides the best view of the renal artery ostia in most patients. Acutely angled takeoffs of the renal artery may require specially shaped catheters or an arm approach entering from above. Atherosclerotic disease of the renal artery usually involves the proximal one third of the renal artery and is seldom present without abdominal atherosclerotic plaques. Delayed imaging to see the nephrogram is essential to exclude accessory renal arteries and to screen for the presence of severe parenchymal disease. Measurement of a pressure gradient across an ostial or proximal lesion is recommended to determine the need for intervention.

A renal artery stenosis alone is rarely the sole determinant for surgery or angioplasty. Refractory hypertension and renal insufficiency are usually the indicators for an interventional (stent) procedure. Renal artery fibromuscular dysplasia may occur and appear as atherosclerotic disease. This finding is often present in middle-aged women with other vessels involved, most commonly cerebral or visceral arteries. In fibromuscular dysplasia the proximal one third of the main renal artery is usually free of disease with distal involvement, in contrast to that of atherosclerotic narrowing.

Angiography of the Thoracic and Abdominal Aorta

Aortography is indicated for suspected aneurysms or dissections that are suggested by clinical, historical, or procedural signs. Injection techniques are the same as for ascending aortography. A lateral projection is commonly needed for anteriorly angulated aneurysm, especially if stent graft repair of abdominal aortic aneurysm is being considered. Evaluation of peripheral lower extremity disease requires identification of iliac bifurcation and common femoral artery patency before subselective injections (see Fig. 4-28).

Angiography of the Lower Extremities

Based on clinical signs and symptoms of arterial insufficiency to the legs, suspected obstructions of vessels are often screened with noninvasive studies (e.g., ankle brachial index) before angiography is performed (Figs. 4-31 and 4-32). Small-diameter (5 F) catheters are satisfactory. Reduced volumes of contrast material (10 to 20 ml over 1 to 2 seconds) are injected during filming with panning down the artery, following the course to the most distal locations. Angulated views may be necessary to open bifurcations and overlying vessels that obscure the vessel origin. When possible, angiographic filming should extend at least to the ankle. Long cut films that cover the entire lower extremity on a moving table are available in

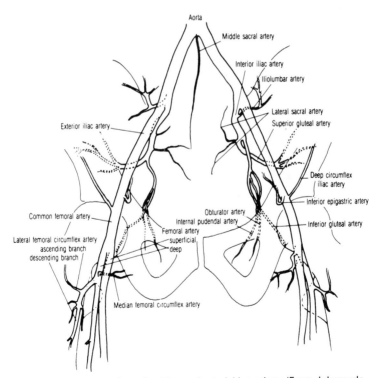

Fig. 4-31 Pelvic and proximal femoral arterial branches. (From Johnsrude IS, Jackson DC, Dunnick NR: *A practical approach to angiography,* ed 2, Boston, 1987, Little, Brown.)

radiologic suites. In cardiac catheterization laboratories, cineangiographic filming with prolonged filming and panning down to the ankle must be tested before final views are obtained. Digital subtraction techniques are available in many modern laboratories. Nonionic contrast agents are less painful than ionic media for peripheral angiography.

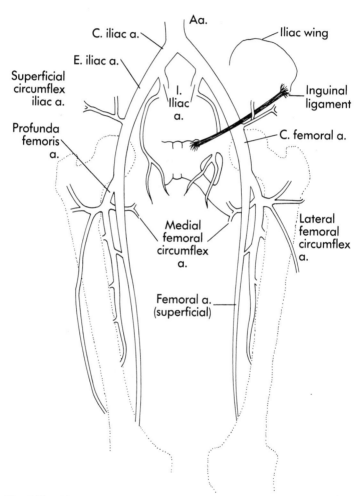

Fig. 4-32   Normal anatomy of the femoral artery, its branches, the distal runoff arteries, and the potential collateral vessels. *Aa,* Aorta; *a,* artery; *I,* internal; *C,* common; *E,* external.

One major challenge encountered with femoroiliac angiography is the contralateral (opposite leg) approach crossing over the aortic bifurcation of the iliac vessels, especially in patients with high bifurcation or prior aortobifurcation graft. To enter the opposite iliac artery, a right Judkins or internal mammary artery graft catheter or other special catheter (e.g., crossover, Simmons catheter) (see Chapter 2) is advanced with a guidewire over the bifurcation and down into the opposite femoral artery. The wire is passed down into the selected artery. The catheter may be advanced and exchanged (over a long 300-cm wire) for an appropriate angiographic or balloon dilation catheter.

The area most frequently involved in peripheral atherosclerotic disease involves the distal superficial femoral artery at the abductor canal. The calf (tibial) and knee (popliteal) arteries are the next most commonly involved vessels after the superficial femoral artery. Disease in the deep femoral artery (femoral profunda) is rare. Pathways of collateralization are often rich and varied in patients with chronic distal femoral artery disease, especially in those with total occlusions of the superficial femoral artery that reconstitutes at or below the knee close to the branching trifurcation of the tibial and deep peroneal arteries. Determining the level of reconstitution of collateralized vessels and distal runoff is crucial in determining the feasibility of revascularization. Magnified images focusing on the area of interest are frequently needed.

X-RAY IMAGE
Generation of the X-ray Image

Cardiac angiography uses a complex interaction of radiographic x-ray elements to transform energy into a visual image. The x-ray image generation chain can be simplified into three major components: (1) the x-ray generator, (2) the x-ray tube, and (3) the image intensifier. The details of x-ray equipment should be familiar to all personnel working in the catheterization laboratory. Figure 4-33 diagrams the x-ray system in a cardiac catheterization laboratory (Fig. 4-34).

X-ray Generator

The x-ray generator provides the power source necessary to accelerate the electrons through the x-ray tube. The duration of

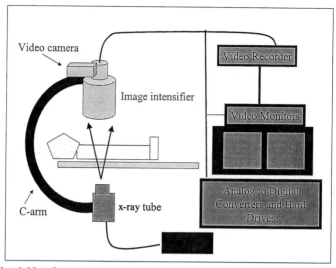

Fig. 4-33   Schematic diagram of an x-ray system. The x-ray tube below the table radiates upward through the patient table to the image intensifier. The video camera transmits the signal to video recorder, monitors, and signal processors.

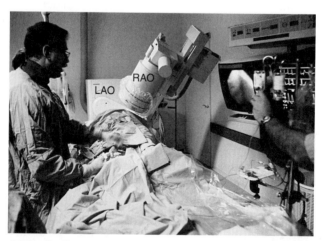

Fig. 4-34   Cardiac catheterization laboratory with C-arm over patient. Operators are observing images on fluoroscopic monitors. *LAO,* Left anterior oblique position; *RAO,* right anterior oblique position.

x-ray exposure is similar to the shutter speed on a regular camera. During the cardiac "photographic" examination the exposure is usually set at a fast enough speed to stop blurring caused by heart movement. During selective coronary arteriography, the shorter the exposure time, the better the image. Exposure times of 3 to 6 ms reduce movement blur. Most modern generators are capable of delivering adequate power and providing precise and automatically adjusted exposure timing. They are equipped with either multiple-phase (alternating on and off) or short and long pulse widths that are adjusted automatically for correct exposure. Manual settings, which are operator selected, are limited to film frame rates (e.g., 30 to 60 frames/sec).

X-ray Tubes

The function of the x-ray tube is to convert electrical energy, provided from the generator, to an x-ray beam. Electrons emitted from a heated filament (cathode) are accelerated toward a rapidly rotating disk (anode) and at contact undergo conversion to x-radiation (Fig. 4-35). This process generates

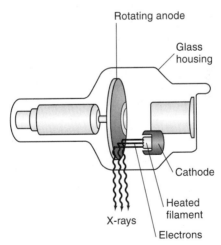

Fig. 4-35 Schematic of x-ray tube and x-ray production. A tungsten rotating anode is the target of high-energy electrons from the cathode and heating elements. The electrons striking the target release x-rays at a 90-degree angle. (Redrawn from Baim DS, Grossman W: *Grossman's cardiac catheterization, angioplasty, and intervention,* ed 6, Philadelphia, 2000, Lippincott, Williams, and Wilkens.)

extreme heat. The heat capacity of the tube is a major limiting factor in the design of x-ray tubes. Only 0.2% to 0.6% of the electrical energy provided to the tube is eventually converted to x-rays.

In addition to the exposure times (controlled by the generator system) and the size of the imaging field (controlled by the x-ray tube), two factors of the x-ray determine the quality of x-ray for proper image exposures:

1. *Electrical current (mA)*—the number of photons (electrical particles) generated per unit of time. The greater the electrical current, the greater the number of photons, resulting in improved image resolution. If the photon volume is marginal, the resulting image may be "mottled" or have a spotty appearance. Increasing the milliamperage improves this result, but the level of milliamperage is limited by the heat capacity of the x-ray tubes. Also, increasing the number of milliamperes markedly increases radiation exposure and scatter to the patient and catheterization personnel.

2. *Level of kilovoltage (kV)*—the energy spectrum (wavelengths) of the x-ray beam. The higher the level of kilovoltage, the shorter the wavelength of radiation and the greater the ability of x-rays to penetrate target tissue. Increased kilovoltage is especially important in obese patients. To obtain better images through more tissue, a higher kilovolt level is required. However, a high kilovolt level also produces lower resolution because of wide scatter, and greater radiation exposure to patients and laboratory personnel occurs. Modern radiographic equipment allows the operator to vary the amperage and voltage to attain optimal quality radiographic images. Results of using high kilovoltage are shown in Box 4-4.

An automatic exposure control system sets exposure times to incorporate changes in voltage and amperage to provide the desired images at the best exposures possible (Fig. 4-36).

Image Intensifier

After the x-rays have penetrated the body (Fig. 4-37), the partially absorbed beams are cast in a shadow fashion on the input screen of the image intensifier. The image intensifier converts the invisible x-ray image into a visual image. Each x-ray photon hits the phosphorus-covered plate of the intensifier,

Box 4-4

Results of High Kilovolt Exposure

Optimal Radiographic Technique
Lowest kilovoltage for penetration
Highest milliamperage for lowest tube heat

High Kilovoltage Yields
Low dose to patient
More mottling
More scatter
More contrast
More operator dose
Remember: Kilovolts plus milliamperes vary inversely
Kilovoltage has greater effect on contrast than milliamperage
Tube heat is less with higher kilovoltage techniques
For example:

70 kV		80 kV
400 mA	= Settings of equal density on film =	200 mA
× 5 sec		× 5 sec
140 heat units		80 heat units

Effect of Kilovolts on Cineangiographic Image
Increased kilovoltage, high energy, short wavelength, uniform penetration—all images tend to become gray at high kilovoltage
Decreased kilovoltage, discriminates among densities, provides contrast

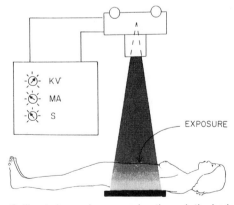

Fig. 4-36   Collimated x-ray beam passing through the body. *KV,* Kilovolts; *MA,* milliamperes; *S,* seconds. (From King SB, Douglas JS Jr: *Coronary arteriography and angioplasty,* New York, 1985, McGraw-Hill.)

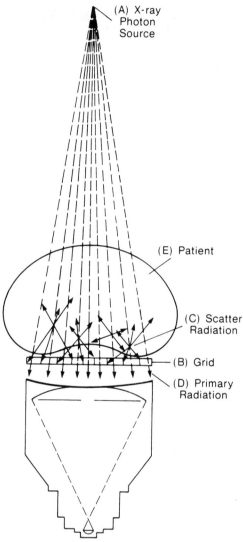

Fig. 4-37 The grid on the image intensifier aligns the beams. *A,* X-ray photon source; *B,* grid; *C,* scatter radiation; *D,* primary radiation; *E,* patient. Scatter radiation is reduced by grid in front of image intensifier. (From King SB, Douglas JS Jr: *Coronary arteriography and angioplasty,* New York, 1985, McGraw-Hill.)

resulting in a light particle, that is detected, the position and intensity of which are noted. The sum of all events produces an image for video. Image intensifiers are equipped with various-sized image fields that alter the image resolution. In general the smaller the input screen diameter, the smaller the image field size and the sharper the resolution. Smaller input screen diameters (5- to 7-inch screens) are better suited for selective coronary cineangiography because of their enhanced resolution. For more detailed work, such as percutaneous trans-luminal coronary angioplasty, even smaller input diameter (4-inch) screens are particularly useful. In contrast, for large-screen (or field) examinations (i.e., left ventriculography, aortography, or peripheral angiography) input screen diameters of 9 to 11 inches are used. The tradeoff is that detailed resolution is impaired.

Image Distortion

Magnification. The x-ray image casts an x-ray shadow onto the input screen of the image intensifier. The distance of the object from the screen determines how sharp or indistinct the image produced is. Figure 4-38 displays the effect of the object-screen distance on image quality. When an object is held close to the surface on which the shadow falls, the image is sharp. The farther the object is moved away from this surface, the larger and more indistinct the image becomes. When the image intensifier is closest to the chest wall and the heart, the image obtained is sharp. When the heart is far away from the image intensifier and closer to the x-ray source, the image is magnified but poorly defined. Increasing the distance of the heart to the image intensifier also requires more kilovoltage to produce the image and further reduces image quality.

Foreshortening. Distortion of the object's perspective is called foreshortening. Figure 4-39 displays the effects of the shadow cast by an object such as a pencil that has a concentric narrowing (similar to an artery stenosis) in the middle portion. The foreshortening (change of true length) of the pencil changes depending on the axis in relation to the beam of the x-ray. When the pencil's long axis is perpendicular to the film plane (parallel to the x-ray beam), all contour details are lost, and the shadow is seen as a dot. When the longitudinal axis is

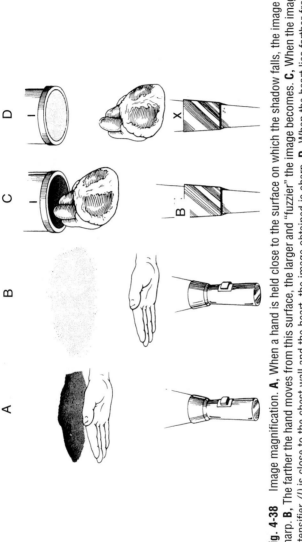

Fig. 4-38 Image magnification. **A**, When a hand is held close to the surface on which the shadow falls, the image is sharp. **B**, The farther the hand moves from this surface, the larger and "fuzzier" the image becomes. **C**, When the image intensifier (*I*) is close to the chest wall and the heart, the image obtained is sharp. **D**, When the heart lies farther from the image intensifier and close to the x-ray source (*X*), the image is magnified but poorly defined and hazy. Increased x-ray source-to-image distances require more kilovoltage, also degrading the image. (From King SB, Douglas JS Jr: *Coronary arteriography and angioplasty*, New York, 1985, McGraw-Hill.)

seen at an oblique angle, the length shadow is foreshortened, and when the axis is perpendicular to the x-ray beam (parallel to the film plane), a full and true image of the length and contour details can be seen. Because of foreshortening, arterial lesions that may appear severe in one projection may not appear at all or may seem significantly less severe in other projections. For this reason, multiple projections are used to identify the severity of lesions within the coronary tree.

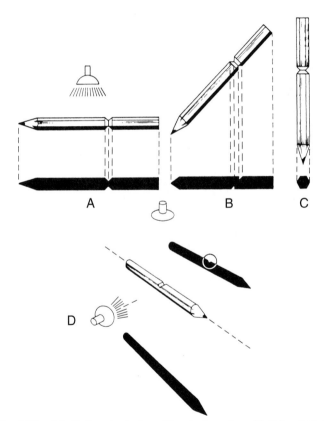

Fig. 4-39   A to C, Foreshortening of the shadow of an object is not parallel with the filming plane. **D,** To evaluate a slitlike lesion accurately, the operator must use a view perpendicular to the longitudinal axis of the vessel but parallel to the longest diameter of the lesion. (From Pujadas G: *Coronary angiography in the medical and surgical treatment of ischemic heart disease,* New York, 1980, McGraw-Hill.)

Videotape Monitors and Recorders

A videotape recorder is used in combination with the angiographic system monitors to record the fluoroscopic images so that they can be reviewed rapidly and information is not lost if something happens to the digital transfer or cineangiographic film. These video recorders commonly use 0.5- to 1-inch tape. Most laboratories now rely on digital cardiac imaging in the laboratory to review angiographic data before a procedure is finished.

X-ray System Preparations by the Angiographic Nurse, Technician, or Assistant

The cineangiography preparations include the establishment of a checklist sequence of steps from x-ray generation to CD or film viewing. A staff member should check the x-ray unit first thing each morning. The following should be checked before the start of a procedure:

1. The staff member ensures the unit powers up and makes fluoroscopic and cineangiographic exposures.
2. A short cineangiographic test strip of a resolution phantom is run to check resolution, known as "line pairs" (smallest distance in millimeters between lines that can be seen).
3. TV monitor screens are cleaned. Contrast and brightness controls are adjusted to optimum.
4. Fluoroscopic times are reset to zero.
5. Proper exposure station is selected.
6. Digital imaging and archiving stations are activated.
7. A patient name plate picture is taken at the start of each procedure.

Technical notes: During the procedure the angiographic technician may be responsible for the angulation of the image intensifier and panning. In some institutions the physician may perform this function. To obtain optimal cineangiograms, the staff should be aware of the following principles:

1. The image intensifier should be as close to the patient's chest as possible. This position optimizes the image detail and decreases scatter radiation.
2. The patient should be instructed to take a deep breath and hold it before the start of cineangiography. This

pulls the diaphragm downward and out of the field of view. The presence of the dense diaphragmatic image in the field can cause poor-quality images. During deep inspiration the x-ray exposure changes automatically (automatic brightness control). It is helpful if a staff member practices breath-holding technique with the patient before the start of the procedure.

3. All ECG electrodes, lead wires, metal snaps on the patient's gown, and jewelry should be out of the field of view before the start of the procedure. Keeping the intravenous lines and wires from hanging down under the table prevents the x-ray tube from pulling out a lead or intravenous tube.

4. Use of the collimators (shutters) should be mandatory. The operator should focus on the exact area of interest to be photographed. This technique eliminates unwanted lung field brightness and helps optimize exposure settings for the automatic brightness control system.

5. During cineangiography the staff member responsible for data recording should note the following information:

   a. Time of each contrast medium injection.

   b. The projection angulation of the cineangiographic unit (right or left obliques and the degree of cranial or caudal angulation). Most x-ray units have a digital readout for these angulations.

   c. The type and French size of the catheter used for each angiogram.

   d. The names and doses of any drugs that are given during the procedure. Drugs that affect coronary dilation or constriction given during the angiogram procedure should be recorded on the film with a lead letter marker.

   e. If LV angiographic volume is to be calculated, a calibrated grid is filmed to calculate a correction factor for ventricular volume analysis. The nurse or technician must record certain data during the ventriculogram that are necessary for grid and image intensifier placement. These data include (1) the position of the image intensifier in relation to the x-ray table top at the time of the left ventriculogram, (2) measurement of the patient's AP diameter so that grid placement can approximate the position of the left ventricle during the angiography, and (3) if a dual or trimode (4-, 6-, or 9-inch) image intensifier is used, the image intensifier magnification for each angiogram.

Imaging Equipment Preventive Maintenance

The x-ray unit should be placed on a program of scheduled preventive maintenance that is performed by trained service technicians. This maintenance should be done at least biannually, with quarterly checks preferred. Maintenance and cleaning schedules should be monitored by the staff so that equipment can be scheduled for routine maintenance (Boxes 4-5 and 4-6).

DIGITAL ANGIOGRAPHY

Digital angiography converts the x-ray image into a quantitative information format for storage and display on a computer. Digital angiography stores x-ray images on magnetic

---

Box 4-5

Optimizing Cineangiographic Techniques
1. Cleaning image chain is important (at least every 1 to 2 months):
   a. Clean cineangiographic camera mirror and lenses
   b. Clean projector lenses, mirrors (every 2 months)
2. Check the following cineangiographic optic chain:
   a. Cineangiographic lens focus tight
   b. f-stop correct (no role in resolution because flat plane)
   c. Image focused on plane of image intensifier
   d. Film magazines secured tightly
3. Cineangiographic film: correct for changing technique if new angiographic equipment installed
4. Processor: fast enough for rapid processing for interventional (percutaneous transluminal coronary angioplasty) procedures when problems need angiographic review
5. Darkroom operator: cross trained for backup staffing
6. Photographic chemistry: corrected for film and techniques
7. Quality control:
   a. Daily, weekly, monthly
   b. Single technician job for high level of reproducibility

Box 4-6

Preventive Maintenance Scheduling for Imaging Equipment

Daily
Clean TV monitor screen
Clean projector screens
Monitor densitometer results
Run a daily cineangiography of resolution phantom and check the line pairs visible

Weekly
Clean lenses on cineangiographic projectors
Clean film debris from cineangiographic camera
Check lens on cineangiographic camera and clean as needed
Clean film processor
Change tapes on videotape decks
Clean heads on videotape decks

tapes, disks, or other electronic media rather than on x-ray film. Digital angiography permits compact storage and quantitative image analysis. Digital imaging also permits various manipulations of the data to enhance the stored images. The contrast image can be amplified or enlarged, or contrast can be adjusted. One image can be subtracted from another, and that image can be subtracted from a third image. Similar contrast adjustments and enlargements are not possible with film radiographs.

Some digital angiography systems may not provide the exquisite resolution of detail found in radiographic films. Digital imaging is now satisfactory for nearly all clinical uses, however. The digital subtraction technique is sensitive to motion, requiring a patient who is alert and can cooperate during the procedure. The durability of some digital archival media has been questioned.

Digital Angiography Systems

Pulsed System. The pulsed system acquires images relatively infrequently. One image per second with a 1026×1026 digital matrix is a typical acquisition rate. Some systems may indicate that 15 images per second can be acquired. (Cineangiographic filming acquisition rates are >30 frames/sec.)

Pulsed systems require special TV cameras and x-ray generators. They operate by pulsing the generator at high-milliamperage currents, which provides a heavy burst of x-ray energy to the image intensifier to obtain sharp images. A single image is scanned by the TV camera, which overcomes the blurring of the x-ray image. Images are stored until after the run is complete.

Fluoroscopic (Real-Time) System. Real-time digital fluoroscopy does not require a special TV camera. Fluoroscopic milliamperage levels from 5 to 20 mA produce satisfactory imaging. The milliamperage required depends on the specific performance of the image intensifier system. A three-phase x-ray generator is not required. Because of the fluoroscopic x-ray requirements and in contrast to pulsed systems, special heavy-duty x-ray tubes are not required. A 300,000–heat unit tube is satisfactory.

The image processing occurs in real time as the data acquisition progresses. For subtraction imaging the operator views the TV monitor as the examination is proceeding. This ability to see the contrast agent passing through the region of interest allows the operator to terminate image acquisition and fluoroscopy as soon as the contrast medium has passed. There is no need for long run-on as there is with pulsed systems.

Digital Subtraction Technique. Many digital angiographic systems use functions of the image processor during fluoroscopy. Subtraction angiography is performed by obtaining a mask imaging without contrast material, then subtracting it from the image with contrast material in the vessel. The resultant image (subtracted) shows only the vessel in detail unobscured by bones and other structures.

Quantitative Coronary Angiography

The degree of coronary stenosis is usually a visual estimation of the percentage of diameter narrowing, with the proximal, assumed normal, arterial segment as a reference. The ratio of normal to stenosis artery diameter is widely used in clinical practice but is inadequate for a true quantitative methodology. The intraobserver variability may range from 40% to 80%, and there is frequently a range of 20% on interobserver differences.

Quantitative methodologies include digital calipers, automated or manual edge detection systems, and densitometric analysis with digital angiography.

RADIATION SAFETY

Radiation protection equipment for all personnel must be available in every cardiac catheterization laboratory. Standards for radiation protection in the cardiac catheterization laboratory have been published by the Society of Cardiac Angiography. Four principles in radiation safety should be self-evident:

1. The less exposure, the less chance of absorbed energy biologic interaction.
2. No known level of ionizing radiation is a permissible dose or absolutely safe.
3. Radiation exposure is cumulative. No washout phenomenon occurs.
4. All participants in the cardiac catheterization laboratory have voluntarily accepted some degree of radiation exposure, but they are obligated to minimize and reduce risks to other personnel and themselves.

The source of radiation in the cardiac catheterization laboratory is the primary x-ray beam that emanates from the undertable tube upward and outward toward the image intensifier. Scatter of this beam exposes all subjects to radiation in a dose *geometrically inverse* to the distance from the source. Radiation scatter is increased when the angle of the tube is set obliquely. A high degree of angulation with large obliquities increases the amount of radiation scatter. Acrylic lead shields and lead table mounted aprons should be used to reduce the amount of scatter.

Fluoroscopy generates x-ray exposure approximately one fifth that of cineangiography. The increased use of cineangiography for complex catheterization procedures has increased the total radiation exposure in the laboratory and should be a consideration in procedures requiring extensive intracardiac manipulation, such as PCI or valvuloplasty.

Personal Radiation Protection

Protection from radiation for the laboratory personnel should include eye, neck, and body protection. Physicians performing cardiac angiography with U-arm systems should be protected by room-installed radiation shields. The exposure with a shield resulting from performing 25 examinations per week on a continuous basis would be within the recommendations of the National Commission on Radiologic Protection and Units.

Radiation exposure is greater during PCI than during diagnostic catheterization. If the protective shields are used carefully, the radiation exposure for single- and double-vessel angioplasty procedures and exposure for diagnostic catheterization procedures may be comparable. Radiation exposures are generally higher for the angioplasty procedures, however, especially when biplane angiography is performed.

During angiographic studies 90% of the x-ray energy entering the body is absorbed. It has been shown that a single exposure of 200 R can produce cataract formation in humans. Thyroid cancers and other carcinomas are associated with x-rays. Techniques often used to improve image quality (e.g., increased amperage, voltage, LAO views) have resulted in increased exposure. A summary of radiation safety for the cardiac catheterization laboratory is provided in Box 4-7 and discussed in Chapter 1.

Box 4-7

Radiation During Catheterization

Radiation to Patient
From the primary x-ray beam
Affects thyroid, eyes, gonads, bone marrow, or gastrointestinal tract
Highest exposure of any diagnostic test

Radiation to Staff
Long-term low dose from scatter, tube leakage
Affects thyroid and eyes
Accepted occupational exposure

Means of Limiting Dose
Maintaining equipment safeguards
Optimizing milliamperage and kilovoltage
Minimizing exposure time
Minimizing scatter with shielding and techniques
Using all protective measures

ANGIOGRAPHIC EQUIPMENT

INJECTORS AND CONTRAST MATERIALS

The angiographic power injector allows the angiographer to administer a precise volume (bolus) of contrast material at a rapid, preset flow rate. Power injectors are necessary for performing most ventricular and vascular angiography. The injector accepts a large syringe for radiographic contrast media. The power injector settings are selected, and on receiving an electronic signal, a calibrated motor discharges the exact amount of contrast material at the predetermined rate through a connecting tube and catheter to the patient. The quantity and type of contrast material (concentration or dilution) and rate of injection are selected by the operator or physician. The signal to the injector to begin contrast material injection is transmitted from a hand- or foot-operated switch.

Power Contrast Injector: Responsibilities of the Nurse or Technician

1. For an off-table freestanding injector, the nurse or technician loads the syringe with contrast media.
2. The nurse or technician sets the volume, flow rate, and rate of pressure rise parameters as instructed by the physician.
3. The nurse or technician presses the inject button that triggers the injection. Releasing the button stops the injection.

The staff member and physicians must be aware of the following points regarding safe power injection.

Clear Air Bubbles. All air must be expelled from the contrast-filled syringe before making the injector available to the physician for the catheter connection. Under no circumstances should the head of the power injector be tilted toward the catheterization table or made available for the physician if air is in the syringe.

Several techniques are used to establish an air-free system when connecting the catheter to the syringe. A running connection is a technique in which a small amount of contrast material is squirted out of the syringe while the catheter is being connected to the syringe. Merging of the fluid streams of blood from the catheter and the forward flow of contrast material from the syringe prevents any large air bubbles from entering the system on connection. After connection the injector operator always aspirates more fluid (usually contrast material in the connector tube) into the syringe to ensure that no air bubbles are present. If air is present, it is expelled, and the clearing procedure is redone.

The operator must be careful when aspirating blood into the contrast syringe for two reasons: (1) a large blood volume in the syringe dilutes the contrast material, and (2) more important, but rarely, after some time the blood may clot in the injector syringe.

Test Injection in Ventricle. When the system is free of air, the injector operator and the physician should be sure that the catheter is cleared of blood. The injector operator squirts a small amount of contrast material out the tip of the catheter under x-ray visualization. This small test injection of contrast material also helps the physician ascertain proper catheter position for ventriculography.

Confirm Injector Settings. The physician should orally confirm the power injector settings for the contrast volume and delivery rate desired. The injector operator should *repeat* the injection parameters back to the physician to eliminate any chance of error in injector setup.

Depending on the type of injector being used, the flow rate may be determined by setting an amount in milliliters per second or by setting the pressure. Regardless of the system, the staff member must ensure that the catheter being used can accept the flow rate that has been entered into the injector.

Safety Features. When the physician has initiated a cine-angiographic run, the injector operator must listen for the physician's command to start the injection. The nurse or technician should be prepared to stop the injection (by hitting or releasing the trigger button) at any time as directed by the physician or at his or her own discretion (e.g., when the catheter is pulled back or a contrast stain in the heart muscle is seen).

Note: All personnel should be watching the power injection setup and injections for small bubbles or other problems. Six (or more) eyes are better than four for seeing catheterization laboratory problems.

Power injectors have many safety features that must be understood by the cardiac catheterization laboratory staff. To ensure patient safety during angiography, staff members must understand all aspects of the operation of the power injector and the built-in safeguards.

Contrast Media

The catheterization laboratory staff provides the technical support with regard to contrast media during angiography in the following areas:

1. Contrast agents should be warmed to body temperature before administration. Commercial warmers are available from the companies that manufacture contrast media. A warm water bath is sometimes used to warm contrast material, but temperature control is difficult to regulate.

2. The nurse or technician preparing the patient for angiography should ask the patient if he or she is aware of any known contrast allergy. Iodine gives contrast material its radiopaque qualities and is a known allergen. Some believe that a history of seafood allergy (iodine is found in certain seafoods, especially shellfish) is significant and the physician should be notified. The physician may wish to give corticosteroids or antihistamines to these patients before performing angiography (see Chapter 1).

3. Before the administration of contrast agents the patient should be prepared for the sensations associated with contrast administration. Some patients have nausea and vomiting. The patient should not have ingested food or water before angiography. If vomiting occurs, the staff member should be quick to respond; the patient's head should be turned (away from the sterile field) to the side to prevent aspiration. This is particularly important when the patient has been heavily sedated for the procedure. Low-osmolality and nonionic contrast agents produce less nausea and vomiting than ionic media.

4. Patients should be told that they may have a hot flushing sensation (caused by artery vasodilation) during bolus

injections of contrast media. This uncomfortable sensation is reduced with the use of nonionic contrast agents. Direct injection of ionic contrast material into peripheral vessels produces a painful burning and cramping sensation in the injected area. The nonionic and low-osmolar agents are highly recommended for peripheral vascular angiography.

During angiography it is important for the nurse to document the type and amount of contrast material delivered. The patient should be observed for any signs of allergy, such as hives, flushed skin, bronchospasm, or laryngeal edema (hoarseness). Appropriate medications for treatment of anaphylaxis, such as epinephrine, and an airway should always be available and easily accessible during administration of contrast agents.

Because hypotension, bradycardia, and arrhythmia are commonly associated with iodinated contrast media administration, the ECG and arterial pressure should be monitored continuously by a laboratory staff member specifically given this responsibility. Atropine, vasopressors, and antiarrhythmic agents should be available for prompt administration.

When ionic contrast material is injected into the coronary artery, transient bradycardia or hypotension may occur. The physician may want the patient to cough after the injection because coughing maintains arterial pressure and cerebral blood flow and influences vagal tone. The staff should instruct the patient on when and how to cough (one or two deep, rapid coughs) before the coronary arteriography. Coughing does not increase coronary blood flow. Increased use of nonionic and low-osmolality contrast agents has reduced greatly the incidence of bradycardia, arrhythmia, hypotension, and the need for coughing during coronary arteriography.

After angiography the nurse or technician should monitor the patient's urine output. An increase in urine output after the procedure is normal. A decrease in urine output after contrast material administration should be documented and the physician notified. Because of increased diuresis caused by the hypertonicity of some contrast agents, the patient should increase fluid intake to replace body fluids lost after contrast material administration. A common practice is the administration of at least 500 to 1000 ml of normal saline IV over 4 to 6 hours after the catheterization.

Selection of Radiographic Contrast Media

The contrast material is selected for the specific examination to be conducted. All contrast materials are x-ray "dense" (as a result of iodine) compared with body structures, which are more x-ray "lucent" and absorb x-rays to provide different gray shades in x-ray images. The quantity and concentration of contrast materials used are specific medical decisions. Factors included in these decisions are the patient's age, size, general health, allergies, and cardiac condition.

All contrast agents contain iodine, an effective absorber of x-rays. Although all agents are derivatives of benzoic acid, the number of iodine molecules and ionic and osmolar composition vary (Fig. 4-40). Osmolarity, viscosity, sodium content, and other additives and properties are different among these agents. Table 4-5 summarizes commonly used contrast agents for coronary and LV angiographic studies. Selection of a contrast agent for the particular laboratory is, to a large extent, a matter of personal preference. Major differences between ionic and nonionic contrast agents include cost, induction of bradycardia and hypotension, and impairment of LV function. Thousands of studies have been performed safely with conventional high-osmolar and ionic agents and pose no major risks. Considerable data exist, however, to suggest that low-osmolar and nonionic agents may be safer and provide satisfactory diagnostic quality, especially for high-risk patients. Indications for low-osmolar/nonionic contrast agents include unstable ischemic syndromes, congestive heart failure, diabetes, renal insufficiency, hypotension, severe bradycardia, history of contrast allergy, severe valvular heart disease, and use for internal mammary artery and peripheral vascular injections.

Ionic contrast media produce hypotension by peripheral arterial vasodilation, transient myocardial dysfunction, and decrease in circulating volume and blood pressure after osmotic diuresis (initially contrast media increase circulating fluid volume by osmotically shifting fluid into the vascular space).

ANGIOGRAPHIC CATHETERS

Many shapes and sizes of catheters are available to the angiographer (see Chapter 2). Basic routine catheters that are preshaped for normal anatomy are available for radial and

Class	Structure	Examples	Iodine	Osm	Viscosity@37°
High Osmolar Ionic Ratio 1.5 (3:2)	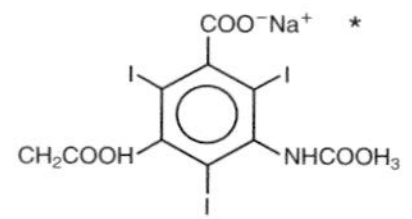	Diatrizoate (Renografin, Hypaque, Angiovist)	370	2076	8.4
Low Osmolar Non-ionic Ratio 3 (3:1)		Iothalmate (Conray)	325	1797	2.8
		Metrizoate (Isopaque)	--		
Low Osmolar Non-ionic Ratio 3 (3:1)	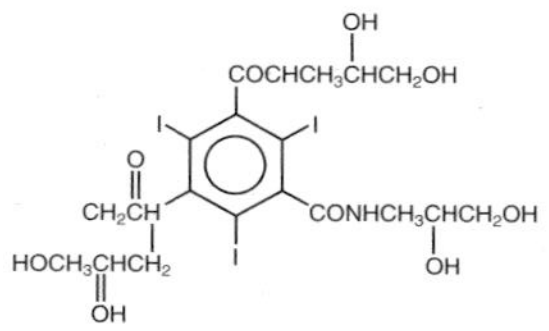	Iopamidol (Isovue)	370	796	9.4
		Iohexol (Omnipaque)	350	844	10.4
		Ioversol (Optiray)	350	792	9.0
		Ioxilan (Oxilan)	350	695	8.1
Low Osmolar Ionic Dimer Ratio 3 (6:2)	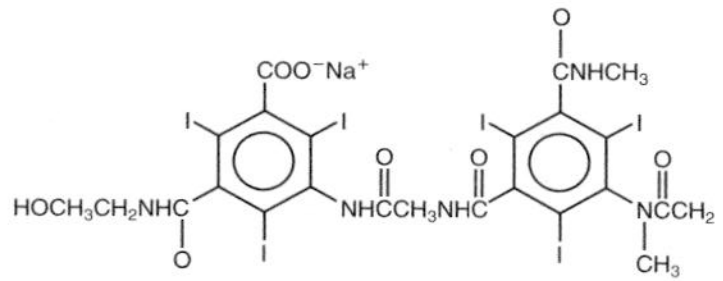	Ioxaglate (Hexabrix)	320	600	7.5
Iso-Osmolar Non-ionic Dimer Ratio 6 (6:1)	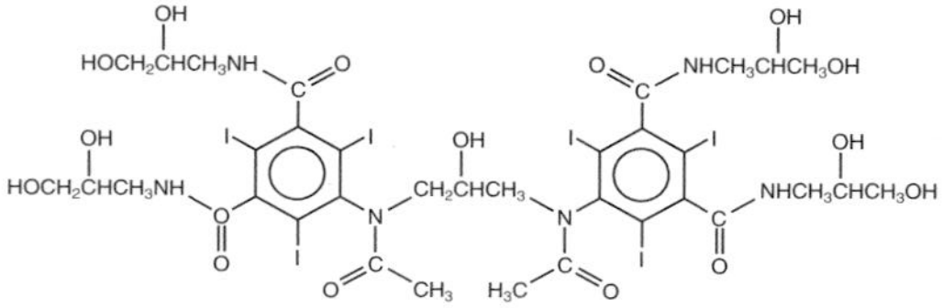	Iodixanol (Visipaque)	320	290	11.8

Fig. 4-40   Properties of radiographic contrast media used in the cardiac catheterization laboratory. (Redrawn from Baim DS, Grossman W: *Grossman's cardiac catheterization, angioplasty, and intervention*, ed 6, Philadelphia, 2000, Lippincott, Williams, and Wilkins.)

Table 4-5

Commonly Used Iodinated Contrast Agents in Cardiac Angiography

Product Category Name	Proprietary Constituent	Generic Active Particles	Ratio of Iodine to Osmotically	Calcium Chelation	Anticoagulation Effect
High-osmolar, ionic	Renografin-76	Diatrizoate and citrate	1.5	(+)	(+++)
High-osmolar, ionic	Hypaque-76	Diatrizoate only	1.5	(−)	(+++)
Low-osmolar, ionic	Hexabrix	Ioxaglate	3.0	(−)	(+++)
Low-osmolar, nonionic	Isovue	Iopamidol	3.0	(−)	(+)
Low-osmolar, nonionic	Omnipaque	Iohexol	3.0	(−)	(+)
Low-osmolar, nonionic	Optiray	Ioversol	3.0	(−)	(+)

(+) = present; (+++) = strongly present; (−) = absent.
From Peterson KL, Nicod P: *Cardiac catheterization: methods, diagnosis, and therapy*, Philadelphia, 1997, WB Saunders.

femoral approaches. The angiographer can select from an array of shapes and sizes when abnormal anatomy is present. The nurse or technician is responsible for knowing the different types of catheters that are available and the indications for their use. The experienced staff member becomes familiar with the different types of difficult anatomy and anticipates what type of catheter may be necessary to achieve proper catheter placement. Anticipation of the physician's needs for special equipment during difficult procedures is not only the mark of a good support staff, but also greatly reduces procedure length and improves patient safety and comfort.

MEDICATIONS USED IN CORONARY ANGIOGRAPHY

Box 4-8 lists medications commonly used during cardiac catheterization.

Coronary Vasodilators

Nitroglycerin. Nitroglycerin is the most commonly used drug during coronary arteriography and ventriculography. Nitroglycerin dilates peripheral arteries, venous beds, and coronary arteries. Nitroglycerin is a safe and short-acting drug. It can be given through the sublingual, IV, intracoronary, or intraventricular route. Sublingual (or oral spray) nitroglycerin (0.4 mg) is frequently given before coronary arteriography. Exceptions include patients in whom coronary spasm is suspected and patients with hypotension (<90 mm Hg systolic pressure). In patients with documented coronary spasm, sublingual or intracoronary nitroglycerin is given to eliminate coronary spasm. In patients with unstable angina, IV infusions of nitroglycerin of up to 250 µg/min with a systolic blood pressure of 90 mm Hg are permissible. In patients in the catheterization laboratory with elevated LV end-diastolic pressure from ischemia or congestive heart failure, intraventricular or IV boluses of 200 µg of nitroglycerin reduce LV end-diastolic pressure and are appropriate before and after ventriculography. Intracoronary nitroglycerin in doses of 50, 100, and 200 µg increases coronary blood flow without a marked reduction in pressure. With doses of more than 250 µg, hypotension without further increases in coronary blood flow may be evident. Care should be used to avoid inducing hypotension when administering nitroglycerin to

Box 4-8

Medications Used in the Cardiac Catheterization Laboratory*

Inotropic Agents
Digitalis 0.125 to 0.25 mg IV >4 hours apart
Dobutamine 2 to 10 µg/kg/min IV drip
Dopamine 2 to 10 µg/kg/min IV drip
Epinephrine 1:10,000 IV
Isoproterenol 1 mg/min IV drip

Antiarrhythmic Agents, Anticholinergic Agents, β-Blockers, Calcium Blockers
Adenosine 5 to 12 mg IV bolus
Atropine 0.6 to 1.2 mg IV
Bretylium 100 to 300 mg IV bolus
Diltiazem 10 mg IV
Esmolol 4 to 24 mg/kg IV drip (β-blocker)
Lidocaine 50 to 100 mg IV bolus; 2 to 4 mg/min IV drip
Procainamide 50 to 100 mg IV
Propranolol 1 mg bolus; 0.1 mg/kg in three divided doses (β-blocker)
Verapamil 2 to 5 mg IV, may repeat dose to 10 mg (calcium channel blocker)

Analgesic Agents, Sedatives
Diazepam 2 to 5 mg IV
Diphenhydramine 25 to 50 mg IV
Meperidine 12.5 to 50 mg IV
Morphine sulfate 2.5 mg IV
Naloxone 0.5 mg IV

Anticoagulants
Heparin 2000 to 5000 U IV; 1000 U/hr IV drip; 40-70 µ/kg for PCI

Vasodilators
Nitroglycerin 1/150 sublingual 100 to 300 µg IC
Nitroprusside 5 to 50 µg/kg/min IV

Vasoconstrictors
Metaraminol 10 mg in 100 ml saline, 1 ml IV
Ergonovine 0.4 mg IV in divided doses
Norepinephrine 1:10,000 IV, 1-ml doses IV

IC, Intracoronary; *IV*, intravenous; *PCI*, percutaneous coronary intervention.
*The list is not meant to be all-inclusive or to exclude emergency life support techniques or standards.

patients with known or suspected severe aortic stenosis, significant LMCA narrowing, or hypertrophic myopathy.

Calcium Channel Blockers. Calcium channel blockers dilate vascular smooth muscle and reduce heart muscle contractility, and some agents block AV nodal conduction. Calcium channel blockers are used to reduce peripheral vascular resistance, decrease blood pressure, block coronary spasm, and increase coronary blood flow. Acute use in the cardiac catheterization laboratory is limited to treating arrhythmias and no-reflow of coronary interventions or to treat radial artery spasm when the transradial approach is used. Doses for calcium channel blockers are as follows: diltiazem, 30 to 60 mg orally, 10 mg IV; verapamil, 120 mg orally, 2.5 to 5 mg IV (for coronary no-reflow, intracoronary bolus of verapamil, 200 µg, to be repeated for two to four doses if needed).

Papaverine. Papaverine is a potent arterial vasodilator used in the investigation of coronary vasodilatory reserve. Intracoronary papaverine causes a marked increase in blood flow in the RCA in doses of 4 to 8 mg and in the LCA in doses of 8 to 12 mg. Doses exceeding these recommended levels do not seem to provide an increase over the maximal blood flow. Papaverine causes QT prolongation. Rare cases of papaverine-induced torsades de pointes have been reported, and antiarrhythmic preparations for this unusual event should be in place before administration of intracoronary papaverine.

Adenosine. Adenosine IV is used for breaking supraventricular tachycardia and is the drug of choice for intracoronary induction of maximal hyperemia for coronary vasodilator reserve. Intracoronary adenosine, 12 to 24 µg for the RCA, and 24 to 40 µg for the LCA, produces optimal results. Adenosine infusions, 140 µg/kg/min IV, produce sustained hyperemia. Adenosine hyperemia lasts less than 60 seconds after drug administration is ended.

Acetylcholine. Acetylcholine dilates normal coronary arteries and constricts diseased vessels. In Japan intracoronary doses of 20, 50, and 100 µg have been used to induce coronary spasm in patients. The drug is short acting and rapidly inactivated, making it suitable for catheterization laboratory use. Marked bradycardia, heart block, and vasospasm are common with acetylcholine. Temporary pacing is required during its administration. Continuous infusions of 0.02 to 2.2 μg (10^{-8}, 10^{-7}, 10^{-6} M) have been used to identify normal endothelial function of coronary vessels (vasodilation, not vasoconstriction).

Nitroprusside. For coronary no-reflow, a 25- to 100-μg bolus of nitroprusside can be used and repeated as needed.

Coronary Vasoconstrictor (for Provocation of Coronary Spasm Only)

Ergonovine. Ergonovine is used to provoke coronary vasospasm in patients with chest pain syndromes and normal or near-normal coronary arteriograms. One commonly used regimen is sequential doses of 0.02, 0.18, and 0.2 mg IV at 3-minute intervals, with ECGs obtained at the end of each dose for a total dose of 0.4 mg. If typical symptoms develop, an ECG is obtained and arteriography performed immediately on the LCA and RCA. Ergonovine-induced diffuse coronary vasoconstriction is a physiologic response. Ergonovine-induced focal coronary constriction (relieved with nitroglycerin) is a positive response for coronary spasm. These angiographic changes should be associated with ECG or symptomatic alterations. Ergonovine-induced coronary vasospasm or physiologic narrowing can be reversed immediately with intracoronary nitroglycerin. Figure 4-41 shows ergonovine-induced coronary spasm.

Anticholinergics for Vagal Reactions

Atropine. Atropine is used to block vagally induced slowing of the heart rate and hypotension. Doses of 0.6 to 1.2 mg IV given immediately reverse bradycardia and hypotension within 2 minutes. In elderly patients and patients who have pacemakers, the heart rate may not slow during vagal episodes in which the only manifestation is low blood pressure. This low blood pressure can be alleviated by the administration of intravenous atropine and normal saline. In the rare patient in whom intravenous access is not immediately available, intraarterial atropine (in the aorta) can be administered.

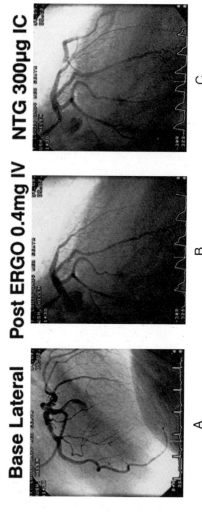

Fig. 4-41 Coronary angiograms depicting the responses to ergonovine in a patient with coronary vasospasm. **A,** Baseline angiogram in the lateral projection. **B,** Coronary vasoconstriction after ergonovine, 0.4 mg intravenously. **C,** Intracoronary nitroglycerin was administered. *Continued*

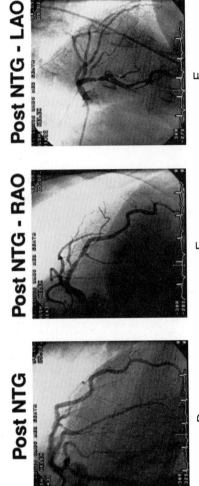

Post NTG   **Post NTG - RAO**   **Post NTG - LAO**

D   E   F

Fig. 4-41, cont'd   **D,** Response after nitroglycerin in the same projection. **E** and **F,** Right anterior oblique and left anterior oblique projections in the postnitroglycerin phase with the coronary artery.

Vasoconstrictors are reserved for persistent hypotension after recovery of heart rate.

Antiarrhythmic Drugs

Lidocaine. Lidocaine is an antiarrhythmic drug used to block or reduce the number of ventricular extrasystoles. Lidocaine can be administered as a bolus of 50 to 100 mg IV before ventriculography if a stable and quiet catheter position within the LV cannot be obtained. In patients in whom myocardial ischemia develops during cardiac catheterization or angioplasty, lidocaine for frequent ventricular ectopy is indicated. A bolus of 50 to 100 mg IV followed by a 1 to 2 mg/min infusion is usually satisfactory.

Amiodarone. Amiodarone is indicated when recurrent ventricular fibrillation or recurrent hemodynamically unstable ventricular tachycardia is nonresponsive to adequate doses of other antiarrhythmics or when alternative agents cannot be tolerated. The loading dose is 150 mg IV over 10 minutes (15 mg/min), then 360 mg intravenously over the next 6 hours (1 mg/min), followed by 540 mg IV over next 18 hours (0.5 mg/min). After the first 24 hours a maintenance IV infusion of 720 mg/24 hr (0.5 mg/min) is continued.

In the catheterization laboratory, amiodarone has been associated with bradycardia, hypotension, arrhythmias, heart failure, heart block, sinus arrest, and edema. Amiodarone may reduce hepatic or renal clearance of certain antiarrhythmics (especially flecainide, procainamide, and quinidine). Use of amiodarone with other antiarrhythmics (especially mexiletine, propafenone, quinidine, disopyramide, and procainamide) may induce torsades de pointes. Amiodarone should be used cautiously with antihypertensives, β-blockers, and calcium channel blockers because of increased cardiac depressant effects and slowing of sinoatrial node and atrioventricular conduction.

Amiodarone may potentiate anticoagulant response with the potential for serious or fatal bleeding. The warfarin dose should be decreased 33% to 50% when amiodarone is initiated. Amiodarone is contraindicated in cardiogenic shock, second-degree or third-degree atrioventricular block, and severe sinoatrial node disease resulting in preexisting bradycardia unless a pacemaker is present.

Cardiac Agonists

Isoproterenol. Isoproterenol is a pure β agonist that increases heart rate and causes peripheral vasodilation. It is indicated during cardiac arrest with refractory bradycardia. Isoproterenol has been used for provocation of cardiac stress (increased heart rate) in patients with valvular heart disease or hypertrophic cardiomyopathy. It is no longer used in the cardiac catheterization laboratory.

Dopamine. Dopamine is a potent vasoconstrictor. In low doses it causes renal vasodilation. In high doses it causes peripheral vasoconstriction, elevating the blood pressure and increasing myocardial contractility. In doses of 2 to 15 μg/min dopamine acts to cause vasoconstriction and tachycardia, elevating the blood pressure for problems resulting in severe hypotension.

Dobutamine. Dobutamine is a potent inotropic agent with no peripheral vasoconstrictor effects. It increases cardiac contractility (inotropy) and is especially useful in patients with low cardiac output or congestive heart failure. Dobutamine may be used in conjunction with a potent vasodilator, such as nitroprusside, in patients with markedly elevated filling pressures and poor cardiac output.

Epinephrine. Epinephrine (1:10,000) is a naturally occurring catecholamine that stimulates cardiac function. It is administered only during cardiac emergencies. This medicine increases heart rate and blood pressure immediately, sometimes to very high levels. Epinephrine should be reserved for patients needing cardiac resuscitation, patients in whom refractory hypotension is present and not responding to peripheral vasoconstrictors, or patients with anaphylactic reactions. Transthoracic administration of epinephrine through a long needle is no longer performed. IV or intraarterial administration of 1 ml of 1:10,000 dilution can increase systemic pressure transiently during hypotension to a safe level until IV vasopressors have been prepared. This dose of epinephrine has a duration of action of 5 to 10 minutes.

Arterial Vasodilators

Nitroprusside. Nitroprusside is a potent, short-acting intravenous arterial vasodilator used to treat aortic insufficiency, mitral regurgitation, hypertensive crisis, and congestive heart failure. Doses administered range from 10 to 100 μg/min and must be monitored by direct arterial pressure measurement.

Recording Medications on Cine Film During Angiography

If drugs that may affect the angiograms are given during the course of the catheterization, the medication may be marked on the film with a cineangiographic exposure of the radiopaque drug marker. Examples of such drugs are sublingual or intracoronary nitroglycerin or ergonovine. A radiographic clock marker may also be used to indicate the time of such events.

PACEMAKERS

Cardiac pacing is a low-risk means of providing emergency cardiac rhythm, especially in cases of symptomatic bradycardia or asystole. Since the introduction of low-osmolar or nonionic contrast media, significant bradycardia and asystole during coronary angiography have been nearly eliminated, obviating the need for prophylactic pacing in this setting. Cardiac pacemakers may be used prophylactically during cardiac catheterization to reduce hemodynamic compromise of heart block and have been used to rescue patients after development of conduction abnormalities associated with hypotension.

The use of pacemakers is not required for routine coronary arteriography and ventriculography and most PCI procedures. External pacing patches are useful for emergency pacing when a temporary pacing wire cannot be positioned immediately. The patient is sedated when pacing patches are used because each electrical stimulation causes chest muscle and heart muscle contraction and may be painful.

Indications

Indications for pacemakers are as follows:
   1. Previously demonstrated high-degree conduction block

2. Symptomatic bradycardia (after contrast administration or angiography of RCA)
3. Preexisting left bundle-branch block with anticipated right-sided heart studies
4. Acetylcholine studies (some ergonovine studies)
5. Acute myocardial infarction with trifascicular block
6. Prophylactic use for rotational atherectomy and thrombectomy procedures, especially those involving the RCA
7. Transluminal alcohol septal artery ablation in patients with hypertrophic obstructive cardiomyopathy

In patients with left bundle-branch block, passage of catheters through the right side of the heart should be performed with great care because the induction of block in the right side of the heart leads to complete heart block, which requires a pacemaker in some patients. Atropine may be used to prevent bradycardia, but a pacemaker should be on standby for patients in whom severe bradycardia develops during coronary injections.

Transvenous Technique

A temporary transvenous pacemaker can be inserted through the internal jugular, subclavian, brachial, or femoral vein route. The easiest access is usually the vein next to the arterial entry site.

In the catheterization laboratory, RV pacing is accomplished with 5 F balloon-tipped pacing catheters. A PA (Zucker) catheter in which pacing electrodes lie along the catheter as it passes through the right ventricle before passing into the PA has been used during coronary angioplasty (see Chapter 2) but is rarely used today. Among the safest catheters is a 5 F balloon-tipped pacing catheter because of a reduced ability to perforate the thin RV free wall or apex when the balloon is inflated. Normal pacemaker position is shown in Figure 4-42.

Setting the Pacemaker

The pacemaker is set in either the "demand" or the "fixed" mode (Fig. 4-43). Demand mode means that the pacemaker paces when the heart rate drops below the level set by the demand rate (e.g., demand set at 50 beats/min). This mode would be useful when a patient has a vasovagal reaction or

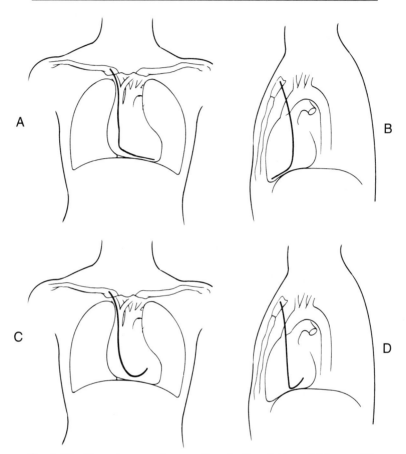

Fig. 4-42 Normal pacemaker position in the right ventricle on (**A**) anteroposterior and (**B**) lateral chest films compared with coronary sinus position in the same views (**C** and **D**). (From Tilkian AG, Daily EK: *Cardiovascular procedures: diagnostic techniques and therapeutic procedures,* St Louis, 1986, Mosby.)

heart block with a heart rate of 40 beats/min. Pacing would start when the pacer detected a rate of less than 50 beats/min; the sensitivity must be lowered to allow the detection of native complexes. Fixed rate mode means that the pacer works continuously at the rate set.

Milliamperes are a measure of the amount of current delivered through the pacing wire to the heart muscle. This

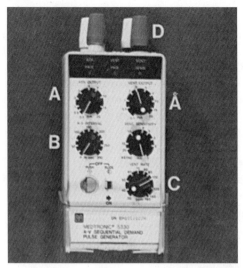

Fig. 4-43 A closeup of pacemaker controls. *A, Å,* Output setting in milliamps for atrial and ventricular channels. *B,* Arteriovenous interval. Opposite *B* is the sensitivity control, which on full counterclockwise to asynchronism is a fixed mode and can be set clockwise to demand rates (see text for details). *C,* Ventricular pacing rate. *D,* Connectors to pacemaker cable.

setting should be three times the threshold value (see next section). A well-positioned pacemaker wire has milliamperage set around 2 to 3 mA. A poorly positioned wire may not pace even with milliamperage of 6 to 7 mA. Repositioning is required.

Determining Pacemaker Threshold

The threshold value is the lowest milliamperage at which the pacemaker will pace. After the wire is positioned, the following procedure should be followed to determine the threshold:

1. Turn the pacer mode fixed at a rate higher than the patient's rate.
2. Set the milliamperage at 5 mA.
3. Turn the milliamperage down in 1-mA increments until the pacing fails. This level is the threshold.
4. Set the milliamperage at three to four times the threshold on demand mode.

Complications

Complications related to the placement of pacemakers are those related to the site of venous access and catheter perforation of the RV. Direct transthoracic pacing should be avoided because of the high likelihood of pneumothorax, hemopericardium, coronary laceration, cardiac tamponade, and major organ or vessel injury.

RV pacing complicated by RV perforation and tamponade occurs in a few patients more commonly when non–balloon-tipped pacing wires are used in patients who are receiving anticoagulants, such as patients who are undergoing PCI. Patients should be selected carefully for prophylactic pacemakers. Perforation of the RV, although uncommon, complicates an otherwise benign yet important procedure for patients with atherosclerotic coronary artery disease.

Other Pacemaker Uses

Pacemakers also are used for (1) provocative testing for ischemia through rapid atrial pacing and (2) ECG signal input and sampling for electrophysiologic studies (see Chapter 5).

Alternatives to Invasive Pacing

External noninvasive cardiac stimulation can be performed with wide patch electrodes placed over the anterior and posterior chest. Although these pacemaker leads may produce some discomfort in the patient who is awake, they create a temporary rhythm when needed.

Suggested Readings

Baim DS, Grossman W, editors: *Grossman's cardiac catheterization, angiography, and intervention,* Philadelphia, 2000, Lippincott Williams & Wilkins.

Balter S, Sones M Jr, Brancato RL: Radiation exposure to the operator performing cardiac angiography with U-arm systems, *Circulation* 58:925-932, 1978.

Dillon JC: Inexpensive radiation protective glasses, *Cathet Cardiovasc Diagn* 5:203-208, 1979.

Gertz EW, Wisneski JA, Gould RG, Akin JR: Improved radiation protection for physicians performing cardiac catheterization, *Am J Cardiol* 50:1283, 1982.

James TN, Bruschke AVG, Bothig S, et al: Report of WHO/ISFC task force on nomenclature of coronary arteriograms, *Circulation* 74:451A-455A, 1986. 1979.

Kardos A, Babai L, Ruda L, et al: Epidemiology of congenital coronary artery anomalies: a coronary arteriography study on a Central European population, *Cathet Cardiovasc Diagn* 42:270-275, 1997.

Kussmaul WG III, Mishra JP, Matthai WH, Hirshfeld JW Jr: Complications of cardiac angiography using low- or high-osmolality contrast agents in patients with left main coronary stenosis, *Cathet Cardiovasc Diagn* 42:376-379, 1997.

Levin DC, Dunham LR, Stueve R: Causes of cine image quality deterioration in cardiac catheterization laboratories, *Am J Cardiol* 52:881-886, 1983.

Mathewson JW: Filmless multimedia display following cardiac catheterization, *Cathet Cardiovasc Diagn* 41:456-466, 1997.

Miller SW, Castronovo FP Jr: Radiation exposure and protection in cardiac catheterization laboratories, *Am J Cardiol* 55:171-176, 1985.

5

ELECTROPHYSIOLOGIC STUDIES AND ABLATION TECHNIQUES

Denise L. Janosik, Antonella Quattromani,
and Lisa Schiller

The electrophysiologic study (EPS) is an invasive procedure that involves the placement of multipolar catheter electrodes at various intracardiac sites. Electrode catheters are routinely placed in the right atrium, across the tricuspid valve annulus in the area of the atrioventricular (AV) node and His bundle (a special part of the conduction system), the right ventricle, the coronary sinus, and sometimes the left ventricle (Fig. 5-1). The general purposes of EPS are to characterize the electrophysiologic properties of the conduction system, induce and analyze the mechanism of arrhythmias, and evaluate the effects of therapeutic interventions. When EPS was introduced in the early 1970s, it was used primarily for diagnostic purposes. Since the late 1990s, the indications and applications of EPS have expanded greatly. EPS is now a technique routinely used in the clinical management of patients who have supraventricular and ventricular arrhythmias (Box 5-1). With the development of safe and effective catheter ablation techniques, an exciting area of interventional electrophysiology has evolved. The field of electrophysiology is a complex subspecialty of cardiology, which is only introduced in this chapter. Individuals seeking a more in-depth discussion of the procedures and concepts described should refer to the Suggested Readings.

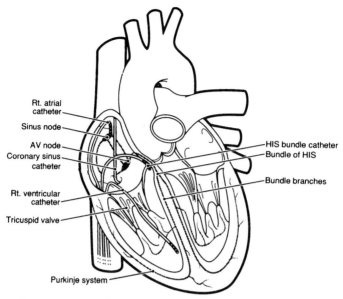

Fig. 5-1 Catheter positions for routine electrophysiologic study. Multipolar catheters are positioned in the high right atrium near the sinus node, in the area of the atrioventricular *(AV)* node and His bundle, in the right ventricular apex, and in the coronary sinus.

TECHNICAL ASPECTS
Personnel

EPS must be performed by appropriately trained personnel. The physician responsible for the performance and analysis of the EPS should be fully trained in clinical cardiology and should have spent a minimum of 1 or preferably 2 additional years training in the subspecialty of electrophysiology. A thorough knowledge of normal and abnormal conduction, refractory periods, activation sequences, and the significance of various responses to programmed electrical stimulation is necessary before clinical judgments and therapeutic recommendations can be based on information obtained from the EPS. The team performing EPS should include at least one electrophysiologist and a well-trained nurse or technician. Because the physician's attention is often focused on the stimulator and electrograms, he or she relies heavily on the

Box 5-1

Clinical Applications of Electrophysiologic Studies

Diagnostic
Diagnose sinus node dysfunction
Determine site of AV nodal block
Define cause of syncope of unclear origin
Differentiate VT from SVT in cases of wide-complex tachycardia
Define mechanism of SVT or VT and map site of origin of tachycardia

Therapeutic
Guide drug therapy for sustained VT, aborted sudden death, or SVT
Select appropriate candidates for cardioverter-defibrillator and antitachycardic
    pacing therapy
Test efficacy of device therapy for ventricular tachyarrhythmias
Select appropriate candidates for catheter ablative and surgical therapy
Test efficacy of ablative and surgical therapies

Interventional
AV nodal ablation or modification for atrial fibrillation
Ablation for atrial tachycardia and atrial flutter
AV nodal modification (slow-pathway or fast-pathway ablation)
Accessory pathway ablation in WPW syndrome
Ablation of ventricular tachycardia

Prognostic
Risk stratification in asymptomatic WPW syndrome
Risk stratification in patients after myocardial infarction
Risk stratification in patients with nonsustained VT

AV, Atrioventricular; *SVT,* supraventricular tachycardia; *VT,* ventricular tachycardia;
WPW, Wolff-Parkinson-White.

nurse to monitor the patient's condition and communicate significant changes. The nurse usually sits between the patient and the cardioverter-defibrillator and crash cart. The nurse monitors the patient's blood pressure, heart rate, rhythm, and oxygen saturation via a pulse oximeter. It is the nurse's responsibility to administer drugs for diagnostic and therapeutic interventions during EPS and to perform cardioversion or defibrillation in response to an induced hemodynamically unstable arrhythmia. Optimally a second nurse is available during procedures to administer medications or to assist in technical aspects of the procedure. Specific guidelines have been published for the training necessary for the physicians and nurses involved in electrophysiologic procedures. In laboratories performing mapping and catheter ablation procedures, an anesthesiologist and cardiothoracic surgeon should be available in case of need for general anesthesia or a rare complication requiring emergency surgery. A biomedical engineer should be readily available to repair equipment that may malfunction and compromise the physician's ability to perform an optimal EPS.

Equipment

The quality of the data collected during an EPS depends partially on the equipment used. An electrophysiology laboratory must be equipped with radiographic equipment, a recording and monitoring system, a stimulator, and all drugs and equipment required for complete cardiopulmonary resuscitation (Fig. 5-2). The reproduction of intracardiac electrical events requires a signal-processing system containing filters and amplifiers that optimize the electrical signals. At least 8 (preferably up to 32) amplifiers should be available to display several surface electrocardiographic (ECG) leads simultaneously with multiple intracardiac electrograms. The number of surface (ECG) leads and intracardiac electrograms displayed varies depending on the type of study being performed. The development of computerized digital recording systems with optical disk storage facilitates collection of large

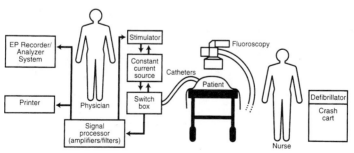

Fig. 5-2   General setup of the equipment used for electrophysiologic studies.

quantities of data that may later be analyzed on system-specific software. The recorder must be able to print hard copy at a variety of paper speeds (10 to 300 mm/sec). Selected segments of the study may be printed on hard copy for off-line analysis and interpretation or for inclusion in the patient's medical record. Some method of obtaining a 12-lead ECG should be available either by standard electrocardiography or through the recording system. Radiographic equipment with a permanent image intensifier capable of a high-quality image is required. It is optimal to have the capacity for multiple views either with a biplane system or with a fluoroscopy unit equipped with a rotating C-arm. Electrical interference may distort intracardiac electrograms and make interpretation of data more difficult. A biomedical or electrical engineer should be involved in the initial design of the electrophysiology laboratory to ensure appropriate shielding, suspension of wires and cables, and proper grounding of equipment.

It is necessary to have a programmable stimulator in the electrophysiology laboratory. The stimulator is equipped with dials or switches by which the pacing intervals and coupling intervals of the extrastimuli may be adjusted (Fig. 5-3). The

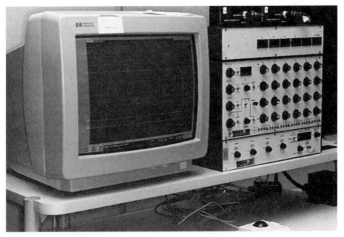

Fig. 5-3 A recording system and monitor *(left)* and commercially available stimulator *(right)*.

stimulator is able to pace over a wide range of rates from two sites simultaneously. It has the ability to introduce a minimum of three extrastimuli (premature beats) coupled to a train of pacing or synchronized to sinus rhythm. A junction box that interfaces with the recording system and stimulator facilitates changes in pacing site without the need to disconnect catheters.

A cardioverter-defibrillator should be close to the patient at all times. A backup defibrillator is optimal in case of a rare but potentially disastrous failure of one defibrillator. The defibrillators should be tested before each study and equipped with an emergency power source. Many laboratories use commercially available R-2 pads, which are placed on the patient before the EPS procedure is begun. One pad is placed under the right scapula and the other on the anterior chest over the left ventricular (LV) apex and connected to the defibrillator with an adaptor. In rare instances in which transthoracic defibrillation fails to convert induced ventricular fibrillation, emergency defibrillation through an intracardiac electrode catheter may be effective in terminating the arrhythmia (Fig. 5-4).

Catheters

A variety of electrode catheters is available for the performance of EPS and catheter-guided ablation (Fig. 5-5). There are many different types of catheters designed for specific purposes, such as steerable and deflectable tip catheters, which facilitate mapping of the atria, AV ring, and ventricles. Special large-tip catheters have been designed for delivery of radiofrequency energy. The catheters are constructed of woven Dacron or synthetic material such as polyurethane and contain 2 to 40 electrodes with 1- to 10-mm spacing between electrodes. Most catheters used in adult patients are 5 F to 7 F in size. The type of catheter selected may vary depending on the intracardiac position desired and the type of data being collected. The preference of catheters varies among operators and depends on properties of the catheter, such as torque, durability, and flexibility, and the experience of the operator.

Bipolar pacing is performed from the distal pair of electrodes, and simultaneous recording of intracardiac electro-

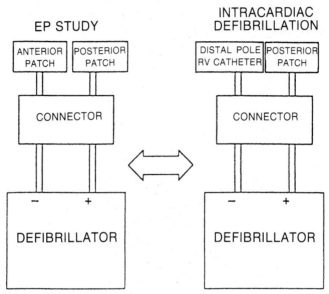

Fig. 5-4 Diagram of intracardiac defibrillation, which may be used when ventricular fibrillation is refractory to multiple transthoracic defibrillations. During the routine electrophysiologic *(EP)* study, anterior and posterior skin patches are attached by a connector to a standard defibrillator. When multiple transthoracic high-energy shocks fail to terminate ventricular fibrillation, the anterior patch may be disconnected and the distal pole of the right ventricular *(RV)* catheter attached to the defibrillator. High-energy shocks are delivered from the right ventricular catheter to the posterior patch. (From Cohen TJ, Scheinman MM, Pullen BT, et al: *J Am Coll Cardiol* 18:1280-1284, 1991.)

grams can be performed from more proximal electrode pairs. For most routine studies, a catheter with two pairs of electrodes (quadripolar catheter) with 5-mm spacing between electrodes is sufficient; pacing is performed from the distal pair of electrodes, and the intracardiac electrogram is recorded from the proximal pair of electrodes. In mapping studies, in which it is important to localize precisely the area of earliest electrical activation, catheters with a greater number of electrodes (up to 40) and smaller inner electrode distances (as little as 1 mm) are optimal.

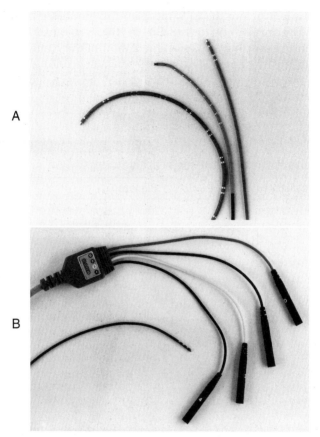

Fig. 5-5 **A,** Several types of multipolar catheters used in routine electrophysiologic studies. Note the difference in the number of electrodes and the differences in spacing between the electrodes among the various catheters. **B,** The proximal end of a hexipolar electrode catheter. The number on each pin corresponds to the electrode position at the tip of the catheter, with *D* representing the most distal electrode.

PROCEDURES
Evaluation and Preparation of the Patient Before Electrophysiologic Study

The results of the EPS must be analyzed in the context of the patient's clinical presentation and cardiac substrate. The physician performing the EPS must comprehensively evaluate the patient before the EPS and plan the procedure based on the information being sought in the individual patient. Whenever possible, ECG documentation of the clinical event, preferably by 12-lead ECG, should be obtained. Some or all of the procedures listed in Table 5-1 may be included in this evaluation.

Table 5-1

Evaluation Before Electrophysiologic Testing*

Procedure	Purpose
History and physical examination	Identify signs and symptoms of cardiac or neurologic disease
	Identify factors known to exacerbate arrhythmias
	Determine details of syncopal events
Neurologic evaluation (if history and physical suggest)	
Electroencephalogram	Rule out seizure disorder
Computed tomography/ magnetic resonance imaging	Identify focal lesion
Carotid ultrasound	Identify significant cerebrovascular disease
12-lead ECG	Identify previous myocardial infarction
	Identify intraventricular conduction delays
	Identify prolonged QT interval
	Identify preexcitation syndromes
24- to 48-hr ambulatory ECG	Correlation of symptoms with ECG events
	Quantitation of ambient ectopy
	Identify diurnal variation in arrhythmia
Event recorder	Correlation of symptoms with ECG events
Head-up tilt-table testing	Diagnose vasovagal/vasodepressor syncope
Echocardiogram and radionucleotide ventriculography	Assessment of left ventricular and right ventricular size and function
	Detection of valvular pathology
Stress test (with or without perfusion scanning)	Detection of reversible ischemia
	Assessment of effects of catecholamines on arrhythmia induction
Cardiac catheterization	Definition of coronary anatomy

ECG, electrocardiogram.
*Selected procedures may vary depending on the clinical presentation.

Any potentially reversible arrhythmogenic factors, such as electrolyte abnormalities or decompensated congestive heart failure, should be corrected before EPS is performed. All anti-arrhythmic medications should be discontinued for at least five half-lives before the baseline study. For supraventricular tachycardia studies medications influencing AV nodal conduction (e.g., β-blockers, digoxin, and calcium channel blockers) should be discontinued. The patient should have nothing by mouth after midnight except for essential cardiac medications, which may be taken with a small amount of water. The patient may be lightly sedated with intravenous (IV) diazepam or midazolam. In long diagnostic studies or in catheter ablation cases, more intensive levels of sedation are usually required. We routinely use IV fentanyl and midazolam to achieve somnolence in the patient during lengthy ablation procedures. Excessive sedation may influence the ability to induce arrhythmias in some individuals, however.

Venous Access

Routine diagnostic EPS involves stimulation and recording of electrical activity from the right side of the heart. Venous access may be obtained from the femoral, subclavian, internal jugular, or antecubital veins. A routine initial diagnostic EPS usually involves insertion of at least three catheters, most commonly via the femoral veins. These large veins easily permit the introduction of two 5- to 7 F catheters per vein. The number of catheters required and venous access selected depend on the type of study being performed and the data being collected. A follow-up study to assess drug efficacy for ventricular tachycardia may be accomplished by the placement of a single quadripolar catheter in the right ventricular (RV) apex via the internal jugular access. Mapping of a left-sided bypass tract may require the insertion of five multipolar catheters, however, and even necessitate catheterization of the left side of the heart for precise mapping.

For patients requiring beat-to-beat assessment of the hemodynamic effects of an induced arrhythmia, an arterial line may be placed. To completely evaluate a patient with Wolff-Parkinson-White syndrome, the physician may have to access the left ventricle for stimulation or recording of intracardiac electrical activity. If arterial catheterization is necessary, administration of IV heparin is mandatory. Patients undergoing prolonged studies involving venous access or with a history of venous thromboembolism should also receive heparin.

Positioning of Catheters

The right atrium is easily accessible by any venous access. The most common site for stimulation and recording is the high posterior lateral wall in the region of the sinus node. The His potential is most easily found with a catheter introduced by the femoral approach and passed into the right atrium across the tricuspid valve and into the right ventricle. The catheter is withdrawn across the tricuspid valve with the application of a slight degree of clockwise torque that tends to keep the catheter in contact with the septum (Fig. 5-6). A hexapolar or octapolar catheter in the His position may be used so that electrical activity from multiple electrode pairs can be recorded, and the one showing the most stable and consistent His potential may be displayed. If multiple attempts to record a His potential with one catheter are unsuccessful, a differently shaped or steerable catheter with a deflectable tip may be used. In most patients a His potential can be recorded successfully.

Usually the left atrium is approached indirectly by recording in the coronary sinus. Cannulation of the coronary sinus os is most often successful from the left subclavian or right or left internal jugular approaches. Catheters introduced through these approaches are more easily deflected off the lateral right atrial (RA) wall toward the coronary sinus os, which lies posteromedially above the tricuspid annulus. The appropriate position of the coronary sinus catheter is verified fluoroscopically in the left anterior oblique and right anterior oblique positions. The catheter curves upward toward the left shoulder in the left anterior oblique projection and is posteriorly oriented in the lateral projection. On the ECG, atrial and ventricular electrograms are recorded with the timing of the left atrial electrograms appearing later than the high RA electrogram. Direct recording of electrical activity from the left atrium is possible in patients with a patent foramen ovale or atrial septal defect or by a transseptal approach.

In most baseline studies the catheter is placed in the RV apex. For ventricular stimulation protocols a second ventricular

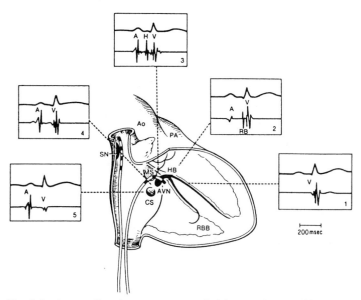

Fig. 5-6 Intracardiac electrograms recorded from various positions on a multipolar catheter positioned across the tricuspid valve. The numbers *1* to *5* refer to the intracardiac location of the catheters along with the corresponding electrograms; 1 represents the most distal location recording a large ventricular electrogram and no atrial electrogram, and 5 represents the most proximal location displaying a large atrial electrogram with a small ventricular electrogram. The His potential is observed when the catheter is in the area of the tricuspid annulus and the atrial and ventricular electrograms recorded are approximately of equal size *(position 3)*. (From Grossman W: *Cardiac catheterization and angiography,* ed 2, Philadelphia, 1974, Lea & Febiger.)

catheter is sometimes placed in the RV outflow tract, although most operators prefer to reposition the catheter from the apex to the outflow tract. The order in which the catheters are placed in the right side of the heart varies among operators, and no particular order is mandatory. In patients with a preexisting left bundle-branch block, it is recommended that the RV apical catheter be positioned first to ensure adequate ventricular pacing in the event of catheter-induced trauma to the right bundle, which may result in complete heart block while the His catheter is being positioned.

Catheterization of the left ventricle may be necessary in patients with ventricular tachycardia or preexcitation syndromes. The left ventricle is most commonly accessed by the retrograde arterial approach for mapping procedures. Fluoroscopy that permits views in multiple planes is essential to ensure accurate positioning of the catheter. Stimulation may also be performed from the left ventricle in cases in which patients with clinically documented sustained ventricular tachycardia have arrhythmias that are noninducible with use of the standard protocol from the right ventricle. The left ventricle may be entered and mapped by the retrograde arterial approach. To avoid inadvertent cannulation of the coronary arteries, the operator safely crosses the aortic valve with a pigtail catheter. In patients with atrial septal defects or patent foramen ovale or in patients undergoing transseptal punctures, the left ventricle may be approached through the left atrium and mitral valve.

Complications

The complications associated with EPS are low, and mortality is extremely rare. Complications of the procedure are usually associated with catheterization and catheter manipulation rather than stimulation and the induction of arrhythmias. The reported complications include hemorrhage, venous thromboembolism (<1%), phlebitis (<1%), cardiac perforation and tamponade, and refractory ventricular fibrillation. Hemothorax and pneumothorax are recognized complications when the subclavian or internal jugular venous approaches are used. Arterial catheterization increases the associated morbidity of the procedure, including vascular complications, stroke, systemic embolism, and protamine reactions. The mortality associated with EPS is extremely low, less than 1 per 25,000 procedures. Most reported deaths have resulted from incessant ventricular fibrillation and have occurred in patients with severe LV dysfunction, active myocardial ischemia, or hypertrophic obstructive cardiomyopathy or because of the proarrhythmic effect of drugs administered during the evaluation. Defibrillation through an intracardiac electrode has been reported to be effective in situations in which transthoracic defibrillation fails and death might otherwise have resulted (see Fig. 5-4).

Study Protocol

Although details of the protocol vary depending on the indication for the EPS and the information being obtained, most studies involve the recording and measurement of spontaneous intracardiac events and observation of the effects of programmed electrical stimulation. An initial study usually takes approximately 2 hours and depends on the complexity of the case. The possible components of the initial comprehensive EPS are listed in Box 5-2.

Measurement of Conduction Intervals

After the catheters are positioned, basic conduction intervals are measured, including the basic sinus cycle length (the A-to-A interval), P wave duration, A-H interval, His spike duration, and H-V interval (Fig. 5-7). Measurements from the surface ECG, including the PR interval, QRS interval, and QT interval, are also recorded. Conduction interval measurements and refractory period measurements should be made at a paper

---

Box 5-2

Possible Components of Comprehensive Initial Electrophysiologic Study*

Measurement of basic intervals

Determination of sinus node function

Determination of atrial, AV nodal, His-Purkinje, and ventricular conduction and refractoriness

Identification of presence of dual AV nodal pathways

Identification of presence, location, and electrical properties of accessory AV pathways

Attempts to induce supraventricular tachycardia

Attempts to induce ventricular tachycardia

Determination of mechanism of induced arrhythmias

Site of origin of induced arrhythmias is mapped

Determination of effect of intravenous antiarrhythmic drugs on induced tachycardia

Determination of efficacy of antitachycardic pacing for induced tachycardia

---

AV, Atrioventricular.

*The actual procedure varies depending on the individual case; not all parameters are assessed in all cases.

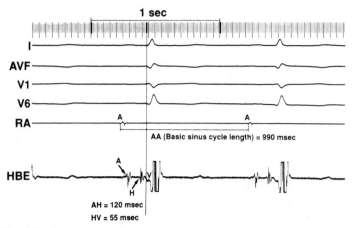

Fig. 5-7   The measurement of the basic sinus cycle length and the AH interval and HV interval. *RA*, Right atrium; *HBE*, His bundle electrogram.

speed of at least 100 mm/sec in routine cases and at speeds of 100 to 200 mm/sec in detailed mapping procedures. All measurements of rate and conduction times are made in terms of milliseconds. The pacing interval can be converted to heart rate by the following formula (Table 5-2):

$$\text{Interval (ms)} = \frac{60{,}000}{\text{Heart rate}}$$

The AH interval represents conduction time from the low right atrium at the interatrial septum through the AV node to the His bundle and approximates AV nodal conduction time. The measurement is made from the earliest reproducible rapid deflection of the atrial electrogram on the His bundle recording to the onset of the His deflection on that electrogram (see Fig. 5-7). Normal values for adults are reported to range from 50 to 140 ms. The AH interval is influenced strongly by the patient's autonomic tone and may vary by 50 ms during a study in a given patient. The AH interval normally increases in response to increases in atrial pacing rates. It may also be altered by drugs that affect AV conduction, and the measurement may be influenced artificially by such factors as gain setting and position of the atrial catheter.

The HV interval represents conduction time from the proximal His bundle to the ventricular myocardium. The measure-

Table 5-2

Pacing Interval Conversion Chart*

Pacing Interval (ms)	Heart Rate (beats/min)
200	300
222	270
231	260
240	250
250	240
261	230
273	220
286	210
300	200
311	193
316	190
333	180
353	170
375	160
400	150
429	140
462	130
500	120
545	110
550	109
600	100
667	90
750	80
857	70
1000	60
1200	50
1500	40
2000	30

*Pulse-to-pulse interval (ms) to beats per minute (beats/min).

ment is made from the earliest deflection of the His spike on the His bundle recording to the earliest onset of ventricular activation recorded from any intracardiac electrogram or surface ECG. Normal values range from 30 to 55 ms. In contrast to the AH interval, the HV interval normally remains relatively constant and is not significantly affected by variations in autonomic tone or atrial pacing rates.

Sequence of Activation

Determination of the sequence of antegrade and retrograde atrial activation during spontaneous rhythms, atrial pacing, ventricular pacing, and induced rhythms is essential in differentiating ventricular tachycardia from supraventricular tachycardia and in defining the reentrant circuit in supraventricular tachycardia. The atrial activation normally begins in the high right atrium, spreads to the low right atrium and His bundle, with left atrial activation, recorded from the coronary sinus catheter, occurring significantly later. When ventriculoatrial conduction is present during ventricular pacing, the earliest retrograde atrial activity is recorded in the His bundle electrogram followed by the RA and coronary sinus recordings. Abnormal or eccentric sequences of retrograde atrial activation occur in the presence of AV accessory pathways (Fig. 5-8). This is discussed in more detail in subsequent sections dealing with supraventricular tachycardia and catheter ablation.

Programmed Electrical Stimulation

Programmed electrical stimulation involves observing the electrophysiologic effects of incremental pacing and the introduction of programmed extrastimuli coupled to normal sinus rhythm or paced rhythms. The major purposes of programmed electrical stimulation are to characterize the electrophysiologic properties of cardiac tissue and to induce and analyze the mechanism of arrhythmias. The most commonly used types of pacing during the EPS are burst pacing, incremental pacing, and programmed stimulation. Fixed burst pacing involves the delivery of a series of impulses at a constant rate. A decremental burst consists of a series of impulses at progressively increasing rates. Programmed stimulation involves the coupling of premature extrastimuli to a short train (six to eight beats) of pacing or to sinus rhythm. The number of extrastimuli may vary from one to four. The pacing train is referred to as S1, first extrastimulus as S2, and second extrastimulus as S3. The coupling intervals are decreased progressively and systematically by 10-ms decrements until an arrhythmia is induced or the first extrastimulus loses capture (the effective refractory period [ERP] of the tissue is reached).

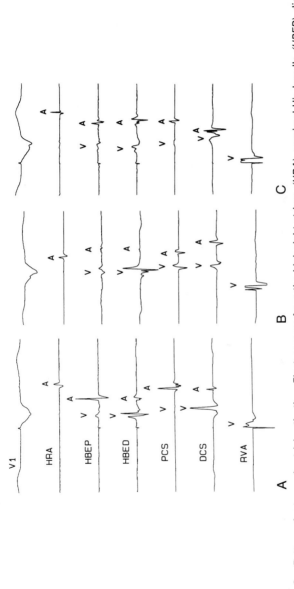

Fig. 5-8   Pattern of retrograde atrial activation. Electrograms from the high right atrium *(HRA)*, proximal His bundle *(HBEP)*, distal His bundle *(HBED)*, proximal coronary sinus *(PCS)*, distal coronary sinus *(DCS)*, and right ventricular apex *(RVA)* are shown. **A,** Normal pattern of retrograde atrial activation through the atrioventricular node. **B,** Sequence of retrograde atrial activation with a right-sided accessory pathway showing earliest activation in the high right atrium. **C,** Sequence of retrograde atrial activation with a left-sided accessory pathway showing earliest activation in the distal coronary sinus.

Assessment of Sinus Node Function

Many studies begin with an evaluation of sinus node and AV node function and assessment of atrial and AV nodal refractoriness. Measurement of sinus node recovery time is performed by pacing the right atrium, most commonly near the region of the sinus node, at a slightly faster rate than the intrinsic sinus rate for approximately 30 seconds, then abruptly terminating pacing. The sinus node recovery time is the time from the last paced atrial complex on the RA recording to the return of the first sinus complex (Fig. 5-9). Generally, the slower the intrinsic sinus rate, the longer the sinus node recovery time. The absolute sinus node recovery time may be corrected for heart rate by subtracting the basic sinus cycle length (corrected sinus node recovery time). Normal values for absolute sinus node recovery time are up to 1.5 seconds and for corrected sinus node recovery time up to 550 ms. Secondary pauses are other indicators of sinus node dysfunction. For

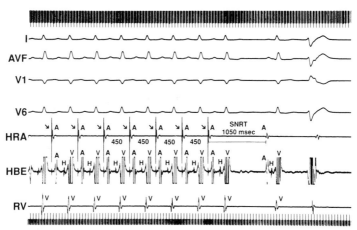

Fig. 5-9 Demonstration of a normal sinus node recovery time in a patient undergoing electrophysiologic study for the evaluation of syncope of unknown cause. After a train of atrial pacing at a cycle length of 450 (approximately 133 beats/min), 1050 ms elapses before return of sinus node activity. The absolute sinus node recovery time is 1050 ms. *HRA*, High right atrium; *HBE*, His bundle electrogram; *RV*, right ventricle; *SNRT*, sinus node recovery time.

most routine studies measurements of sinus node recovery time are sufficient for assessment of sinus node function. The interested reader may consult the Suggested Readings for further description of techniques used in the assessment of sinus node function.

Assessment of Atrioventricular Nodal and His-Purkinje System Function

AV nodal function is assessed by determining the point at which 1:1 AV conduction ceases and AV nodal Wenckebach begins. The normal response to incremental atrial pacing at progressively faster rates is to develop a longer AH interval and, ultimately, block in the AV node (Fig. 5-10). Most normal individuals develop AV nodal Wenckebach at paced atrial cycle lengths of 500 to 350 ms (heart rates of 120 to 170 beats/min). AV nodal Wenckebach cycle length normally increases with age. AV nodal Wenckebach does not usually occur during exercise when similar heart rates are achieved because catecholamines enhance conduction through the AV node. The point at which Wenckebach occurs in response to atrial pacing may be influenced by drugs that affect AV nodal conduction and by autonomic tone. Wenckebach occurs at longer cycle lengths (slower pacing rates) in patients with enhanced vagal tone and at shorter cycle lengths (faster pacing rates) in patients with enhanced sympathetic tone. In contrast to the AH interval, the HV interval remains relatively constant during decremental atrial pacing, and block below His (intra-Hisian block) is considered pathologic at pacing cycle lengths greater than 400 ms (rates <150 beats/min).

Determination of Refractory Periods

The refractoriness of cardiac tissue is defined by the response of the tissue to the introduction of premature stimuli. For most routine EPS the ERP is defined as the longest coupling interval between the basic drive and the premature stimulus that fails to propagate through the tissue. Normal values for AV nodal, atrial, and ventricular refractory periods have been established (Table 5-3). The ERP of cardiac tissue may be affected by the current strength used, the pacing rate, medications, and autonomic tone in the AV node.

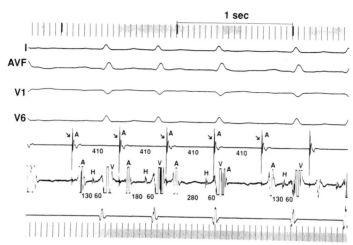

Fig. 5-10 Type I second-degree atrioventricular (AV) block (Wenckebach) in the AV node induced by atrial pacing at a cycle length of 410 ms. Each paced atrial depolarization is followed by a progressively longer AH interval until the fourth atrial depolarization is blocked in the AV node (no His depolarization is seen after the atrial electrogram). The AH interval after the blocked atrial depolarization is shorter (130 ms) compared with the AH interval preceding the block beat (280 ms). The HV interval remains constant despite the progressive increase in AH interval during the Wenckebach sequence.

Table 5-3

Normal Intervals and Refractory Periods

Parameter	Normal Duration (ms)
AH	50-150
HV	30-55
His	10-25
Atrial ERP	150-360
AV nodal ERP	230-430
HPS ERP	330-450
Ventricular ERP	170-290

AV, Atrioventricular; *ERP,* effective refractory period; *HPS,* His-Purkinje system.

Atrioventricular Nodal Function Curves

AV nodal function curves can be constructed by plotting of the coupling interval of the premature stimulus (A_1A_2 interval) on the horizontal axis versus the AH interval (AV nodal conduction time) of the premature stimulus (A_2H_2 interval) on the vertical axis. In individuals without dual AV nodal pathways a progressive and gradual increase occurs in the AH interval before the premature stimulus blocking in the AV node, and the function curve is continuous (Fig. 5-11, A). A sudden large increase (at least 50 ms) in the AH interval (often referred to as a jump) in response to a small decrement (10 ms) in the coupling interval of the premature beat is evidence of

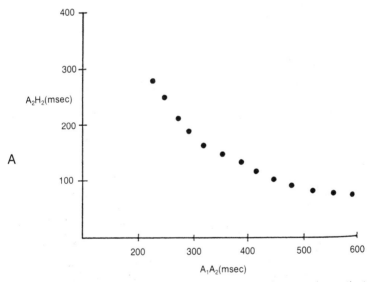

Fig. 5-11   A, Normal atrioventricular (AV) nodal function curve in a patient without functional dual AV nodal pathways. In this graph the conduction intervals (A_1A_2) are displayed on the X axis and the resulting AH interval (A_2H_2) is displayed on the Y axis. With progressively shorter coupling intervals, premature atrial beats are followed by progressively longer AH intervals (A_2H_2), which represents progressive conduction delay in the AV node. The normal AV nodal conduction curve is smooth and continuous. (From Forgoros RN: *Electrophysiologic testing,* Cambridge, Mass, 1991, Blackwell Scientific.)   *Continued*

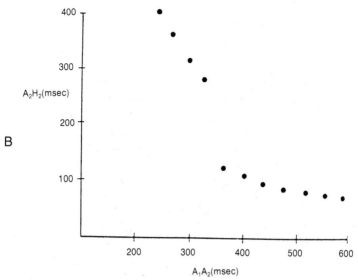

Fig. 5-11, cont'd B, A typical AV nodal function curve in a patient with functional dual AV nodal pathways. Premature atrial impulses with longer coupling intervals conduct down the fast pathway and have short AH intervals. With progressively earlier premature atrial impulses, the refractory period of the fast pathway is reached, and conduction shifts to the slow pathway. The jump from the fast pathway to the slow pathway is manifested by a sudden lengthening of the A_2H_2 interval and discontinuity in the AV nodal function curve.

functional dual AV nodal pathways (Fig. 5-12). This represents a shift from conduction over the fast AV nodal pathway to conduction over the slow AV nodal pathway (with a longer AH interval), and the AV nodal function curve is discontinuous (see Fig. 5-11, *B*). During programmed stimulation in patients with dual AV pathways, supraventricular tachycardia is often initiated when the jump to the slow pathway occurs. Multiple extrastimuli may be used in patients with suspected or known supraventricular tachycardia in an attempt to induce a clinically significant tachycardia. Drugs that modify refractoriness and conductive velocity in the AV node, such as isoproterenol or atropine, may be given in attempts to induce a clinically significant supraventricular tachycardia.

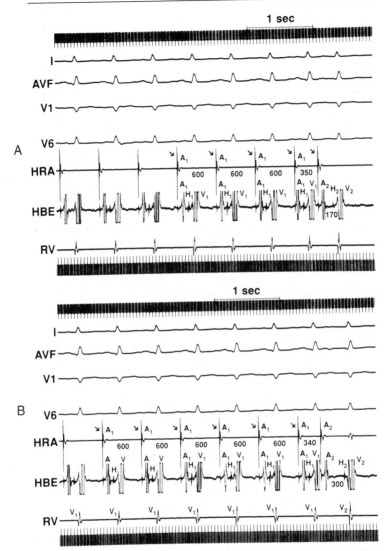

Fig. 5-12 A 130-ms jump in atrioventricular nodal conduction in a patient with functional dual atrioventricular nodal pathways. Premature atrial stimuli are coupled to a train of atrial pacing at a cycle length of 600 ms. **A,** At a coupling interval of 350 ms the premature atrial stimulus has an AH interval of 170 ms. **B,** At a coupling interval of 340 ms the AH interval of the premature impulse suddenly increases to 300 ms, representing a shift to the slow pathway. *HRA,* High right atrium; *HBE,* His bundle electrogram; *RV,* right ventricle.

Ventricular Stimulation

The safety and efficacy of programmed electrical stimulation in the diagnosis and treatment of patients with ventricular arrhythmias have been well established. The reported sensitivity and specificity of ventricular stimulation vary depending on the stimulation protocol used, the presenting arrhythmia, and the underlying cardiac disease. The sensitivity and specificity of programmed ventricular stimulation have been defined best in patients with coronary artery disease whose arrhythmia is spontaneous sustained monomorphic ventricular tachycardia. In these individuals the yield (and sensitivity) of the EPS increases with the addition of up to three extrastimuli; the addition of more extrastimuli provides little or no added benefit. In most patients the clinical ventricular tachycardia is initiated reproducibly by programmed electrical stimulation. The clinical significance of arrhythmias induced by programmed electrical stimulation must be interpreted with regard to the specific arrhythmia for which a patient is being evaluated. With more aggressive stimulation protocols polymorphic ventricular tachycardia or ventricular fibrillation that may represent a nonclinical (or false-positive) response may be initiated. Even in normal individuals, at close coupling intervals of the extrastimuli (usually <180 ms), ventricular fibrillation or polymorphic ventricular tachycardia may be induced. In contrast, sustained monomorphic ventricular tachycardia is considered a specific response to programmed electrical stimulation and generally occurs only in patients with previous spontaneous ventricular tachycardia or a pathologic substrate known to predispose to ventricular tachycardia.

Although ventricular stimulation protocols vary slightly among different laboratories, the minimal complete protocol usually involves the introduction of three extrastimuli coupled to ventricular pacing at two cycle lengths from two RV sites, typically RV apex and RV outflow tract (Box 5-3). LV stimulation may be performed in some individuals who have documented sustained monomorphic ventricular tachycardia but whose arrhythmia is noninducible from the right ventricle. The yield is relatively low from LV stimulation, and LV stimulation may increase the morbidity of the procedure. In individuals with exercise-induced ventricular tachycardia or catecholamine-

Box 5-3

Ventricular Stimulation Protocol

Standard Protocol

Single extrastimulus coupled to ventricular pacing at cycle lengths of 600 and 400 ms from RV apex and RV outflow tract

Double extrastimuli coupled to ventricular pacing at cycle lengths of 600 and 400 ms from RV apex and RV outflow tract

Rapid ventricular pacing (400 ms to loss of 1:1 ventricular capture)

Triple extrastimuli coupled to ventricular pacing at cycle lengths of 600 and 400 ms from RV apex and RV outflow tract

Additional Maneuvers That May Be Performed

Extrastimuli may be coupled to sinus rhythm or other paced cycle lengths

A fourth extrastimulus may be coupled to ventricular pacing at cycle lengths of 600 and 400 ms from both RV sites

Stimulation may be performed at additional RV sites or from the left ventricle

Isoproterenol may be infused and the stimulation protocol repeated

Intravenous procainamide may be infused and the stimulation protocol repeated

RV, Right ventricular.

dependent ventricular tachycardia, isoproterenol may be infused and programmed stimulation repeated.

To perform the stimulation protocol , the operator systematically decreases the coupling interval between the last beat of the pacing train and the extrastimuli until the tissue reaches refractoriness (the first extrastimulus fails to capture) or an arrhythmia is induced (Fig. 5-13). If the patient is hemodynamically stable, a 12-lead ECG of the induced ventricular tachycardia is recorded before attempts to terminate the tachycardia. The morphology of the ventricular tachycardia is noted, and the cycle length is obtained. The most common method of terminating the ventricular tachycardia is ventricular burst pacing at a cycle length less than that of the tachycardia. The cycle length of the burst pacing is decreased gradually until the tachycardia either terminates (Fig. 5-14) or accelerates and results in hemodynamic compromise, at which point cardioversion or defibrillation is performed on the patient. An initial 200 J shock is routinely used for sustained ventricular tachycardia and a 360-J shock (or equivalent biphasic) for subsequent shocks.

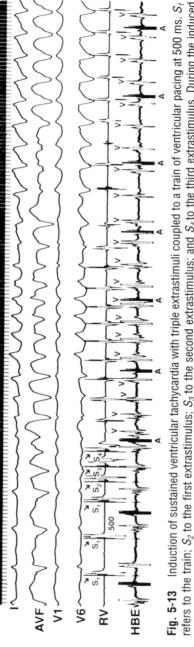

Fig. 5-13 Induction of sustained ventricular tachycardia with triple extrastimuli coupled to a train of ventricular pacing at 500 ms. S_1 refers to the train; S_2 to the first extrastimulus; S_3 to the second extrastimulus; and S_4 to the third extrastimulus. During the induced ventricular tachycardia, the atrial activity is dissociated from the ventricular activity. This may be observed on the His channel (*HBE*) by the atrial electrogram (*A*) marching randomly through the tachycardia. *RV*, Right ventricle; *HBE*, His bundle electrogram.

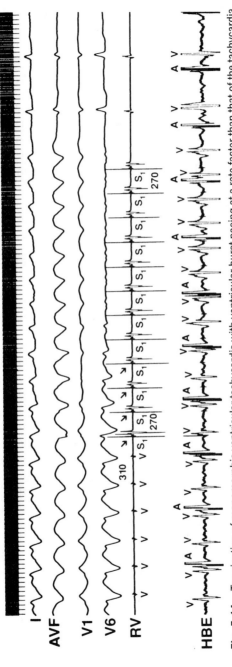

Fig. 5-14 Termination of monomorphic ventricular tachycardia with ventricular burst pacing at a rate faster than that of the tachycardia. On the right ventricular channel (*RV*), the cycle length of the monomorphic ventricular tachycardia is measured at 310 ms. Ventricular burst pacing (indicated by the *arrows* and S_1) at a cycle length of 270 ms terminates the tachycardia. *HBE*, His bundle electrogram.

The most specific end point of the ventricular stimulation protocol is the induction of a sustained monomorphic ventricular tachycardia that is identical to a patient's clinical ventricular tachycardia. Sustained ventricular tachycardia is commonly defined as ventricular tachycardia lasting at least 30 seconds or requiring termination because of hemodynamic collapse before 30 seconds. Noninducibility by ventricular stimulation refers to the failure to induce sustained ventricular tachycardia after the use of at least three extrastimuli at two pacing rates from two RV pacing sites. The arrhythmia may be noninducible on the initial EPS or may be rendered noninducible by antiarrhythmic drug therapy. Partial drug efficacy refers to significant lengthening (>100 ms) of the cycle length of the induced tachycardia or rendering a previously intolerable tachycardia hemodynamically stable.

UTILITY OF ELECTROPHYSIOLOGIC STUDY FOR SPECIFIC DIAGNOSIS
Sinus Node Disease

The clinical applications of EPS in sinus node disease are limited. Although abnormal sinus node recovery times and sinoatrial conduction times have been reported to have a specificity of 90% to 100% in patients documented to have spontaneous sinus node dysfunction, the sensitivity is significantly less. In contrast to most induced tachyarrhythmias on EPS, it is difficult to correlate symptoms with an abnormal sinus node recovery time. In symptomatic patients with sinus bradycardia an abnormal sinus node recovery time has been reported to predict which patients may benefit from cardiac pacing. The finding of an abnormal sinus node recovery time in an asymptomatic patient who is being studied for tachyarrhythmias may influence a decision to use certain medications or, in device candidates, to select a cardioverter-defibrillator with backup pacing.

Disorders of Atrioventricular Conduction

Abnormalities of AV conduction are classified as first-degree, second-degree, or third-degree AV block (Table 5-4). Clues to the site of AV block can be derived by observing serial changes in PR interval in sequences of block that are less than 2:1

Table 5-4

Types of Atrioventricular Block

Type	Characteristics	Site of block
First-Degree AV Block	All P waves conducted, prolonged conduction manifested by long PR interval	Delay may be above, within, or below His
Second-Degree AV Block	P waves are intermittently blocked	
Type I	Progressive prolongation of PR interval before blocked P wave	Usually within AV node
Type II	Sudden failure of conduction; prolonged conduction manifested with no change in PR interval	Usually within or below His bundle
Third-Degree AV Block	No P waves are conducted to ventricle; ventricular escape rhythm may occur	May be within AV node, within or below His

AV, Atrioventricular.

(i.e., 3:2 or 4:3), the rate and duration of the QRS of the escape rhythm, and the presence or absence of underlying intraventricular conduction delays on ECG. Compared with prolonged conduction in the AV node, conduction disease within or below the His bundle is associated with a high likelihood that complete AV block will develop. Complete AV block that occurs within or below the His bundle is associated with a slower and less stable escape rhythm than occurs with complete AV block situated within the AV node. EPS can confirm the site of spontaneous AV block or conduction delay and assess the response of the conduction system to various pacing rates and the introduction of premature impulses. EPS may identify indications for permanent pacemaker implantation in individuals with syncope of unknown cause. Long HV intervals

(>80 to 100 ms) and block below the His bundle at atrial pacing rates of less than 150 beats/min indicate disease in the His-Purkinje system and are associated with a relatively high incidence of subsequent complete heart block.

Sustained Ventricular Arrhythmias

For more than two decades, EPS was used to determine the efficacy of antiarrhythmic drug therapy in patients with sustained ventricular tachycardia and survivors of cardiac arrest. This practice was based on the supposition that (1) the induced ventricular arrhythmia represents the patient's clinical arrhythmia and (2) the inability to induce the arrhythmia after drug treatment in a patient whose arrhythmia was previously inducible correlates with freedom from the clinical recurrence of the arrhythmia. The predictive accuracy of serial EPS is highest in patients with previous myocardial infarction and spontaneous sustained monomorphic ventricular tachycardia. There may be a significant number of false-negative results with EPS in patients with nonischemic cardiac disease or polymorphic ventricular tachycardia or ventricular fibrillation as a presenting clinical arrhythmia. Another important limitation of the technique is that even in patients whose arrhythmia is rendered noninducible by antiarrhythmic therapy there is a significant clinical recurrence rate of sustained ventricular arrhythmia and cardiac arrest, reported to be as high as 50% over 4 years. Data indicate that survivors of cardiac arrest or sustained ventricular tachycardia derive a significant survival benefit from an implantable cardioverter-defibrillator (ICD) compared with antiarrhythmic drug therapy. In most centers, most patients surviving a hemodynamically unstable ventricular arrhythmia receive an ICD without a preceding EPS. In rare cases bundle-branch reentry tachycardia or atrial fibrillation with rapid ventricular response (in the setting of Wolff-Parkinson-White syndrome) may precipitate a patient's cardiac arrest or unstable ventricular arrhythmia. If these circumstances are suspected, EPS may be useful because these arrhythmias are potentially curable by radiofrequency catheter ablation, which may obviate the need for an ICD. In patients with hemodynamically stable monomorphic ventricular tachycardia in whom drug or ablative therapy is being considered, EPS is indicated.

Primary Prevention of Sudden Death

The survival rate after out-of-hospital cardiac arrest is extremely low, and attention has been directed at identifying high-risk patients who may benefit from prophylactic treatment as a means of primary prevention of sudden cardiac death. Two primary prevention trials indicated that patients with coronary disease, significant LV dysfunction (LV ejection fraction 35% to 40%), spontaneous nonsustained ventricular tachycardia, and inducible sustained ventricular arrhythmia by EPS experienced a survival benefit from prophylactic ICD implantation. There is no evidence that EPS-guided antiarrhythmic drug therapy is effective as preventive therapy for sudden cardiac death in high-risk individuals. A primary prevention trial, which did not require spontaneous or induced ventricular arrhythmias as entry criteria, concluded that prophylactic ICD implantation benefited patients with coronary artery disease and an LV ejection fraction less than 30%. This study suggests that poor LV function alone is a strong predictor of subsequent sudden cardiac death. Whether EPS could be used for further risk stratification of these patients to select the highest risk individuals for prophylactic ICD implantation is not known.

Patients with Implantable Cardioverter-Defibrillator

Discussion regarding the function of the ICD is beyond the scope of this chapter, and interested readers are referred to comprehensive textbooks on this subject. Briefly the ICD is a device capable of sensing ventricular tachycardia or fibrillation and rapidly delivering a shock. All devices also incorporate antitachycardic and antibradycardic pacing. ICD pulse generators and lead systems evolved in the 1990s, resulting in a simple system comprising an active can and a single lead placed at the RV apex. The role of EPS in patients with ICDs includes selection of appropriate patients, intraoperative testing of the lead systems to ensure appropriate rate sensing and defibrillation threshold, and, frequently, postoperative testing to ensure adequate function of the device for all induced arrhythmias. Postoperative testing of devices may be indicated when antitachycardic pacing is used or in sudden death survivors who receive an ICD without a preceding EPS. When a patient with an ICD undergoes a change in his or her antiarrhythmic drug regimen, the device should be retested because changes in rate of the tachycardia may necessitate reprogramming of the device's rate detection criteria and changes in the defibrillation threshold may be caused by certain medications. Atrial defibrillators for treatment of paroxysmal atrial fibrillation are now also available.

Syncope of Unknown Cause

Syncope is a common clinical disorder, the workup of which can be expensive and nonproductive. The diagnostic utility of EPS in patients with recurrent syncope has been reported to range from 12% to 79%. The reported abnormalities are listed in Box 5-4. The yield is highly dependent on the prevalence of structural heart disease in the population being studied. In patients with structurally normal hearts and no suggestion of ischemia, EPS has a low yield and an increased likelihood of false-positive results. In patients with a history of coronary artery disease and segmental wall motion abnormality or conduction disease on ECG, the EPS has a relatively high yield and may rule out potentially life-threatening causes of syncope, such as sustained ventricular arrhythmia. In an unwitnessed

---

Box 5-4

Reported Abnormalities in Patients with Syncope on Electrophysiologic Study

Sinus Node Dysfunction
Prolonged sinus node recovery time
Prolonged sinoatrial conduction time
Secondary pauses

Abnormalities of AV Conduction
Prolonged AV nodal refractory period
Prolonged AV nodal Wenckebach cycle length
Prolonged HV interval
Block induced within or below the His bundle

Induced Tachyarrhythmias
Rapid supraventricular tachycardia
Sustained ventricular tachycardia

AV, Atrioventricular.

syncope episode the cause of the patient's syncope is never certain, and there is always the potential for inaccurately attributing the patient's syncope to an abnormality detected on EPS. It is desirable that a patient's symptoms be reproduced by the induced arrhythmia.

Supraventricular Tachycardia

The treatment of supraventricular tachycardia has undergone dramatic change because radiofrequency catheter ablation offers a high probability of cure with a low complication rate for many reentrant tachycardias. Although the relationship between the QRS complex and P waves on the 12-lead ECG may suggest the mechanism of supraventricular tachycardia, performance of a detailed EPS is the only method of accurately characterizing the mechanism of tachycardia and defining the anatomic substrate.

The most frequently observed mechanism of narrow-complex supraventricular tachycardia is AV nodal reentrant tachycardia, which usually involves slow- and fast-conducting pathways within or near the AV node. Although it was previously thought that AV nodal reentry occurred entirely within the compact AV node, experience from radiofrequency catheter ablation indicates that extranodal tissue may be involved in the reentrant circuit. Dual AV nodal pathways are characterized by discontinuous AV nodal conduction curves (see Fig. 5-11, *B*). In typical AV nodal tachycardia, which constitutes more than 90% of AV nodal reentrant tachycardia, antegrade conduction occurs over the slow pathway and retrograde conduction occurs up the fast pathway (slow-fast tachycardia) (Fig. 5-15). The retrograde ventriculoatrial conduction time is usually short, and the atrial depolarization often occurs simultaneously with or immediately after the ventricular depolarization. On surface ECG the P waves either are not visible or occur in the ST segment with a short RP interval.

Another common mechanism of supraventricular tachycardia is AV reciprocating tachycardia, using an extranodal AV bypass tract (also referred to as an accessory pathway). The most common type of accessory pathway is the bundle of Kent, which occurs in Wolff-Parkinson-White syndrome. The accessory pathway may be between the right atrium and ventricle or left atrium and ventricle. In an individual patient an accessory

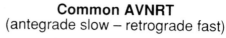

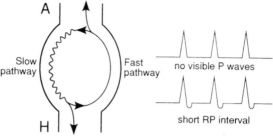

Fig. 5-15 Schematic representation of the common form of atrio-ventricular (AV) nodal reentrant tachycardia. In the typical form of AV nodal tachycardia, antegrade block occurs in the fast pathway, forcing antegrade conduction down the slow pathway. If antegrade conduction down the slow pathway is slow enough to allow retrograde conduction to occur up the previously refractory fast pathway, reentrant tachycardia ensues. Although previously it was thought that the limbs of the tachycardic circuit were contained within the compact AV node, more recent studies using radiofrequency ablation for AV nodal tachycardia suggest that perinodal tissue is contained in the reentrant circuit.

pathway may be capable of antegrade conduction, retrograde conduction, or both. Individuals with antegrade conduction over an accessory pathway exhibit a short PR interval and a wide QRS complex because of ventricular preexcitation (this is also referred to as a delta wave). The axis of the delta wave and morphology of the QRS depend on the position of the accessory pathway and the amount of tissue depolarized through accessory pathway conduction compared with conduction over the normal AV node. During sinus rhythm, activation of the ventricle can occur over the accessory pathway and through the normal conduction pathway using the AV node (Fig. 5-16, A). The QRS morphology results from fusion of the two mechanisms of ventricular activation. Pathways capable of only retrograde conduction are referred to as concealed pathways, and no ventricular preexcitation (or delta wave) is present on the ECG.

Wolff-Parkinson-White syndrome is characterized by the presence of ventricular preexcitation (short PR interval and delta wave on ECG) and the clinical occurrence of arrhythmias.

In patients with Wolff-Parkinson-White syndrome the most common type of supraventricular tachycardia is orthodromic tachycardia, in which antegrade block occurs in the accessory pathway and a reentrant circuit is established with antegrade conduction occurring over the AV node and retrograde conduction up the accessory pathway (Fig. 5-16, *B*). In orthodromic tachycardia the QRS is narrow unless aberrancy occurs and there is a short RP interval on the surface ECG. A less common type of tachycardia in patients with Wolff-Parkinson-White syndrome is antidromic tachycardia, which is a reentrant

Possible Rhythms in WPW Syndrome

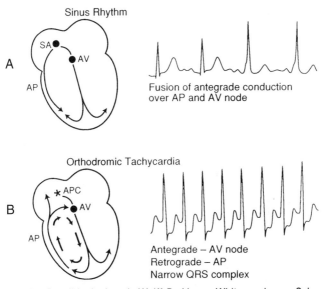

Fig. 5-16 Possible rhythms in Wolff-Parkinson-White syndrome. Schematic representation of possible rhythms in a patient with an accessory atrioventricular (AV) bypass tract. **A,** During sinus rhythm the ventricle may be activated by conduction over the accessory pathway *(AP)* and through the normal AV conduction system. The QRS complex may be narrow if the ventricle is activated primarily by conduction through the AV node. The QRS complex is wide and preexcited if activation of the ventricle occurs primarily via the accessory pathway. **B,** During orthodromic reentrant tachycardia antegrade conduction occurs through the AV node and normal conduction system, whereas retrograde conduction occurs via the accessory pathway. The resulting tachycardia has a narrow QRS morphology. *Continued*

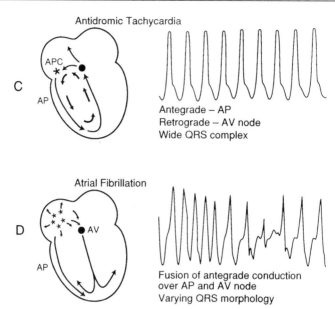

Fig. 5-16, cont'd   C, Antidromic tachycardia uses the accessory pathway as the antegrade limb of the reentrant circuit and the AV node and normal conduction system as the retrograde limb. The resulting tachycardia has a wide QRS complex. **D,** When atrial fibrillation occurs in a patient with manifest accessory pathway, antegrade conduction to the ventricle may occur through the AV node or over the accessory pathway. Morphology of the QRS complex may be narrow, which occurs primarily through the AV node, or wide and preexcited if conduction occurs over the accessory pathway. The morphology of the QRS complex may vary beat by beat during atrial fibrillation.

tachycardia with antegrade conduction occurring over the accessory pathway and retrograde conduction through the AV node (Fig. 5-16, *C*). Antidromic tachycardia is a regular wide-complex tachycardia that may resemble ventricular tachycardia on surface ECG. Compared with the general population, patients with Wolff-Parkinson-White syndrome have an increased incidence of atrial fibrillation and conduction to the ventricle may occur over the accessory pathway and the AV node (Fig. 5-16, *D*). The QRS morphology depends on the relative amount of conduction occurring through the accessory pathway compared with the normal conduction system. In patients with pathways capable of antegrade conduction and atrial fibrillation, rapid ventricular responses may occur with a potential for degeneration to ventricular fibrillation. During EPS in patients with Wolff-Parkinson-White syndrome, it is important to induce atrial fibrillation and observe the shortest R-R interval that shows ventricular preexcitation to assess the antegrade ERP of the accessory pathway and the risk of sudden cardiac death. Patients who have Wolff-Parkinson-White syndrome and are resuscitated from ventricular fibrillation usually have inducible atrial fibrillation with a rapid ventricular response and shortest preexcited R-R interval of less than 250 ms. Programmed atrial stimulation with single premature extrastimuli defines the antegrade ERP of the accessory pathway. Programmed stimulation of the ventricle shows the retrograde conduction properties of the accessory pathway and defines retrograde ERP.

CATHETER ABLATION

Catheter ablation is an interventional discipline within electrophysiology whereby an arrhythmogenic focus or critical portion of an arrhythmia circuit is identified, localized, and subsequently destroyed by means of a percutaneous transcatheter technique. Arrhythmias that are currently amenable to ablative therapy include atrial fibrillation, atrial flutter, ectopic atrial tachycardias, supraventricular tachycardias caused by AV nodal reentry or accessory bypass tracts, and ventricular tachycardia. Many modalities have been used for ablation. Historically, direct current energy was the initial energy source used for ablative procedures, dating back to the early 1980s.

More recently, radiofrequency energy has become the energy source most commonly used for ablative therapy. Radiofrequency energy uses a frequency range from 200 to 1200 kHz. Application of radiofrequency current causes tissue desiccation in a well-localized region at the point of catheter contact, resulting in a small discrete lesion approximately 0.5×0.5 cm^2. The localized nature of radiofrequency energy–induced lesions has made it the energy source of choice for most ablative procedures. Thermistor-tip catheters allow regulation of temperature at the electrode-tissue interface, ensuring adequate contact and preventing sudden impedance rises. Other energy sources for ablation, such as microwave and ultrasound, are being investigated.

New cardiac mapping technologies have recently been developed. The CARTO system is an electromagnetic navigation system that provides a three-dimensional reconstruction of the mapped heart chambers with a color-coded visualization of the endocardial activation sequence. The EnSite system uses a noncontact mapping balloon probe that can be deployed in the atrium or ventricle. It creates a three-dimensional computer model of the heart chamber with virtual electrograms. This system allows the mapping of hemodynamically unstable patients because the arrhythmia need be present for only one to two beats.

Indications for Ablative Therapy

Atrial Fibrillation. Catheter destruction of the AV junction has been used to treat patients with atrial fibrillation and rapid ventricular responses refractory to medical therapy. Patients who are intolerant of medical therapy and patients not desiring lifelong medical therapy are also candidates for this procedure. In the procedure complete heart block is created and a permanent ventricular pacemaker is required to normalize the heart rate.

Ablation procedures have been developed in an attempt to "cure" atrial fibrillation. Initial attempts were to create linear lesions in the left and right atria, similar to the surgical Maze procedure. More recently, attention has turned to the pulmonary vein ostia, which have been identified as the sites for electrical discharges that can initiate atrial fibrillation. Focal ablation of these sites has been performed with a high success rate in acute cases. There is also a high recurrence rate, however, with patients often needing two or more procedures. Another option is the anatomic approach, which consists of mapping around the left atrial–pulmonary vein border and ablating connections to these structures (pulmonary vein isolation).

Atrial Flutter. A crucial segment of the reentrant circuit of atrial flutter has been localized to the low posterior septum of the right atrium. Radiofrequency application to this area may eliminate the arrhythmia and is indicated in patients with medically refractory atrial flutter or in patients who are intolerant of medical therapy.

Ectopic Atrial Tachycardias. Ectopic atrial tachycardia, also known as automatic atrial tachycardia, may be mapped and ablated. This procedure is now a front-line therapy for medically resistant ectopic atrial tachycardias as a more economical and less invasive alternative to the traditional surgical isolation procedures.

Atrioventricular Nodal Reentry Tachycardia and Wolff-Parkinson-White Syndrome. The usefulness of catheter ablation is described best in the category of reentrant tachycardias that includes the more common mechanisms of supraventricular tachycardias: AV nodal reentrant tachycardia and tachycardias associated with accessory bypass tracts. The indication for catheter ablation in this group of arrhythmias includes recurrent symptomatic tachycardias that are medically refractory or situations in which medical management is not well tolerated or desired by the patient. Ablation therapy has become a front-line therapeutic option for patients with paroxysmal supraventricular tachycardia, obviating the need for therapy with antiarrhythmic agents. Another important indication for radiofrequency ablation is atrial fibrillation in the setting of an accessory pathway capable of conducting in an antegrade manner. These pathways have the potential for extremely rapid conduction, resulting in dangerously rapid ventricular responses with rates exceeding 250 beats/min. In this clinical setting degeneration to ventricular fibrillation is possible. Patients with a history of syncope and an accessory pathway capable of antegrade conduction present another indication for curative ablation therapy.

Ventricular Tachycardia. Ventricular tachycardia presents a challenge to the interventional electrophysiologist in terms of applications of catheter ablation techniques. The extremely variable site of tachycardia origin and the diffuse nature of the arrhythmia circuit make localizing successful sites for energy application difficult. Initial applications of ablation therapy in ventricular tachycardia were undertaken in patients with recurrent ventricular tachycardia and structurally normal hearts (idiopathic ventricular tachycardia). Catheter mapping and ablation have abolished recurrent ventricular tachycardia successfully with a remarkably low recurrence rate. However, only a small portion of patients have idiopathic ventricular tachycardia with sustained recurrent ventricular tachycardia. Other candidates for radiofrequency ablation are patients with non-ischemic cardiomyopathy and bundle-branch reentry tachycardia. In these patients ablation of the right bundle may eliminate the ventricular tachycardia.

Patients with coronary artery disease represent most patients with recurrent ventricular tachycardia. Patients with sustained hemodynamically stable ventricular tachycardia and relatively well-maintained LV function seem to be the best candidates for mapping and ablation procedures. Another relative contra-indication to ablative therapy is the induction of multiple ventricular tachycardia morphologies during initial EPS.

Technical Aspects of Specific Ablation Procedures

General Aspects. Before ablation procedures the patient is prepared in a manner similar to that for a general EPS. All anti-arrhythmic drugs are discontinued. Catheters are placed in the same manner described earlier. Systemic heparinization during the ablation procedure is required. When ablations that require retrograde approach via the aorta/left ventricle are performed, activated coagulation times should be monitored regularly and full anticoagulation (activated coagulation times >300 seconds) maintained throughout the procedure. In many laboratories prophylactic broad-spectrum IV antibiotics are administered before and during the procedure.

In addition to the standard catheters, special steerable tip catheters have been designed to facilitate mapping and ablation procedures (Fig. 5-17). They are constructed with a large platinum tip (4 to 8 mm), which can produce adequate lesion size in the endocardial surface. An energy source is also necessary. In radiofrequency energy ablations a generator capable of delivering a continuous unmodulated sine wave at approximately 500 kHz is standard. These generators also continuously monitor energy output and catheter impedance. The circuit is completed by a large indifferent skin electrode, usually positioned in the infrascapular region on the patient's back. A sophisticated electrogram monitoring and storage system is necessary for mapping and ablation procedures. Multiple computer-based multichannel recording systems are available that allow for real-time data analysis and facilitate the

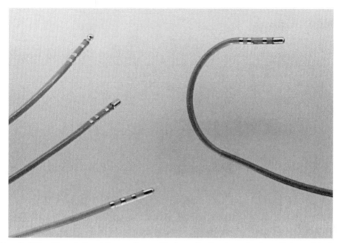

Fig. 5-17 Specialized large-tip catheter electrodes designed for ablative procedures.

mapping-ablation procedure. Radiologic equipment capable of multiplane views is necessary for optimal catheter placement.

When the patient has been prepared properly and catheters are placed, a baseline EPS is undertaken to document the properties of the tachycardia and the inducibility of the tachycardia. After the characteristics of the tachycardia have been evaluated fully, the mapping and ablation procedures are begun. Techniques used in this part of the procedure are unique to the tachycardia to be studied. Specific mapping techniques are discussed as follows. When the optimal site for ablation has been localized, radiofrequency current is applied to the distal pole of the mapping catheter. Typically, 15 to 35 W of current is applied over 30 to 60 seconds to achieve a target temperature of 60° C while the rhythm and intracardiac electrograms are monitored closely (Fig. 5-18).

After ablation there is typically a 30- to 60-minute waiting period during which repeat EPS is undertaken. This EPS is used to document successful ablation or signs of early recurrence. If no evidence of recurrent tachycardia is seen during approximately 60 minutes after ablation, the procedure can be terminated and the patient returned to his or her hospital room. The patient should be hospitalized and observed with cardiac monitoring for approximately 24 hours after the procedure.

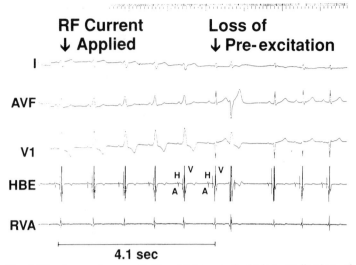

Fig. 5-18 Loss of preexcitation (delta wave) during application of radiofrequency current. Surface leads I, aVF, and V₁ are displayed. *HBE,* His bundle electrogram; *RVA,* right ventricular apex electrogram. Note the loss of the delta wave and lengthening of the PR interval after 4.1 seconds of radiofrequency *(RF)* energy application, signifying successful ablation of the accessory pathway.

During this time early recurrence can be detected or iatrogenic conduction abnormalities observed. The patient can be watched for complications from the procedure, including pneumothorax, the development of postprocedure fever, or vascular injury associated with the ablation procedure. The patient can typically be discharged the morning after the procedure with few physical limitations.

Atrioventricular Node Ablation. A temporary pacing wire is placed in the RV apex for pacing support during the procedure. A 4- to 8-mm deflectable tip electrode is placed across the tricuspid annulus and positioned where a prominent His potential is recorded. The catheter is slowly withdrawn into the atrium (Fig. 5-19). When the ablation catheter is positioned so that equal atrial and ventricular electrograms are recorded with a small His potential present, radiofrequency energy can be applied. Success is indicated by an accelerated junctional rhythm that is observed soon after the onset of radiofrequency

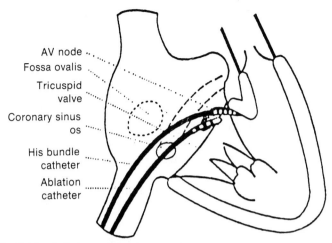

Fig. 5-19 Catheter position during atrioventricular (AV) junction ablation represented in the right anterior oblique view. The position of the His bundle recording catheter is used as a reference. The ablation catheter is positioned on the atrial side of the tricuspid valve just below the diagnostic catheter. (From Haines DE, Di Marco JP: *Curr Probl Cardiol* 27:409-477, 1992.)

energy delivery and is followed by high-degree AV block. Immediately after AV nodal ablation a permanent ventricular pacemaker must be implanted to ensure an adequate ventricular rate. Alternatively, the pacemaker may be implanted before the ablation procedure. The efficacy of radiofrequency-induced AV block is approximately 95% with a 5% to 10% recurrence rate of AV conduction. Significant complications occur in 1% to 2% of patients. There also is a rare but recognized complication of sudden malignant ventricular arrhythmias occurring hours to days after AV node ablation. The mechanism is poorly understood but may be related to inhomogeneous dispersion of repolarization. This complication has largely been eliminated by programming of the pacemaker rate to at least 80 beats/min for the first several months.

Atrial Fibrillation. Focal ablation of pulmonary vein ectopic beats must be performed during sinus rhythm. The feasibility of this technique is limited by the difficulty in mapping the focus if the patient is in atrial fibrillation or has no consistent firing. The anatomic approach, in which circumferential radiofrequency lesions are created around the ostia of each pulmonary vein, may be more expedient. Both approaches necessitate one or more transseptal punctures and use several multipolar mapping catheters. Newer mapping and ablation catheters (balloon and lasso-shaped) have been developed to facilitate these procedures in the left atrium. At present these procedures have mediocre long-term success rates and significant complications, including pulmonary vein stenosis, and should be considered only for select patients and at centers where a high volume of these procedures are performed.

Atrial Flutter. Atrial flutter has been ablated successfully with application of radiofrequency current in the area of the isthmus (between the inferior vena cava, coronary sinus, and tricuspid annulus). Mapping of the sequence of activation in the atrium and septum and documentation of block are necessary for successful ablation. High success rates have been achieved with the use of a large-tip catheter and long sheaths that help stabilize the catheter tip in the low right atrium (Fig. 5-20). Initial success rates are 80%, although recurrence of atrial flutter or atrial fibrillation is common.

Ectopic Atrial Tachycardia. Extensive mapping of the atria is crucial in ablation of ectopic atrial tachycardia. A coronary sinus catheter is necessary for initial mapping of the left atrium. A multipolar (20-polar) catheter is positioned in the right atrium. Activation mapping is performed to localize the region of earliest atrial activation. More precise mapping is undertaken with a deflectable-tip mapping catheter until the earliest site of atrial activation is located. If during initial testing the tachycardia is localized to the left atrium, mapping is undertaken with a transseptal approach via a patent foramen

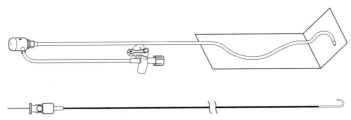

Fig. 5-20 Long (60-cm) introducer sheath (Daig, Minnetonka, Minn.) used to stabilize catheter tip during atrial flutter ablation.

ovale or transseptal puncture technique. For mapping of the left side of the heart, meticulous anticoagulation must be maintained to reduce the risk of procedure-related embolic events.

Radiofrequency energy application to atrial endocardium can be painful for the patient. Using the lowest energy output capable of terminating the tachycardia can maximize the patient's comfort.

Atrioventricular Nodal Reentrant Tachycardia. In AV nodal reentry the circuit consists of a slowly conducting pathway and a rapidly conducting pathway. Anatomically, these pathways are located in the perinodal interatrial septum and compact AV node, respectively. The current approach to ablation for AV nodal reentry, termed AV nodal modification, is selective ablation of the slow pathway. In rare cases a fast or intermediate pathway ablation must be performed for successful AV nodal modification.

Mapping of the slow pathway is performed around the inferior and posterior perinodal area in the posterior septal region of the right atrium extending inferiorly to the os of the coronary sinus. Radiofrequency energy is delivered along the tricuspid annulus where low-amplitude fragmented atrial electrograms are recorded (Fig. 5-21). Radiofrequency energy can be delivered during AV nodal reentrant tachycardia or in sinus rhythm. Successful ablation is heralded by termination of the tachycardia when energy is delivered during supraventricular tachycardia or by development of accelerated junctional rhythm when ablating in sinus rhythm.

Complete elimination of the slow pathway results in the inability to induce AV nodal reentrant tachycardia or show conduction along the slow AV pathway. After ablation, routine programmed electrical stimulation is repeated to evaluate for the presence of slow pathway conduction or inducible AV nodal reentry. If the slow pathway is not functional in the drug-free state, isoproterenol should be infused to validate noninducibility. Success rates for AV nodal modification are 95% or greater, and the risk of major complication is estimated to be 1% to 5%. Potential complications include iatrogenic high-degree AV block, pericarditis, cardiac perforation with tamponade, and vascular complications related to access. The estimated recurrence rate is 5%.

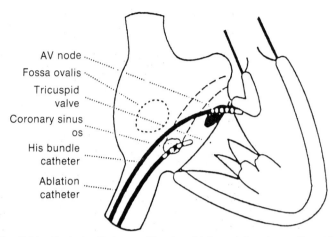

AV node
Fossa ovalis
Tricuspid valve
Coronary sinus os
His bundle catheter
Ablation catheter

Fig. 5-21 Typical catheter position for ablation of the slow pathway for atrioventricular (AV) nodal reentry tachycardia. The ablation catheter is positioned on the atrial side of the tricuspid valve in the vicinity of the coronary sinus os. The ablation catheter is inferior and posterior to the His bundle catheter. (From Haines DE, Di Marco JP: *Curr Probl Cardiol* 27:409-477, 1992.)

Accessory Pathways. The technique used for ablating accessory pathways is different depending on the location and the conduction properties of the accessory pathways. Before the ablation the patient undergoes a comprehensive EPS to determine the presence and electrical properties of the accessory pathways. The pathways that conduct antegrade in sinus rhythm and exhibit a delta wave (manifest preexcitation) can be mapped during sinus rhythm. The general location of the accessory pathway can be identified by the axis of the delta wave on the 12-lead ECG. EPS and mapping are required, however, to localize precisely the site of the accessory pathway. With a manifest accessory pathway the mapping catheter is maneuvered slowly along the valve annulus to locate the optimal electrode placement that will result in the earliest ventricular activation during sinus rhythm or atrial pacing (Fig. 5-22). Discrete electrical potentials from the accessory pathway have frequently been recorded at the successful ablation site and are referred to as pathway potentials. For pathways capable only of retrograde conduction, mapping is performed by determining the site of earliest retrograde atrial activity during ventricular pacing or induced orthodromic reciprocating tachycardia. Accessory pathways on the left side of the heart can be ablated by a transseptal approach using a patent foramen ovale, the Brochenbrough technique

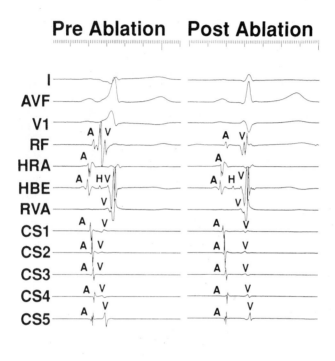

Fig. 5-22 Sequence of antegrade ventricular activation before and after radiofrequency ablation of a left-sided accessory pathway. Surface leads 1, aVF, and V_1 are displayed. *HRA,* High right atrial electrogram; *HBE,* His bundle electrogram; *RVA,* right ventricular apex electrogram; CS_1 to CS_5, recordings from the coronary sinus, with CS_1 representing the most proximal coronary sinus recording and CS_5 representing the most distal. The earliest ventricular activation during sinus rhythm occurs in the mid–coronary sinus (CS_2 to CS_3) region. Electrograms recorded from the ablating catheter at the successful ablation site *(RF)* show early ventricular activation and a short atrioventricular interval. Postablation, a normal sequence of antegrade activation is shown. Note lengthening of the A-to-V interval in the coronary sinus electrograms and the electrogram recorded from the ablation catheter.

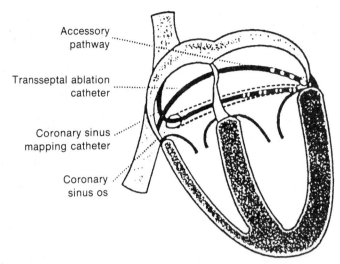

Accessory pathway

Transseptal ablation catheter

Coronary sinus mapping catheter

Coronary sinus os

Fig. 5-23 Catheter position for ablation of a left free wall pathway using a transseptal approach. The catheter is passed through a sheath that has been placed through the atrial septum, then positioned above the mitral valve annulus in close proximity to the accessory pathway, which is located near the coronary sinus catheter. (From Haines DE, Di Marco JP: *Curr Probl Cardiol* 27:409-477, 1992.)

(Fig. 5-23), or the more conventional retrograde approach, in which the ablating catheter is prolapsed across the aortic valve (Fig. 5-24).

The overall success of radiofrequency ablation for accessory pathways depends on operator experience and the location of the accessory pathway. Success rates of greater than 95% are reported for left-sided pathways. Right-sided pathways are usually reported to be less successful with efficacy rates greater than 90%. The complication rate for accessory pathway abla-tion is estimated to be 1% to 2%, and most complications result from catheter manipulation and not from the delivery of the radiofrequency energy. Complications include iatrogenic high-degree AV block (most commonly seen with anteroseptal accessory pathway ablations), pericarditis, cardiac perforation with tamponade, and vascular complications related to access associated with radiofrequency ablation of accessory pathways. Mortality is rare but has been reported as approximately 0.3%. Complications, including procedure-related deaths, are higher

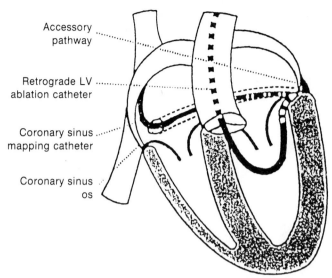

Accessory pathway

Retrograde LV ablation catheter

Coronary sinus mapping catheter

Coronary sinus os

Fig. 5-24 Catheter position for ablation of left free wall accessory pathway via the retrograde approach. The ablation catheter is prolapsed across the aortic valve and positioned under the mitral valve leaflet in close proximity to the accessory pathway located near the coronary sinus catheter. *LV,* Left ventricular. (From Haines DE, Di Marco JP: *Curr Probl Cardiol* 27:409-477, 1992.)

in low-volume laboratories (<20 ablations per year) than in high-volume laboratories (>50 ablations per year). The estimated recurrence rate after ablation for an accessory pathway is 3% to 17%; the higher recurrence rates are seen with right-sided accessory pathways. Patients who remain asymptomatic for 3 months after the procedure have an extremely low incidence of recurrence thereafter.

Ventricular Tachycardia. Several mapping techniques are used to target radiofrequency application during treatment for ventricular tachycardia. These techniques usually are used in combination to locate the optimal site of energy delivery. They can be used for idiopathic ventricular tachycardias (the most common being RV outflow tract tachycardia) or ventricular tachycardias associated with coronary artery disease. Initially a gross estimation of tachycardia origin can be made from the 12-lead ECG of ventricular tachycardia. This estimate helps to direct mapping efforts to the right or left ventricle and to specific regions within the appropriate ventricle.

During activation time mapping the mapping catheter is maneuvered to an endocardial location that shows the earliest activation time in tachycardia (Fig. 5-25). The presence of

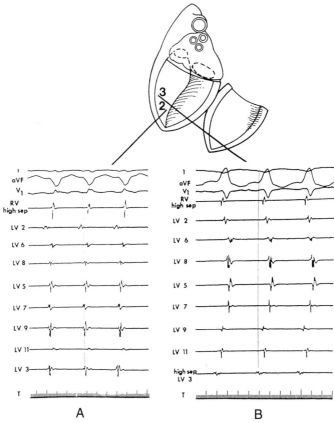

Fig. 5-25 Endocardial catheter mapping of two different ventricular tachycardia morphologies. **A,** Ventricular tachycardia with a right bundle-branch morphology and right superior axis. A reference right ventricular *(RV)* catheter is shown along with multiple ventricular recordings. The earliest ventricular activation is recorded at LV$_2$, which corresponds with the RV apex. **B,** Ventricular tachycardia with a left bundle-branch block pattern in right inferior axis. The earliest ventricular activation occurs near LV$_3$, which corresponds to the high septal area. *T,* Time line. (From Josephson ME: *Clinical cardiac electrophysiology: techniques and interpretations,* Philadelphia, 1993, Lea & Febiger.)

mid-diastolic potentials identifies optimal ablation sites. Pace mapping, in which pacing from the ablation catheter duplicates the QRS morphology of the clinical ventricular tachycardia, is also used to identify the appropriate site for ablation energy application. After the ablation procedure, ventricular stimulation is undertaken again to ensure that the tachycardia is no longer inducible. Ablation of idiopathic ventricular tachycardia seems to have a higher success rate (approximately 85%) than ablation of ventricular tachycardia associated with coronary artery disease (approximately 60%). A survey by the North American Society of Pacing and Electrophysiology reported a low complication rate and mortality associated with radiofrequency catheter ablation despite its use in a relatively high-risk patient population. Ventricular tachycardia associated with ischemic heart disease is an extremely variable entity and must be assessed on an individual basis.

Suggested Readings

Antiarrhythmics Versus Implantable Defibrillators (AVID) Investigators: A comparison of antiarrhythmic-drug therapy with implantable defibrillators in patients resuscitated from near-fatal ventricular arrhythmias, *N Engl J Med* 337:1576-1583, 1997.

Calkins H, Yong P, Miller JM, et al: Catheter ablation of accessory pathways, atrioventricular nodal reentrant tachycardia, and the atrioventricular junction, *Circulation* 99:262-270, 1999.

Cohen TJ, Scheinman MM, Pullen BT, et al: Emergency intracardiac defibrillation for refractory ventricular fibrillation during routine electrophysiologic study, *J Am Coll Cardiol* 18:1280-1284, 1991.

Feld GK, Fleck RP, Chen PS, et al: Radiofrequency catheter ablation for the treatment of human type 1 atrial flutter: identification of a critical zone in the reentrant circuit by endocardial mapping techniques, *Circulation* 86:1233-1240, 1992.

Fogoros RN: *Electrophysiologic testing*, Oxford, 1991, Blackwell.

Forcinito M: Guidelines for clinical intracardiac electrophysiologic studies: a report of the American College of Cardiology/American Heart Association Task Force on Assessment of Diagnostic and Therapeutic Cardiovascular Procedures (Subcommittee to Assess Clinical Intracardiac Electrophysiologic Studies), *J Am Coll Cardiol* 14:1827-1842, 1989.

Haines DE, DiMarco JP: Current therapy for supraventricular tachycardia, *Curr Probl Cardiol* 27:409-477, 1992.

Horowitz LN, Kay HR, Kutalek SP, et al: Risks and complications of clinical cardiac electrophysiologic studies: a prospective analysis of 1,000 consecutive patients, *J Am Coll Cardiol* 9:1261-1268, 1987.

Jackman WM, Beckman KJ, McClelland JH, et al: Treatment of supraventricular tachycardia due to atrioventricular nodal reentry by radiofrequency catheter ablation of slow-pathway conduction, *N Engl J Med* 327:313-318, 1992.

Jackman WM, Wang X, Friday KJ, et al: Catheter ablation of accessory atrioventricular pathways (Wolff-Parkinson-White syndrome) by radiofrequency current, *N Engl J Med* 324:1605-1611, 1991.

Josephson ME: *Clinical cardiac electrophysiology: techniques and interpretations,* Philadelphia, 1993, Lea & Febiger.

Mason JW, for the ESVEM Investigators: A comparison of seven antiarrhythmic drugs in patients with ventricular tachyarrhythmias, *N Engl J Med* 329:452-458, 1993.

Morady F, Harvey M, Kalbfleisch SJ, et al: Radiofrequency catheter ablation of ventricular tachycardia in patients with coronary artery disease, *Circulation* 87:363-372, 1993.

Moss AJ, Hall WJ, Cannom DS, et al: Improved survival with an implanted defibrillator in patients with coronary artery disease at high risk for ventricular arrhythmia, *N Engl J Med* 335:19331940, 1996.

Moss AJ, Zareba W, Hall WJ, et al: Prophylactic implantation of a defibrillator in patients with myocardial infarction and reduced ejection fraction, *N Engl J Med* 346: 877-883, 2002.

Munawar M, Hanafy M, Rachman OJ, Harjowasito S: Successful radiofrequency catheter ablation of idiopathic left ventricular tachycardia using both retrograde and transseptal approach, *Cor Europaeum* 6:52658, 1997.

Pappone C, Rosanio S, Oreto G, et al: Circumferential radiofrequency ablation of pulmonary vein ostia, *Circulation* 102:26192628, 2000.

Scheidt S: Basic electrocardiography, West Caldwell, NJ, 1986, CIBA-GEIGY Pharmaceuticals.

Scheinman MM: Patterns of catheter ablation practice in the United States: results of the 1992 NASPE survey, *Pacing Clin Electrophysiol* 17:873-875, 1994.

Waller TJ, Kay HR, Spielman SR, et al: Reduction in sudden death and total mortality by antiarrhythmic therapy evaluated by electro-physiologic drug testing: criteria of efficacy in patients with sustained ventricular tachyarrhythmia, *J Am Coll Cardiol* 10:83-89, 1987.

6

RESEARCH TECHNIQUES

Steve C. Herrmann, Morton J. Kern, and Sanjeev Puri

Research techniques are commonly performed in catheterization laboratories in which cardiology fellows train. Such techniques have been of great value in understanding common problems in cardiology. This chapter is an overview of commonly used research procedures in the cardiac catheterization laboratory. Many clinical methods were once research techniques that have been incorporated into the routine of diagnostic cardiac catheterization. Tables 6-1 and 6-2 show the most commonly used research techniques and their functions.

The support staff in the cardiac catheterization laboratory may view clinical research as unnecessary, unimportant, or dangerous to the patient. These commonly held misconceptions should be dispelled by the physician, who should explain the utility and safety of the procedure. Only skilled physicians with directed goals and institutional research board approval should apply these research techniques. The data have been invaluable in identifying new therapies and advancing the frontiers of treatment for cardiac disease. It is most helpful for nurses and catheterization laboratory physicians to appreciate this problem and convey a sense of confidence and enthusiasm to the patient. The most common research catheterization techniques described in this chapter may be used alone or combined with others, as follows:

1. Quantitative angiographic analysis
2. Coronary sensor pressure guidewire and flow velocity measurements
3. Myocardial blood flow determination
4. Myocardial metabolism measurement
5. High-fidelity hemodynamic studies

Table 6-1

Research Techniques

Objective	Method
I. Ventricular Function	
1. Systolic function	Ventricular P-V relationship (simultaneous LV pressure with LV volume by echocardiogram, contrast angiogram, nuclear angiogram, or impedance catheter)
	Variables derived: end-systolic P-V slope, intercept; contractility (+ dP/dt)
2. Diastolic function	Ventricular P-V relationship (as above)
	Variables derived: end-diastolic P-V slope, intercept; relaxation ($- dP/dt$, τ, K)
3. Exercise studies	
4. Combined hemodynamic and echocardiographic studies	
II. Myocardial Blood Flow (Coronary Vasodilatory Reserve, Effects of Drugs)	Indicator dilution; inert gas (xenon, nitrogen); thermodilution
	Doppler flow velocity
	Digital radiographic studies
III. Endothelial Function	
1. IVUS	
2. Doppler flow	
3. QCA	
IV. Electrical Function (Abnormal Conduction, Excitation)	Electrophysiologic studies
	His bundle
	Atrial and ventricular refractory periods
	Conduction abnormalities
	Inducible ventricular ectopy
	Bypass tracts

LV, Left ventricular; *P-V*, pressure-volume; *IVUS*, intravascular ultrasound; *QCA*, quantitative coronary angiography.

Table 6-2

Additional Research Techniques in the Catheterization Laboratory

LV Function	Methods
Pressure-Volume Relationships	
End systole	High-fidelity pressure
End diastole	LV volume
	LV-gram (cineangiographic, digital)
	RV-gram
	Two-dimensional echocardiogram
	Impedance catheter
Wall Stress	
LV mass	Quantitative ventriculography
Diastolic function	High-fidelity pressure
	Doppler mitral inflow
Ventricular interaction	RV/LV high-fidelity pressures
Aortic impedance	Aortic flow velocity, high-fidelity pressure
Coronary Physiology	
Coronary blood flow, coronary reserve, coronary vasodilation (response to drugs)	Pharmacologic studies with papaverine and adenosine, acetylcholine
	Physiologic flow responses during interventional procedures such as angioplasty or hemodynamic studies
Ischemia Testing	
Induced tachycardia	Electrical pacing
Isoproterenol, dopamine	Pharmacologic infusion
Transient coronary occlusion	Coronary angioplasty

LV, Left ventricular; *RV,* right ventricular.

6. Combined hemodynamic-echocardiographic methodologies
7. New imaging modalities such as optical coherence tomography

QUANTITATIVE CORONARY ANGIOGRAPHY AND VENTRICULOGRAPHY

Quantitative coronary angiography and ventriculography are sophisticated approaches to analyzing coronary images and routine ventriculographic techniques. A precise angiographic method and computer analysis facilitate quantitative measurements.

TIMI Frame Count

Myocardial blood flow has been assessed angiographically by use of the Thrombolysis in Myocardial Infarction (TIMI) score for qualitative grading of coronary flow. TIMI flow grades 0 to 3 have become a standard description of coronary blood flow in clinical trials. TIMI grade 3 flows have been associated with improved clinical outcomes.

The method uses cineangiography with 6 F catheters and filming at 30 frames/sec. The number of cine frames from the introduction of dye into the coronary artery to a predetermined distal landmark is counted. The TIMI frame count for each major vessel is standardized according to specific distal landmarks. The first frame used for TIMI frame counting is that in which the dye fully opacifies the artery origin and in which the dye extends across the width of the artery, touching both borders with antegrade motion of the dye. The last frame counted is when dye enters the first distal landmark branch. Full opacification of the distal branch segment is not required. Distal landmarks commonly used in analysis are as follows: (1) for the left anterior descending (LAD) coronary artery, the distal bifurcation of the LAD artery; (2) for the circumflex system, the distal bifurcation of the branch segments with the longest total distance; and (3) for the right coronary artery, the first branch of the posterolateral artery.

The TIMI frame count can be corrected further for the length of the LAD coronary artery. The TIMI frame count in the LAD artery requires normalization or correction for comparison with the two other major arteries. This is called corrected TIMI frame count (CTFC). The average LAD coronary artery is 14.7 cm long, the right is 9.8 cm, and the circumflex is 9.3 cm according to Gibson and colleagues. CTFC accounts for the distance the dye has to travel in the LAD artery relative to the other arteries. CTFC divides the absolute frame count in the LAD artery by 1.7 to standardize the distance of dye travel in all three arteries. Normal TIMI frame count and CTFC for the LAD artery are 36 ± 3 and 21 ± 2, respectively; for the circumflex artery, TIMI frame count is 22 ± 4; for the right coronary artery,

TIMI frame count is 20 ± 3. TIMI flow grades do not correspond to measured Doppler flow velocity or the CTFC. High TIMI frame count may be associated with microvascular dysfunction despite an open artery. CTFCs of less than 20 frames were associated with low risk for adverse events in patients after myocardial infarction. A contrast injection rate increase of greater than or equal to 1 ml/sec by hand injection can decrease the TIMI frame count by two frames. The TIMI frame count method provides valuable information relative to clinical responses after coronary interventions.

MYOCARDIAL BLOOD FLOW

Techniques for determining myocardial blood flow include coronary sinus thermodilution, intracoronary Doppler velocity measurement, and digital coronary angiographic blood flow velocity. These techniques, for the most part, are used in well-defined research protocols.

Indications

Indications for techniques for determining myocardial blood flow are as follows:

1. Study of coronary flow reserve and the microcirculation identification of syndrome X (chest pain with normal coronary arteries)
2. Effects of drugs or interventions on myocardial blood flow or metabolism
3. Coronary endothelial function
4. Study of coronary physiology during percutaneous coronary intervention (PCI) (e.g., stents, atherectomy, Rotablator).
5. Examination of collateral flow

Coronary vasodilator reserve (maximal coronary blood flow/resting coronary blood flow) can be measured by coronary sinus blood flow with the use of continuous thermodilution technique or, more accurately, with intracoronary arterial flow velocity using miniaturized Doppler-tipped angioplasty guidewires. This methodology involves measurement of coronary blood flow velocity at rest and during stimulation with hyperemic agents such as adenosine (intracoronary or intravenous [IV]), papaverine, or dipyridamole (IV). When abnormal coronary vasodilatory responses are associated with abnormal myocardial metabolism (i.e., lactate generation) in patients with chest pain syndromes and normal coronary arteries, the diagnosis of syndrome X is probable. Coronary reserve is affected by epicardial and microvascular circulatory abnormalities (Fig. 6-1).

The measurement of volumetric changes in coronary blood flow (velocity, mm/sec · cross-sectional area, $mm^2 = mm^3/sec$) should be combined with measurement of myocardial oxygen consumption (arterial and coronary sinus blood) to identify whether increases in blood flow are caused by increased myocardial oxygen demand (metabolic regulation) or by pharmacologic changes independent of myocardial demand (primary artery vasodilation or constriction). The coronary sinus thermodilution catheter is ideally suited for metabolic studies. For determination of myocardial oxygen extraction, a second catheter may be placed in the coronary sinus to measure transmyocardial oxygen values.

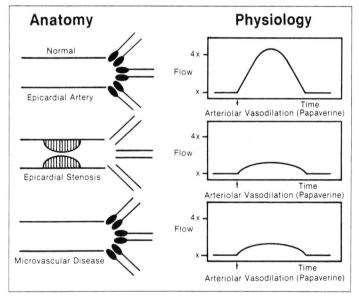

Fig. 6-1   Normal epicardial coronary artery and microvascular bed. Coronary vasodilatory reserve is normal. Coronary vasodilator reserve can be abnormal because of either epicardial artery narrowing or microvascular disease. (From White CW, Wilson RF: *Am J Cardiol* 67:44D-56D, 1991.)

MYOCARDIAL METABOLISM
Measurement of Specialized Blood Products

Transmyocardial (arterial and coronary vein blood) blood sampling is used to study myocardial metabolism. Measurements of pyruvate, lactate, and oxygen extraction are the most common products. The transmyocardial extraction of drugs after systemic delivery can also be determined. Specialized collection tubes for lactate and heparinized syringes for arterial and coronary sinus oxygen blood samples should be prepared in advance. Myocardial catecholamines (norepinephrine, epinephrine) and other specialized products (e.g., prostaglandin) require special handling but can also be obtained with this technique.

Measuring of specialized blood products requires that the sampling tubes should be prepared in advance so that the physician can pass the drawn blood quickly to the technicians for insertion into the collecting tubes. In addition to sample tube preparation, ice, a centrifuge, or a series of dilutional tubes may be required. These techniques are not complicated, but correct labeling and anticipation of which samples will be obtained at which point in the procedure reduce errors without unnecessarily prolonging the study.

CORONARY SINUS CATHETERIZATION
Technique

Coronary sinus (CS) catheterization is generally performed from the left brachial venous approach or through the right internal jugular vein. The ostium of the CS is located inferior and posterior to the tricuspid valve.

A specially shaped catheter is inserted through a percutaneously placed venous sheath. After careful insertion in the right atrium, the catheter is directed toward the tricuspid valve and in a posterior direction. Gentle medial advancement with a 1- to 2-ml flush of contrast medium enables the physician to know when the catheter has entered the CS. Ventricular ectopy indicates contact with right ventricular wall or septum. The catheter is withdrawn and readvanced after slight rotation.

The CS catheter is usually positioned in the anteroposterior view with the catheter seen passing upward across the tricuspid valve and spine. In the left anterior oblique position the catheter appears to be coming directly in plane toward the observer. In the right anterior oblique position it should pass away from the ventricular apex (i.e., not into the right ventricle). This technique is particularly difficult from the inferior vena cava, and this approach should probably be avoided unless specifically shaped catheters are available (confirm position by oxygen saturation [<35%]).

Care should be taken not to cannulate the inferior cardiac vein and to avoid perforation of the CS, right ventricle, or atrium. The catheter must be secured once it is positioned. If a brachial approach is used, the patient's arm should also remain fixed during the study.

Coronary Sinus Thermodilution Catheter Setup

After the catheter position is secured, the electrical connections from the catheter to the CS temperature-sensing device are made, and connections to the physiologic recorder are calibrated. Thermistor signals (i.e., patient's body temperature) are set to the baseline. The indicator solution (5% dextrose in water at room temperature) is injected through the catheter at a rate of 25 to 50 ml/min by use of a Harvard pump or Medrad injector.

DOPPLER CORONARY FLOW VELOCITY TECHNIQUES

The Doppler coronary flow velocity technique allows quantitative measurement of coronary flow by the use of pulsed sound waves (12 to 15 mHz) and measurement of the returning signal reflecting off moving red blood cells (Fig. 6-2). Measurement of the physiologic response of the coronary circulation to various drugs, maneuvers, and interventions and assessment of the significance of coronary obstructive lesions are examples of useful applications.

The Doppler guidewire is superior to earlier Doppler catheters (Fig. 6-3). Some of the clinical uses of the Doppler guidewire are listed in Box 6-1. The FloWire is small enough (0.014 to 0.018 inch in diameter) to assess coronary flow velocity across most coronary stenoses. After diagnostic angiography, the Doppler guidewire can detect flow velocity impairment caused by an intermediately severe angiographic lesion and can help direct PCI. It can also determine whether normal blood flow velocity has been restored after PCI and monitor flow changes thereafter.

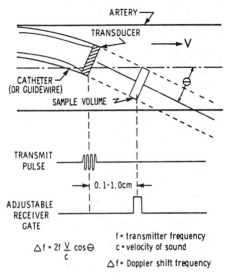

Fig. 6-2 Coronary Doppler principles. The catheter or guidewire emits high-frequency sound from the tip-mounted crystal, which reflects off moving red blood cells passing through the sample volume. The velocity of the blood flow is calculated using the Doppler shift formula. (Modified from Hartley CJ, Cole JS: *J Appl Physiol* 37:626-629, 1974.)

Method of Use of the Doppler FloWire

The 15-MHz crystal on the tip of the guidewire sends and receives ultrasound waves. The timing of the reflected sound waves is used to measure blood flow velocities from moving red blood cells in a sample area 5 mm from the tip of the wire (and 2 mm across), far enough away that the blood velocity is not affected by the wake of the wire. The returning signal is transmitted in real time to the display console. The gray-scale spectral scrolling display shows the velocities of all the red blood cells within the sample volume. The key parameters are derived from the automatically tracked peak blood velocities, making them less position sensitive (Fig. 6-4).

The Doppler angioplasty guidewire has a forward-directed ultrasound beam that diverges in a 27-degree arc from the long axis (measured in the −6 dB roundtrip points of the ultrasound beam pattern). The pulse repetition frequency of greater than 40 Hz, pulse duration of +0.83 second, and sampling delay of

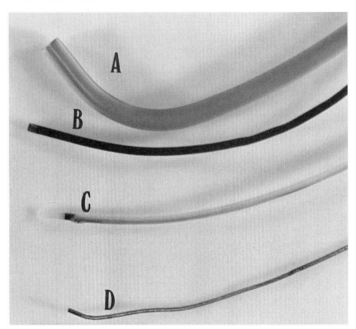

Fig. 6-3 Intracoronary Doppler catheters. **A,** Judkins Doppler (Cordis Corp., Miami, Fla.). **B,** Millar 3 F end-mounted crystal Doppler (Millar Instruments, Houston, Tex.). **C,** NuMed 3 F side-mounted catheter (NuMed, Hopkinton, N.Y.). **D,** FloWire 0.018-inch Doppler-tipped angioplasty guidewire (Jomed, Inc., Cordova, Calif.). (From Ofili EO, Kern MJ, Labovitz AJ, et al: *J Am Coll Cardiol* 21:308-316, 1993.)

Box 6-1

Uses of the Doppler FloWire

Intermediate (40% to 70%) Lesion Assessment
Collateral Flow Studies
Coronary Vasodilatory Reserve Assessment
Syndrome X
Transplant coronary arteriopathy

Coronary Flow Research Studies
Pharmacologic and endothelial function studies
Intraaortic balloon pumping
Coronary physiology of vascular disease
Ischemic test correlation

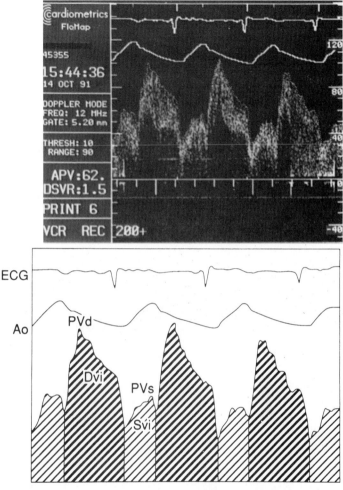

Fig. 6-4 Normal coronary flow velocity spectra showing small systolic and large diastolic velocity components. The diagram of measurements in the lower panel shows a darkly hatched diastolic velocity integral *(Dvi)*, a lightly hatched systolic velocity integral *(Svi)*, and peak systolic *(PVs)* and peak diastolic *(PVd)* velocities. The means of diastole and systole can be computed and total cycle variables. *Ao,* Aortic pressure; *DSVR,* diastolic-to-systolic velocity ratio; *ECG,* electrocardiogram; *APV,* average peak velocity (mean). (From Ofili EO, Kern MJ, Labovitz AJ, et al: *J Am Coll Cardiol* 21:308-316, 1993.)

6.5 seconds are standard for clinical use. The system is coupled to a real-time spectrum analyzer, videocassette recorder, and video page printer. The spectrum analyzer uses on-line fast-Fourier transformation (see Fig. 6-4) to process the Doppler audio signals. Simultaneous electrocardiographic and arterial pressure data are also displayed. During in vivo testing the Doppler guidewire–measured velocity showed excellent correlation with electromagnetic measurements of flow velocity and volumetric flow.

Before the Doppler guidewire is placed into an artery, the patient should be given IV heparin (40 to 60 µ/kg with target activated coagulation time >200 seconds). Pressure and velocity signals should be recorded continuously during hyperemia (Figs. 6-5 and 6-6).

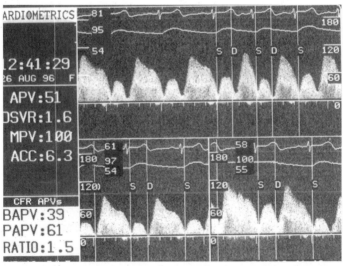

Fig. 6-5 Doppler flow velocity screen is split into continuous phasic signals *(top)* and base and hyperemic signal storage areas *(below)*. Electrocardiogram and aortic pressure are at top of each signal area. Scale is 0 to 120 cm/sec at far right. Numbers in dark boxes in upper left corner are heart rate and systolic and diastolic blood pressure. *S,* Systolic marker; *D,* diastolic marker; *APV,* average peak velocity; *DSVR,* diastolic-to-systolic velocity ratio; *MPV,* maximal peak velocity; *ACC,* acceleration; *B,* base; *P,* peak coronary reserve ratio.

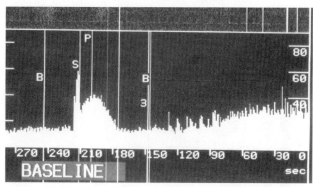

Fig. 6-6   Doppler flow velocity continuous trend plot of average peak velocity panel. Baseline value *(B)* is obtained. Intracoronary adenosine is injected (note artifact before S, [search]). Hyperemia is stimulated, and peak *(P)* hyperemia is captured and stored.

Measurement of Translesional Velocity

After diagnostic angiography or during angioplasty the Doppler guidewire is passed through a standard angioplasty Y connector attached to either a 6 F diagnostic or guiding catheter. The guidewire is advanced into the artery and beyond the stenosis by a distance equivalent to at least 5 to 10 times the arterial diameter (approximately 2 cm). Placement in any side branches is avoided. Distal flow velocity data are obtained at rest and during hyperemia.

Flow Reserve

Hyperemic measurements are obtained by intracoronary injections of adenosine (24 to 30 μg in the right coronary artery and 24 to 40 mg in the left coronary artery). Papaverine (10 to 12 mg intracoronary injection), has rarely caused ventricular tachycardia or ventricular fibrillation. Coronary flow reserve is computed as the ratio of hyperemic and basal mean flow velocities. Coronary flow reserve and fractional flow reserve and correlations with ischemic stress testing are shown in Table 6-3.

Setting up of the FloWire system usually takes less than 10 minutes, and use of the system is easily incorporated into

Table 6-3

Comparison of Stress (Ischemia) Testing and Directly Measured Coronary Blood Flow Physiology

Author	(n)	Ischemic Test	Physiologic Threshold	Sensitivity	Specificity	PV+	PV–	Accuracy
Poststenotic CVR/rCVR								
Miller	33	Adeno/Dipy MIBI	<2.0	82	100	100	77	89
Joye	30	Exercise thallium	<2.0	94	95	94	95	94
Deychack	17	Exercise thallium	<1.8	94	94	100	91	96
Heller	100	Exercise thallium	<1.8	89	92	96	89	92
Danzi	30	Dipy echo	<2.0	91	84	—	—	87
Schulman	35	Exercise ECG	<2.0	95	71	—	—	86
Donahue	50	Exercise/Pharm thallium	<2.0	98	76	88	88	—
Duffy	43	Stress echo	<2.0, rCVR<0.75	80	93	—	—	88
				100	76	—	—	81
Chamuleau	127	Dipy MIBI	CVR <0.2, rCVR <0.75	—	—	—	—	69
				—	—	—	—	75
El Shafei	53	Exercise/Pharm thallium	CVR <0.2, rCVR <0.75	71	83	81	74	—
				63	88	83	70	—

Author	(n)	Ischemic Test	Physiologic Threshold	Sensitivity	Specificity	PV+	PV–	Accuracy
FFR								
Pijls	45	4-test standard*	<0.75	88	100	100	88	93
de Bruyne	60	Exercise ECG	<0.72	100	87	—	—	—
Bartunek	37	Dobu/Exercise echo	<0.68	95	90	—	—	—
Chamuleau	127	Dipy MIBI	<0.75	—	—	—	—	75
Caymaz	30	Exercise thallium	<0.75	90	100	91	100	95

Adeno/Dipy MIBI, Adenosine or dipyridamole sestamibi scan; *CVR*, coronary vasodilatory reserve; *Dobu*, dobutamine; *ECG*, electrocardiogram; *Echo*, echocardiography; *FFR*, fractional flow reserve; *Pharm*, pharmacologic; *PV+/PV–*, predictive value positive/negative.
*Four tests were ECG, Echo, pacing, nuclear stress tests.

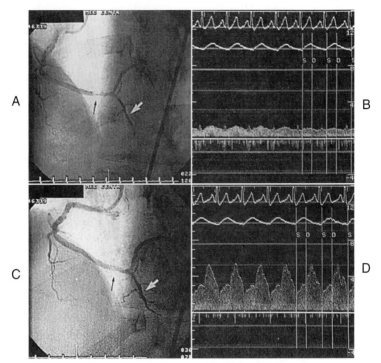

Fig. 6-7 Distal coronary flow velocity, **A,** before and, **C,** after successful percutaneous transluminal coronary balloon angioplasty of the distal right coronary artery 90% stenosis. **B,** Distal prepercutaneous transluminal coronary balloon angioplasty flow velocity is 12 cm/sec with reduced phasic pattern. **D,** After percutaneous transluminal coronary balloon angioplasty the mean flow velocity is 35 cm/sec with normal phasic pattern. The black arrows show percutaneous transluminal coronary balloon angioplasty sites, and white arrows show Doppler guidewire sample volume location.

routine procedures. Figure 6-7 shows coronary flow velocity before and after percutaneous transluminal coronary angioplasty in the right coronary artery.

Methodologic Difficulties. Doppler coronary velocity measures only relative changes in velocity. For measurement of absolute blood flow, the following assumptions must be made:

    1. The cross-sectional area of the vessel being studied remains fixed during hyperemia.

2. The velocity profile across the vessel is not distorted by arterial disease.

3. The angle between the crystal and sample volume remains constant and less than 30 degrees from the horizontal flow stream.

Measurement of Collateral Circulation

Coronary collateral flow can be measured with the use of the Doppler-tipped flow wire (Fig. 6-8) and pressure wire. A 0.014-inch pressure wire is set at 0, calibrated, and advanced through a balloon catheter and positioned in the vessel of interest. Collateral flow is measured by simultaneous measurement of mean aortic pressure (P_{ao}, mm Hg), coronary occlusion pressure (P_{occl}, mm Hg) and central venous pressure (CVP, mm Hg). Collateral flow is calculated as ($P_{occl} - CVP/P_{ao} - CVP$).

Intravascular Ultrasound Imaging

High-frequency, two-dimensional coronary ultrasound imaging uses catheters of 2.9 F or smaller with either mechanically or electronically rotating 20- to 40-MHz echo crystals, which produce cross-sectional images of the artery (Fig. 6-9). Ultrasound catheters are introduced over guidewires in a monorail fashion. In mildly diseased arteries a characteristic three-layered image is normally observed. These images are more accurate than angiography in identifying the amount of atherosclerotic material inside a vessel, as well as identifying other characteristics, such as calcium. Research studies using this tool are investigating endothelial function, progression and regression of plaque, responses to new pharmacologic agents, and results of catheter-based interventional techniques (e.g., atherectomy, laser, or rotoblator).

Coherence Tomography

In the future, use of fiberoptic technology will provide topographic, real-time images of the coronary artery. The glass fibers that transmit the light for imaging constitute a fiberoptic array with a distal lens that serves to focus the transmitted light. A reduction in fiberoptic size with increased flexibility and improved signal analysis will permit optical coherent tomographic studies with 10- to 20-μm level resolution (Fig. 6-10).

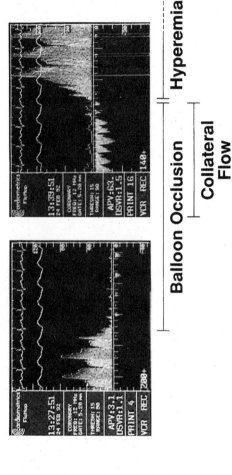

Fig. 6-8 Time sequence of flow velocity during coronary balloon occlusion in a patient with a left anterior descending (LAD) coronary artery filled with collaterals originating from the right coronary artery. Note the retrograde collateral flow velocity below the baseline in a phasic pattern appearing after 15 seconds of coronary occlusion. On release of balloon occlusion, immediate anterograde hyperemia can be observed in the distal bed with a loss of the retrograde flow pattern, corresponding with successful angioplasty. See Fig. 6-4 for abbreviations. (From Kern MJ, Donohue TJ, Bach RG, et al: *Am J Cardiol* 71:34D–40D, 1993.)

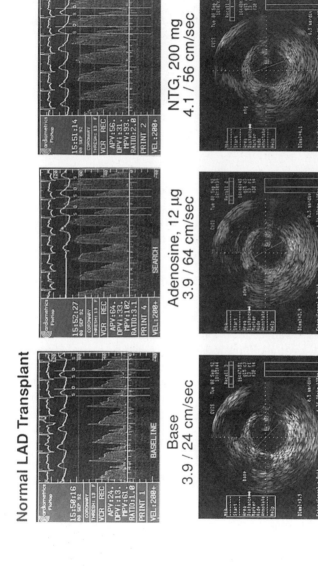

Fig. 6-9 *Top,* Doppler guidewire flow velocity and 4.3 F two-dimensional coronary ultrasound images. *Bottom,* Cross-sectional artery images show a normal lumen with a diameter of 3.9 mm and minimal changes to adenosine or nitroglycerin *(NTG). LAD,* Left anterior descending artery; *APV,* average peak velocity; *DPVi,* diastolic peak velocity integral; *MPV,* maximal peak velocity; *Ratio,* coronary reserve ratio; *VEL,* velocity scale.

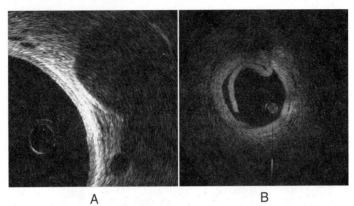

A   B

Fig. 6-10   Images from optical coherent imaging system. **A,** In vivo artery showing fine arterial structure. **B,** Dissection flap in vitro human artery.

The optical catheter is introduced into the artery and a small, compliant balloon is inflated to block antegrade blood flow. A flush system replaces blood to clear the viewing field. This technique allows identification of thrombus, arterial dissection, and plaque characteristics.

COMBINED HEMODYNAMIC AND ECHOCARDIOGRAPHIC METHODOLOGIES

Two-dimensional or M-mode echocardiography of left ventricular (LV) wall motion provides detailed information of myocardial contractile responses, which can be recorded with simultaneous hemodynamic measurements. The echocardiogram provides continuous observation of LV geometry and wall motion or valvular flow functions during study interventions without additional radiation. Transesophageal echocardiography has been used to guide transseptal balloon placement and improve the results during mitral valvuloplasty.

Some echocardiographic machines used for studies in the cardiac catheterization laboratory can be modified to accept pressure and other signals from the physiologic recorder (Figs. 6-11 and 6-12). Specialized input amplifiers for echocardiographic machines are available, facilitating the recording of pressures simultaneously with echocardiographic parameters. Use of Doppler echocardiography and simultaneous hemodynamics has advanced the understanding of cardiac

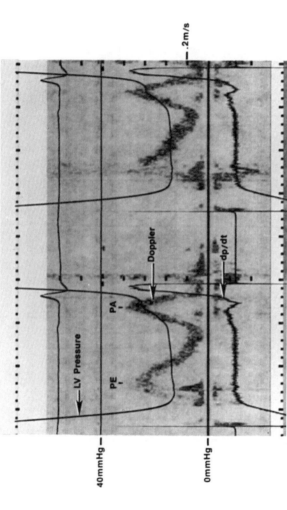

Fig. 6-11 Simultaneous high-fidelity left ventricular *(LV)* pressure (0 to 40 mm Hg scale) superimposed on Doppler echocardiogram showing peak early *(PE)* and peak atrial *(PA)* filling waves of the mitral valve inflow. Also superimposed is the dP/dt signal from the left ventricular pressure tracing and the electrocardiogram. These combined methods permit analysis of function not available by a single technique.

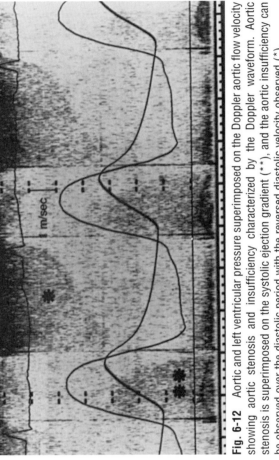

Fig. 6-12 Aortic and left ventricular pressure superimposed on the Doppler aortic flow velocity showing aortic stenosis and insufficiency characterized by the Doppler waveform. Aortic stenosis is superimposed on the systolic ejection gradient (**), and the aortic insufficiency can be observed over the diastolic period with the reversed diastolic velocity observed (*).

function and provides a means of examining questions previously unanswered with the use of other techniques.

HIGH-FIDELITY MICROMANOMETER-TIP PRESSURE MEASUREMENTS
Indications

High-fidelity transducer-tipped catheter measurements are made for studies requiring precise pressure waveforms for accurate analysis of small changes in absolute pressure and rates of upstroke and downstroke slopes used for assessment of contractility. High-fidelity pressure measurements are useful for studies of cardiac contractility, afterload reduction, or myocardial metabolism. In addition, high-fidelity pressures combined with quantitative volume measurements are used to determine myocardial function. The most precise hemo-dynamic studies use this technique.

Assessment of Ventricular Function from High-Fidelity Pressure Catheters

Contractility is the force or rate of myocardial muscle activity and often is measured by the electronically derived rate of rise (the first derivative dP/dt, i.e., change in pressure, dP, divided by change in time, dt) of pressure in the left ventricle (Fig. 6-13). This measurement is obtained with a micromanometer-tipped (high-fidelity) catheter because of its precise and instantaneous pressure transmission. The frequency responses of fluid-filled systems are too slow for research data. Various other iso-volumetric measurements are also derived from the dP/dt taken at different pressure levels (e.g., pressure at 40 mm Hg or at end diastole).

Measurement of Diastolic Function

A simple measure of active myocardial relaxation during isovolumetric diastole is measured by the rate of fall of LV pressure. A high-fidelity micromanometer catheter is used to generate a pressure signal from which the physician can calculate maximal negative dP/dt. Peak negative dP/dt is sensitive to loading conditions. The afterload dependence of peak negative dP/dt is eliminated by calculation of the time constant of isovolumic relaxation called tau (τ). Calculation of "τ" is based on the observation that the pressure fall during

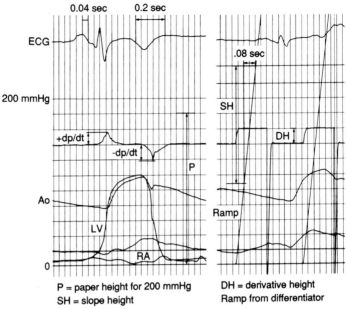

P = paper height for 200 mmHg
SH = slope height
DH = derivative height
Ramp from differentiator

Fig. 6-13 High-fidelity, micromanometer-tipped hemodynamic tracings of aortic and left ventricular pressures with differentiated dP/dt signal showing method of calculation of dP/dt. See text for details. To compute dP/dt:

1. SH: mm deflection from *ramp* over 80 m
2. DH: mm deflection of *square* box of derivative
3. Compute K:K = (12.5 × SH)/DH
4. Scale factor P = mm paper deflection of 200 mm Hg

5. Compute dP/dt:

$$dP/dt = \frac{200 \text{ mm Hg}}{P}(K)$$

Peak dP/dt positive or negative deflection; normal value range: 1500 to 1800 mm Hg/sec

isovolumic relaxation is roughly exponential. τ is approximately 40 ms in a normal left ventricle.

PHYSIOLOGIC MANEUVERS IN THE CATHETERIZATION LABORATORY
Exercise During Cardiac Catheterization

Exercise evaluation of cardiac function is helpful to relate symptoms of fatigue or dyspnea to hemodynamic changes of cardiac dysfunction, especially for patients with valvular heart disease (e.g., mitral stenosis). Hemodynamic data are measured at rest and during peak exercise with bicycle ergometry, repeated leg or arm lifts, and occasionally arm bicycle ergometry. Adequate response to exercise includes the following:

1. Normal minute ventilatory responses to exercise
2. Normal oxygen extraction
3. Normal heart rate increase in response to increases in cardiac output
4. Normal ventricular volume responses (decrease in filling pressures)
5. Adequate metabolic substrate use (i.e., glucose metabolism without lactate production)

Exercise may be dynamic or isometric. Measurement of each type shows different features of LV function.

Dynamic Exercise. Dynamic exercise measures the ability of the cardiovascular system to supply oxygen in keeping with the demands of the heart. Oxygen consumption and workload increases should be parallel until the maximal oxygen consumption for the patient is reached. Dynamic exercise in the cardiac catheterization laboratory requires simultaneous pressure measurements of the right and left sides of the heart during exercise (e.g., treadmill device mounted on the catheterization table). The patient's oxygen consumption is also measured by artery and vein oxygen saturations and is compared with the normal hemodynamic responses. Supine exercise in the catheterization laboratory differs from normal upright exercise in several ways:

1. Ventricular volumes are larger when the patient is supine rather than upright.
2. Heart rate and diastolic arterial pressure are higher when the patient is upright rather than supine.
3. Pulmonary and intracardiac filling pressures are lower when the patient is upright.
4. Stroke volume increases 100% with maximal exercise when the patient is upright and only 20% to 50% when the patient is supine.
5. Upright exercise and supine exercise are normally associated with increases in LV end-diastolic volume and decreases in end-systolic volume with concomitant

increase in ejection fraction. In patients with coronary artery disease, these findings may not occur.

Method. The performance of a dynamic exercise test in the catheterization laboratory is as follows:

1. With the patient in a supine position, resting hemo-dynamic data are obtained.
2. Exercise begins. Heart rate and changes in hemo-dynamics are recorded during the 6 minutes of exercise at constant load with bicycle ergometry.
3. At minute 4 exercise hemodynamic data collection is begun.
4. At minute 5, peak cardiac output measurements are obtained.
5. Exercise is terminated at minute 6. Fick oxygen consumption is obtained over minutes 4 to 6.

Data are analyzed with respect to change in hemodynamics (valve gradients), cardiac output, and oxygen consumption. Patients may be unable to exercise because of leg weakness, depressed cardiac function, peripheral vascular disease, or severe deconditioning. These factors may preclude determination of accurate exercise results in the catheterization laboratory and should be considered before the study is undertaken.

Measurements of Response to Exercise.

1. Cardiac output (CO) (a useful measurement for studying practically all types of heart disease) predicts a normal response and allows categorization of a given patient's response.

Dexter index: The predicted cardiac index (CI) with exercise is equal to $2.99 + 0.0059 \times$ (measured oxygen [O_2] consumption index with exercise). The measured CI is the CO divided by body surface area (BSA). The normal Dexter index equals the measured CI with exercise divided by the predicted CI and should be greater than 1.

Normal exercise factor: For every 100 ml/min increase in oxygen consumption with exercise, the CO should increase by at least 600 ml/min, thus normal exercise factor:

$$= \frac{\text{ml/min CO}}{\text{ml/min } O_2 \text{ consumption}} \geq 6$$

Note: Exercise factor is calculated directly from observed changes in CO and O_2 consumption; it is normalized to BSA.

2. Appropriate increases in arterial blood pressure and heart rate should be noted.

3. Compute LV volumes (useful in myopathic, coronary, and valvular disease). Changes in LV end-diastolic volume or LV end-diastolic pressure (more commonly used) with exercise may be plotted against observed changes in some parameter of LV systolic function (stroke volume or stroke work) to define a modified LV function curve.

4. Changes in filling pressures or valvular gradients are useful in valvular, myopathic, and coronary disease.

Isometric Exercise. Isometric exercise consists of skeletal muscle contraction without shortening. In the cardiac catheterization laboratory isometric exercise is commonly performed using a handgrip with a graded hand dynamometer. Measurements of hemodynamic data and ventricular function are obtained during sustained handgrip at a predetermined range (15% to 50% of the maximal handgrip contraction) for 3 to 4 minutes. The size of the involved muscle group is unimportant, provided that maximal voluntary contraction is maintained to increase oxygen demand during the isometric exercise period. Isometric exercise is easy to perform and easy to repeat and requires inexpensive equipment. It does not involve body motion that may interfere with hemodynamic measurements. An involuntary Valsalva maneuver during straining may occur during unsupervised isometric exercise. Careful monitoring, patient cooperation, and practice in use of the handgrip dynamometer minimize false hemodynamic information. In patients with coronary artery disease, isometric exercise rarely precipitates ischemia but may induce new LV wall motion abnormalities, a decrease in LV ejection fraction, and an increase in end-systolic volume with no change in diastolic volume. Stroke volume (SV) and CO may decline during isometric exercise. In patients with congestive heart failure, heart rate and systemic pressure may rise appropriately with a fall in SV and CO resulting in increase in LV end-diastolic volume and pulmonary artery pressure.

Valsalva Maneuver. The Valsalva maneuver is performed by having the patient forcibly expire against a closed glottis and strain as if having a bowel movement. The magnitude of the Valsalva maneuver can be quantitated by measuring the pressure against which the patient must expire. The Valsalva maneuver can be performed safely and without complications by almost every type of patient. The four phases of the normal Valsalva maneuver (strain, hypotension, release, and pressure overshoot) (Fig. 6-14) may be absent in patients with specific cardiac diseases (congestive heart failure, coronary artery disease, and obstructive cardiomyopathy). In addition, the hemodynamic data shown for different types of valvular lesions may be more pronounced during the Valsalva maneuver because of changes in ventricular filling (see Chapter 3).

Muller Maneuver. The patient performs the Muller maneuver by inspiring against a closed glottis, and this maneuver is considered the inverse or opposite of the Valsalva maneuver. The subject inhales, and the force of inhalation is measured with a manometer, usually −30 to −60 mm Hg for 30 seconds. Hemodynamic alterations of the Muller maneuver include increased right ventricular filling, increased period of diminished filling as a result of the collapse of the venae cavae at thoracic inlets, increasing LV afterload with increase in LV end-diastolic and end-systolic volumes, diminished SV, reduced CO, and reduced ejection fraction. This maneuver is used to augment right-sided heart murmurs and to decrease the physical findings of obstructive cardiomyopathy by a reduction in LV outflow gradient. A reduction in the intensity of the systolic murmur in patients with echocardiographic evidence of anterior mitral valve leaflet motion also can be shown with this maneuver.

Cold Pressor Testing. Cold pressor testing is an α-adrenergic stimulus, mediated by cold-induced pain in the forearm, hand, or forehead. Hemodynamic findings occurring with cold pressor testing include an increase in heart rate (5% to 15%), an increase in systolic and mean arterial pressure (15% to 20%), and a mild increase in CO. These responses usually occur within 2 minutes of application of the cold stimulus. In normal subjects cold pressor testing increases coronary blood

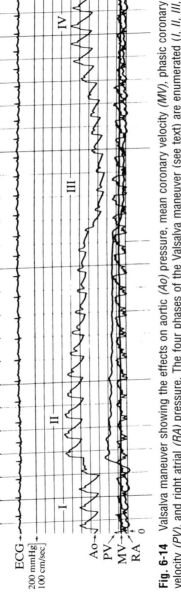

Fig. 6-14 Valsalva maneuver showing the effects on aortic *(Ao)* pressure, mean coronary velocity *(MV)*, phasic coronary velocity *(PV)*, and right atrial *(RA)* pressure. The four phases of the Valsalva maneuver (see text) are enumerated (*I, II, III,* and *IV*).

flow and reduces coronary vascular resistance. Cold pressor testing in some patients with coronary artery disease causes coronary vasoconstriction, which may be potentiated by a β-adrenergic blockade. Angina is rarely precipitated, although changes in regional LV function have been identified. Coronary vasospasm has also been reported during cold pressor testing.

Hyperventilation. Hyperventilation has been used to induce coronary spasm. Deep breathing (30 breaths/min for 5 minutes) is a commonly used method. Ischemia is rarely precipitated during hyperventilation but may commonly occur at the termination of rapid breathing. Heart rate, oxygen consumption, arteriovenous oxygen difference, and arterial pH increase during hyperventilation. Arterial pressure, pulmonary artery pressure, and arterial PCO_2 fall. Peripheral vascular resistance, CO, and left ventricular stroke volume are unchanged with the increase in LV ejection fraction seen in normal patients. These abnormalities may not be observed in patients with stable or variant angina.

Pharmacologic Stress. Pharmacologic stresses are used to assess alterations of ventricular function (see Chapter 5).

Nitroglycerin. Nitrates decrease systolic and mean arterial pressure and often produce a reflex increase in heart rate. Preload is reduced markedly with nitrates. There is no demonstrable effect on LV performance unless a profound decrease in systemic arterial pressure occurs, resulting in a marked reflex stimulation. Nitroglycerin relieves coronary ischemia and coronary vasospasm and may improve LV function through this mechanism.

Amyl Nitrite. Amyl nitrite acts in a similar fashion to that of nitroglycerin. Its pronounced effects, quick onset, and rapid resolution make this drug an ideal agent for the study of brief but intense changes in preload (dose).

Dobutamine. Dobutamine is a synthetic catecholamine that increases contractility and reduces vascular resistance. IV infusions and two-dimensional echocardiographic examination of LV wall motion are used to screen for severe coronary artery narrowings.

Nurse and Technician Viewpoint

The nursing and technical staff should be presented with a clear, concise project protocol. The protocol should include the following:

1. Overview of the project with clearly delineated objectives
2. Patient safety
3. Special equipment if necessary
4. Additional staffing if required
5. Data sheets (prepared to facilitate study periods)

If additional sterile equipment is necessary, a "protocol pack" with all additional equipment aids with setup. Many research techniques require the use of special catheters that must be interfaced with various flowmeters, computers, and other equipment. Personnel must be careful not to contaminate the sterile field when connecting the catheter to the interface cable. There are two ways to approach this situation. One is to sterilize all interface cables. The other is to wrap the nonsterile cable in a sterile drape. If the latter technique is used, the physician must be careful not to pull the nonsterile cable into the sterile field. If medications are involved, dose calculation worksheets aid the staff in drug preparation.

Suggested Readings

Chapman CB, editor: Physiology of muscular exercise, *Circ Res* 20(suppl 1):I1-I255, 1967. (Also available as Monograph 15 from American Heart Association.)

Kass DA, Maughan WL: From 'Emax' to pressure-volume relations: a broader view, *Circulation* 77:1203-1212, 1988.

Kern MJ, De Bruyne B, Pijls NHJ: From research to clinical practice: current role of intracoronary physiologically based decision making in the cardiac catheterization laboratory, *J Am Coll Cardiol* 30:613-620, 1997.

Kern MJ, Dupouy P, Drury JH, et al: Role of coronary artery lumen enlargement in improving coronary blood flow after balloon angioplasty and stenting: a combined intravascular ultrasound Doppler flow and imaging study, *J Am Coll Cardiol* 29:1520-1527, 1997.

McLaurin LP, Grossman W: Dynamic and isometric exercise during cardiac catheterization. In Grossman W, editor: *Cardiac catheterization and angiography,* Philadelphia, 1974, Lea & Febiger.

Mirsky I: Assessment of diastolic function: suggested methods and future considerations, *Circulation* 69:836-841, 1984.

Mitchell JH, Harris MD: Exercise and the heart: physiologic and clinical considerations. In Willerson JT, Sanders CA, editors: *Clinical cardiology,* New York, 1977, Grune & Stratton.

Ofili EO, Kern MJ, Labovitz AJ, et al: Analysis of coronary blood flow velocity dynamics in angiographically normal and stenosed arteries before and after endoluminal enlargement by angioplasty, *J Am Coll Cardiol* 21:308-318, 1993.

Sagawa K, Suga H, Shoukas AA, Bakalar KM: End-systolic pressure-volume ratio: a new index of contractility, *Am J Cardiol* 40:748-753, 1979.

Seiler C, Fleisch M, et al: Coronary collateral quantitation in patients with coronary artery disease using intravascular flow velocity or pressure measurements, *J Am Coll Cardiol* 32:1272-1279, 1998.

Sheehan FH, Schofer J, Mathey DG, et al: Measurement of regional wall motion from biplane contrast ventriculograms: a comparison of the 30 degree right anterior oblique and 60 degree left anterior oblique projections in patients with acute myocardial infarction, *Circulation* 74:796-804, 1986.

Weiss JL, Frederiksen JW, Weisfeldt ML: Hemodynamic determinants of the time-course of fall in canine left ventricular pressure, *J Clin Invest* 58:751-760, 1976.

7

Special Techniques

Morton J. Kern, Saad Bitar, and Sanjeev Puri

TRANSSEPTAL HEART CATHETERIZATION

Retrograde left-sided heart catheterization for aortic or mitral stenosis or prosthetic valve dysfunction may not be suitable for or accurate in all patients. Transseptal access across the thin atrial septal membrane at the fossa ovalis into the left atrium and left ventricle is an established technique.

Indications

Indications for transseptal heart catheterization include the following (Box 7-1):

1. Conditions that require direct left atrial (LA) or left ventricular (LV) measurement of pressure (e.g., mitral stenosis, pulmonary venous disease, left intraventricular gradient, aortic stenosis, or hypertrophic cardiomyopathy).
2. Access for mitral balloon catheter valvuloplasty.
3. Access for deployment of atrial septal defect closure devices.
4. Prosthetic aortic or mitral heart valve dysfunction. Retrograde crossing of the minor orifice of a tilting disk-type prosthetic valve in the aortic position has been performed with varying success, although death from entrapped catheters has been reported.

Contraindications

Contraindications for transseptal heart catheterization include the following:

1. Patients who cannot lie flat
2. Anticoagulant therapy, low platelet count, or other abnormalities of hemostasis (warfarin [Coumadin] should

411

Box 7-1

Indications for Transseptal Left-Sided Heart Catheterization

Measurement of Left Atrial or Left Ventricular Hemodynamics
Mitral valve
Precise hemodynamic measurement for valvular stenosis
Prosthetic mitral valve
Previous mitral valve surgery
Pulmonary venoocclusive disease

Aortic valve
Retrograde catheterization not possible
Mechanical prosthetic valve
Inconclusive echocardiographic data
Hypertrophic obstructive cardiomyopathy

Left Ventricular Angiography
To assess mitral regurgitation when retrograde catheterization not possible

Valvuloplasty
Mitral approach
Antegrade aortic approach

Electrophysiology Studies
Left-sided radiofrequency ablation atrioseptostomy

---

be discontinued several days before transseptal puncture so that the international normalized ratio is ≤1.5)
3. Left or right atrial thrombus
4. Atrial myxoma
5. Inferior vena cava mass or obstruction

Transseptal left-sided heart catheterization should be considered carefully for patients with distorted cardiac anatomy resulting from congenital heart disease, dilated aortic root, marked atrial enlargement, or thoracic skeletal deformity.

Procedural Highlights

Several methods exist to cross the atrial septum. The one used most often in our laboratory is described here. Crossing of the interatrial septum is performed in the anteroposterior (AP) projection after the transseptal Mullen catheter and sheath system or Brockenbrough catheter has been correctly positioned. Steps to perform transseptal catheterization are as follows:

1. A pigtail catheter is placed in the sinus of Valsalva of the aorta for anatomic reference and measurement of aortic pressure.

2. A guidewire is advanced to the superior vena cava (SVC) via the right femoral vein.

3. The transseptal catheter (and sheath) is advanced over the guidewire to the SVC.

4. The wire is withdrawn. The catheter is flushed. A transseptal needle is advanced through the catheter, permitting free rotation of the needle. The needle is positioned in the SVC at the 12 o'clock position, and the needle tip is kept within the catheter. The needle is connected to a pressure transducer to permit continuous observation during septal crossing.

5. The catheter and needle assembly is withdrawn into the right atrium with a clockwise rotation, with the needle angle indicator pointing posteriorly between 3 and 5 o'clock (Fig. 7-1).

6. On withdrawal downward into the right atrium the catheter assembly passes over the aortic knob with a forward motion, and on further withdrawal passes under the aortic indentation into the fossa ovale. Slight advancement until contact is made with the atrial septum

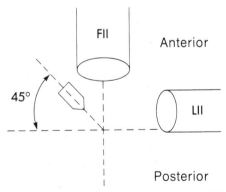

Fig. 7-1 Transseptal arrow is oriented approximately 45 degrees posteriorly. *FII,* Frontal image intensifier; *LII,* lateral image intensifier. (From Weiner RI, Maranhao V: *Cathet Cardiovasc Diagn* 15:112, 1988.)

is performed at this point. Approximately 15% to 20% of patients have a patent foramen ovale, which allows unobstructed passage of the catheter assembly into the left atrium without puncture.

7. The technique described by Croft and others is used to precisely localize the point of puncture on the interatrial septum (Fig. 7-2). This technique consists of right anterior oblique angulation and identification of the pigtail catheter within the sinus of Valsalva in the aorta and right atrial (RA) posterior wall. A line is drawn from the lower end of the pigtail catheter horizontally to the vertical line of the RA border. The operator moves the needle to 1 cm below the line at the midpoint. This point usually is centered within the fossa ovale.

8. After the needle makes contact with the interatrial septum, the operator maintains firm pressure on the

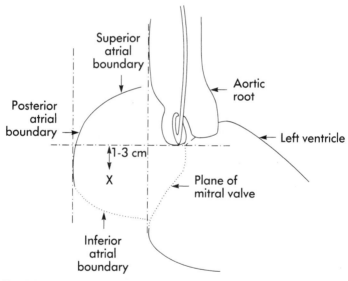

Fig. 7-2 The optimal spot for transseptal puncture. Diagrammatic representation of the structures visualized in 40 degrees right anterior oblique projection. The limits of the atria are depicted behind the aorta. The pigtail catheter positioned in the noncoronary aortic cusp defines the posterior boundary of the aortic root. The point of intended atrial septal puncture is delineated by *X*. (From Croft CH, Lipscomb K: *J Am Coll Cardiol* 5:904-910, 1985.)

needle and advances it into the septum while continuously monitoring pressure waveforms. Entry of the needle into the left atrium is signified by observation of left atrial pressure waveforms. If the operator is in doubt about the location of the needle tip, blood may be aspirated for determination of oxygen saturation (which should be arterial) or a small amount of contrast material may be injected under fluoroscopy. After the operator confirms the proper positioning of the needle in the left atrium, it is advanced slightly and the catheter is advanced over the needle with a counterclockwise rotation of the needle, which permits the transseptal catheter to turn anteriorly into the mitral valve orifice area. The needle is withdrawn, and the transseptal catheter is *carefully* aspirated and connected to pressure. (Left-sided injections of thrombus or bubbles can enter the systemic circulation.) After the transseptal catheter is positioned in the left atrium the sheath can be advanced over the catheter into the left atrium. A small amount of contrast material may be injected to identify catheter position and to avoid advancing the catheter into pulmonary veins.

9. A guidewire is inserted into the transseptal catheter or sheath and advanced across the mitral valve and into the left ventricle. In some cases a balloon catheter can be passed through the transseptal sheath and floated into the left ventricle. The catheter (or sheath) is advanced over the guidewire or balloon catheter into the left ventricle.

Preparatory Notes

1. The transseptal catheter must be measured against the transseptal needle to identify the position at which the needle extends outside the catheter (Fig. 7-3, *A*). This measurement is done before insertion of the catheter-needle assembly. The operator places the catheter over the needle, notes at what point the needle leaves the catheter end, and marks this distance with the fingertip. Keeping the needle inside the catheter protects the wall of the atrium from inadvertent needle damage.

2. As the transseptal needle is passed through the transseptal catheter to the SVC, it is rotated at three points

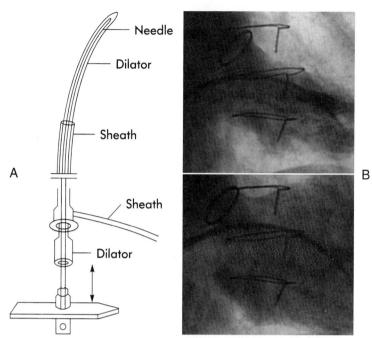

Fig. 7-3 **A,** Transseptal catheter assembly. The distance between the transseptal needle and the dilator hub *(arrow)* is noted so that the needle lies just inside the dilator. **B,** Frames of left ventricular cine angiogram using transseptal sheath and Berman catheter in left ventricle. *Top,* Systolic frame; *bottom,* diastolic frame. Note ring of prosthetic aortic valve. (**A** from Weiner RI, Maranhao V: *Cathet Cardiovasc Diagn* 15:112, 1988.)

along its course. The first is the iliac crest, the second is over the spine near the renal vein, and the third is at the inferior junction of the cardiac silhouette. The needle should rotate freely over these three segments and slide smoothly up through the transseptal catheter. Damage to the catheter or injury to the patient can occur if the needle does not rotate freely.

3. Left ventriculography through the transseptal catheter should be performed at low volume (20 ml) and moderate flow rates (<10 ml/sec) because of the end-hole configuration of the catheter. A small test injection of contrast medium should be performed to avoid catheter malposition. Perforation of the left ventricle with end-hole

catheters has been reported. It is preferable to exchange the transseptal catheter for a pigtail catheter or use a Berman catheter through the Mullin sheath (Fig. 7-3, *B*).

4. The fossa ovalis is located in the middle third of the atrial septum and is concave toward the left atrium in a normal heart. Valvular disease may significantly alter the location of the fossa ovalis. In aortic valve disease the dilated ascending aorta may displace the fossa superiorly and anteriorly. In mitral valve disease the left atrium usually enlarges posteriorly and inferiorly and displaces the fossa ovalis inferiorly. In severe mitral disease the fossa may become everted and displaced into the lower third of the septum. This makes the fossa difficult to locate on catheter descent, and the transseptal puncture technique must be modified accordingly.

Risks of Transseptal Catheterization

Punctures of the aortic root, the coronary sinus (CS), or the posterior free wall of the atrium are potentially lethal problems (Box 7-2). In patients who have not been given anticoagulants the 21-gauge tip of the needle rarely causes a problem. However, if the large transseptal catheter is advanced into these spaces cardiac tamponade may occur. The catheter-needle combination should not be advanced if the operator is not satisfied with the position of the transseptal catheter in the right atria. If the catheter assembly is not in the correct position, the

---

Box 7-2

Risks Related to Transseptal Catheterization
Cardiac perforation
- Right atrium
- Posterior left atrium
- Left atrial appendage
- Pulmonary vein
- Left ventricle

Puncture into the aortic root
Pericardial tamponade*
Embolus from the left atrium

---

*Almost all deaths related to transseptal catheterization are a result of tamponade.

operator must remove the transseptal needle, reinsert the guidewire to the SVC, reposition the catheter, and reposition the needle with withdrawal and turning to the fossa ovalis as indicated earlier.

DIRECT TRANSTHORACIC LEFT VENTRICULAR PUNCTURE

The development of retrograde arterial catheterization and transseptal catheterization has enabled clinicians to obtain hemodynamic data without direct transthoracic puncture techniques except in unusual situations. This technique carries a high potential of risk and should be performed only by experienced operators.

Indications

Transthoracic LV puncture is required to measure LV pressure or to perform LV angiography when no other access is available. This occurs mainly in patients who have had combined mitral and aortic valve replacement with mechanical tilting disk prostheses. Although several investigators report techniques for crossing mechanical tilting disks, retrograde complications have been reported involving catheter entrapment and occlusion of the ball valves or tilting disks with disastrous results. When ventricular pressure and angiography are required in a patient who has had double-valve replacement, direct puncture with echocardiographic guidance can be performed at relatively low risk.

Before the procedure two-dimensional echocardiography from the apical window is helpful in locating the true LV apex and determining the direction of the long axis of the left ventricle. After the arterial and right-sided heart catheters have been placed, an 18-gauge, 4.25 inch–long needle with a Teflon sheath connected to a pressure transducer is inserted at the apical area through the intercostal space close to the upper border of the lower rib in this space. It is directed posteriorly toward the right shoulder. The pressure tracing is continuously monitored while the needle is advanced. After the needle enters the ventricle, it is removed, leaving the Teflon sheath in place through which pressure recordings and angiography are performed. Alternatively a guidewire can be inserted and a 4 F pigtail catheter can be advanced into the left ventricle for hemodynamic and angiographic data. Figs. 7-4 and 7-5

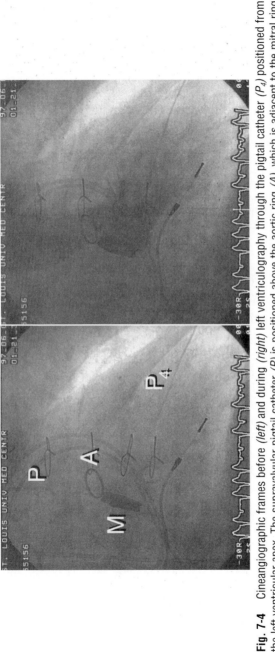

Fig. 7-4   Cineangiographic frames before (*left*) and during (*right*) left ventriculography through the pigtail catheter (*P₄*) positioned from the left ventricular apex. The supravalvular pigtail catheter (*P*) is positioned above the aortic ring (*A*), which is adjacent to the mitral ring (*M*). There are multiple pacing leads and two pulmonary artery catheters positioned near the supraaortic pigtail catheter. Contrast injection during ventriculography shows no mitral regurgitation.

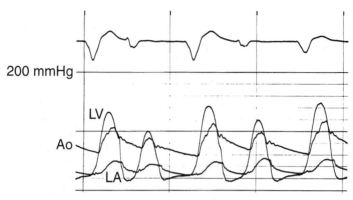

Fig. 7-5 Left ventricular *(LV)*, left atrial *(LA)*, and aortic *(Ao)* pressures (0 to 200 mm Hg scale) showing the aortic and mitral prosthetic valve gradients. Note the influence of the paced beats on the valve gradients.

illustrate a typical case of direct LV puncture and associated hemodynamics.

Complications

The patient should be watched carefully for hemopericardium, hemothorax, or pneumothorax. Should any of these complications occur they can be treated with direct aspiration or surgery as needed. A vasovagal reaction with bradycardia and hypotension may be encountered. Bleeding complications may result from laceration of the left anterior descending (LAD) or intercostal arteries. Patients who have had previous cardiac surgery usually have obliterated pericardial space, which decreases the likelihood of cardiac tamponade.

Embolism may occur if an LV clot is displaced from the apex. The detailed methodologic approach to insertion of the direct LV needle can be found in the reference texts. Direct LV puncture is contraindicated in a patient who is receiving anticoagulants.

Use of Pressure Sensor Guidewire to Assess Pressure Across Prosthetic Heart Valves

An alternative method to obtain LV pressure across a mechanical prosthetic valve in the aortic (or mitral) position is the use of a 0.014-inch pressure sensor guidewire. Although the use of a catheter to cross a prosthetic valve retrogradely is generally prohibited because of the potential for catheter entrapment, a fine-diameter (0.014-inch) guidewire with a high-fidelity pressure sensor has been used safely in many cases. This technique is novel and under examination. Caution should be used when passing the guidewire through the valve and retrieving it. The minimal mass of the guidewire prevents its entrapment. An example of the pressure guidewire used to cross an aortic prosthetic valve is shown in Figure 7-6.

ENDOMYOCARDIAL BIOPSY

Endomyocardial biopsy is an increasingly common procedure in the catheterization laboratory. At least 50,000 endomyocardial biopsy procedures were performed in the United States in 2000, mostly for monitoring of cardiac transplant rejection.

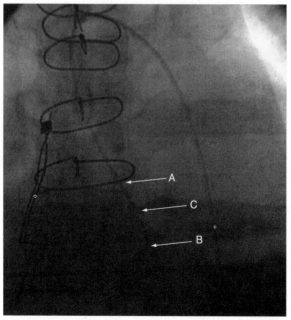

Fig. 7-6   Cine frame shows St. Jude valve with Radi 0.014 pressure wire across valve advanced through a multipurpose catheter. The tilting disk valve in mitral position *(DV)* made a transseptal approach impossible. *A,* 6 F multipurpose catheter; *B,* Radi pressure wire; *C,* leaflet of St. Jude valve.

Indications

Monitoring for cardiac transplant rejection and monitoring for anthracycline cardiotoxicity are the only two definitive indications for endomyocardial biopsy (Box 7-3). Other indications include diagnosis for secondary causes of cardiomyopathy, myocarditis (when there is a history of congestive heart failure in the past 6 months), and differentiation between restrictive and constrictive cardiomyopathies.

Contraindications

Contraindications to endomyocardial biopsy are anticoagulation and anatomic abnormality.

Complications

Complications of endomyocardial biopsy include the following:

1. Access site related (3%)
2. Biopsy related (3%)
3. Arrhythmia (1%)
4. Conduction abnormalities (1%)
5. Perforation (0.7%)
6. Death (0.4%)

Note: Complication rates are higher for patients with cardiomyopathy than for heart transplant recipients.

Box 7-3

Indications for Endomyocardial Biopsy

Definitive
Cardiac transplantation follow-up
Monitoring of anthracycline cardiotoxicity

Possible
Viral myocarditis
Secondary cardiomyopathies (sarcoidosis, hemochromatosis, amyloidosis)
Differentiation of restrictive versus constrictive cardiac disease
Endocardial fibrosis
Hypereosinophilic syndrome
Malignancies involving the heart

Biopsy Devices

There are two basic types of bioptomes: (1) stiff shaft (pre-shaped) devices (Konno, Kawai, and Stanford bioptomes) (Fig. 7-7) and (2) floppy shaft devices (King and Cordis bioptomes) (Fig. 7-8) that are positioned with the aid of a long sheath. The femoral sheath dilator is 94 cm long, and the long sheath is 85 cm long. Biopsy sheaths come in 5- and 7-cm curves (for hearts with large right atria or transplanted hearts).

Technique

Endomyocardial biopsy can be performed under fluoroscopic or echocardiographic guidance from the femoral or internal jugular approach.

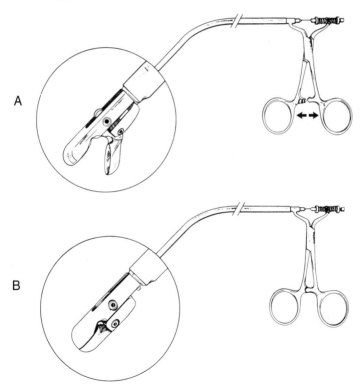

Fig. 7-7   Scholten bioptome. **A,** open; **B,** closed. (From Tilkian AG, Daily EK: *Cardiovascular procedures: diagnostic techniques and therapeutic procedures,* St Louis, 1986, Mosby.)

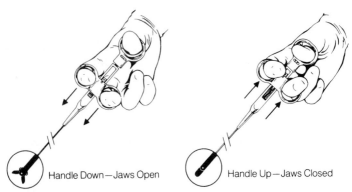

Handle Down—Jaws Open   Handle Up—Jaws Closed

Fig. 7-8 Disposable biopsy forceps with formable tip, pivoting jaws, a clear wire–braided body, stainless-steel cutting jaws, a stainless-steel wire coil, and a spring-loaded, three-ring plastic handle that controls the operation of the jaws. The thumb ring of the handle is flexible and rotates to accommodate any thumb position, reducing manual stress. (Courtesy of Cordis Corporation, Miami, Fla.)

Femoral Approach. After the patient is given local anesthesia, the right or left femoral vein is punctured by the modified Seldinger technique and a 0.038-inch guidewire is advanced into the femoral vein. A 7 F biopsy sheath with a 7 F dilator is advanced over the guidewire. A large-curve (7-cm) sheath is used when the atrium is dilated, as in cardiac transplantation. In some systems the dilator is not completely radiopaque. The sheath and dilator are advanced into the right atrium. The dilator is withdrawn into the sheath. With the help of the guidewire the sheath is advanced across the tricuspid valve and into the right ventricle. The biopsy sheath is equipped with a valve and a side arm for flushing. The sheath is flushed and connected to the pressure monitor, and a right ventricular (RV) pressure tracing is identified. A floppy shaft biopsy forceps is advanced through the sheath and into the right ventricle. The sheath is pointed horizontally toward the intraventricular septum, which should be confirmed in the left anterior oblique projection to ensure that the bioptome has not inadvertently entered the CS. The RV outflow tract (upward sheath angle) and (usually) the inferior (downward sheath angle) and RV free wall should be avoided.

To reduce the chance of perforation, the operator always opens the bioptome jaws inside the sheath before the bioptome exits the sheath. The bioptome is carefully advanced with the jaws fully open until contact with the ventricular wall is made and the bioptome shaft is slightly bent. The bioptome jaws are then closed. After 2 to 3 seconds, to permit tissue excision, the "bite" is slowly withdrawn into the sheath as the sheath is advanced. A tugging sensation is often felt by the operator on full extraction of the bioptome into the sheath. After the bioptome is removed from the patient the sheath should be aspirated and flushed to eliminate air bubbles. (Flushing can be minimized if saline is free to flow into the sheath as the bioptome is being withdrawn. Otherwise, air fills the negative space of the bioptome through the valve.) The procedure is repeated until an adequate number of specimens (usually four to six) are obtained. RV pressures are measured before and after the biopsy. The biopsy sheath is removed, and hemostasis is secured.

For heterotopic heart transplantation (i.e., piggyback hearts), the right atrium of the donor's heart is located in the right hemithorax. Its connection to the atrium of the recipient's heart may be marked with a radiopaque ring. The biopsy sheath is advanced over the guidewire and into the right ventricle of the donor's heart, and biopsy samples are taken as described.

Internal Jugular Approach with Echocardiographic Guidance. Extensive experience in performing endomyocardial biopsies under echocardiographic guidance and fluoroscopy has been reported (Figs. 7-9 and 7-10). An 8 F short sheath is inserted into the right internal jugular vein by the standard Seldinger technique. A rigid, curved bioptome is inserted through the venous sheath and into the right atrium. The tricuspid valve leaflets are readily visible with the use of two-dimensional echocardiography, which helps the operator pass the bioptome across the valve with minimal trauma. A counterclockwise (anterior) rotation helps guide the bioptome past the tricuspid valve. Further counterclockwise rotation straightens the curve and orients the bioptome toward the central ventricular septum. Under echocardiographic guidance biopsy samples can be obtained safely from the intraventricular septum, apex,

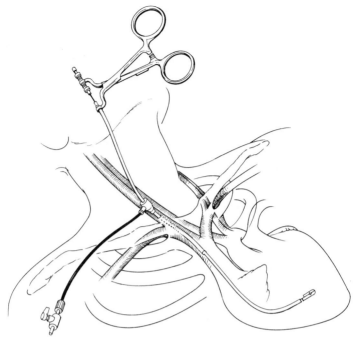

Fig. 7-9 Internal jugular approach. The bioptome tip is in the right ventricular apex, pointing toward the ventricular septum. (From Tilkian AG, Daily EK: *Cardiovascular procedures: diagnostic techniques and therapeutic procedures*, St Louis, 1986, Mosby.)

and free wall. The sheath is removed, and hemostasis is secured.

The advantages of echocardiographically guided endo-myocardial biopsy include the following:

1. It does not require the use of the angiographic suite.
2. The patient or operator are not exposed to radiation.
3. Because two-dimensional echocardiography equipment is portable the procedure can be performed in the intensive care unit or the patient's room.
4. Biopsy samples can be obtained from multiple areas including the intraventricular septum, apex, and free wall, which may increase the diagnostic yield.
5. More accurate positioning of the bioptome is achieved with two-dimensional echocardiography than with fluoroscopy, especially in heart transplant recipients. At

St. Louis University as of 1990 only two significant complications occurred in 4700 biopsies performed under echocardiographic guidance over a 5-year period.

If cardiac tamponade from RV perforation is present, it is apparent 20 to 30 minutes after biopsy. Conduction block and tricuspid leaflet damage have been reported.

Internal Jugular Approach with Fluoroscopic Guidance. The same technique and principles are used as those described for echocardiographic guidance except that fluoroscopic guidance is substituted for the echocardiogram.

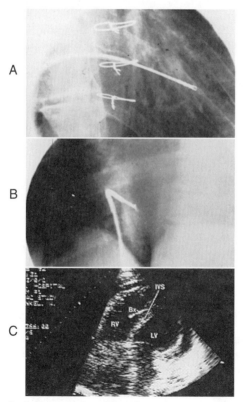

Fig. 7-10   A, Anteroposterior cineangiographic image of femoral endo-myocardial bioptome location. **B,** Corresponding left anterior oblique view. **C,** Simultaneous two-dimensional echocardiographic image shows position of bioptome *(Bx)* against the right ventricular side of the interventricular septum *(IVS). LV,* Left ventricle; *RV,* right ventricle.   *Continued*

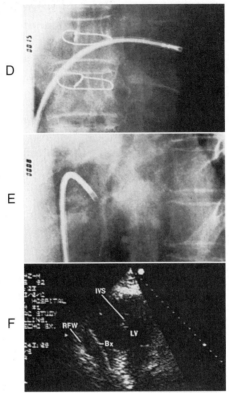

Fig. 7-10, cont'd **D** to **F,** Same views in another transplant recipient show nearly identical angiographic location but positioning of bioptome and sheath against the right ventricular free wall *(RFW).* (**A** to **C** from Bell CA, Kern MJ, et al: *Cathet Cardiovasc Diagn* 28:291-294, 1993.)

CORONARY SINUS CATHETERIZATION (See Chapter 6)

The coronary sinus (CS) is located in the inferoposterior aspect of the tricuspid valve on the RA side. The CS ostium is approximately 0.5 to 1 cm in diameter and proceeds in a caudal-posterior then superior direction (see Chapter 6).

Indications

Indications for CS catheterization are as follows:

1. Electrophysiology studies (particularly for localization of accessory conduction pathways)

2. Collection of transmyocardial oxygen, lactate catecholamines, and other cardiac metabolites
3. Measurement of CS thermodilution blood flow
4. Retroperfusion in the CS as an investigational technique

Techniques

The approach to the CS is typically from the right internal jugular vein, the left subclavian vein, or the antecubital veins from either arm (as described previously). The CS can be entered from the femoral vein with specific and at times difficult catheter manipulations. Most catheters used for CS blood flow measurement and oxygen and metabolite extraction are large-diameter (>6 F), relatively stiff catheters that do not lend themselves to CS cannulation from the femoral approach.

PERICARDIOCENTESIS
Indications

Pericardiocentesis may be required for diagnosis and management of acute and chronic pericardial effusions. In cardiac tamponade this is a lifesaving technique. An operator must have sufficient skill to prevent further damage to the heart and pericardium.

Procedure

Pericardiocentesis is usually preceded by echocardiographic confirmation of pericardial fluid. In cases in which a large pericardial effusion is known or suspected with hemodynamic compromise in which tamponade is acute, echocardiographic assessment is not required and may be detrimental in that it may delay needed intervention. Although monitoring of pericardial pressure is not essential for elective procedures, it is important to document evidence of cardiac tamponade and to resolve pericardial pressure restricting cardiac output.

Route to Pericardium. In the catheterization laboratory a long 16- or 18-gauge needle connected to a stopcock and tubing to a pressure transducer can be used. The preferred approach is the subxiphoid route, but other sites are acceptable depending on the location and volume of the pericardial effusion (Fig. 7-11). The advantage of the subxiphoid approach is a decreased likelihood of coronary and internal thoracic artery laceration. At least a finger-width below the edge of the rib is needed to avoid difficulty in advancing the catheter through fibrous tissue near the xiphoid process (Fig. 7-12).

Setup and Positioning. The patient is positioned at a 30- to 45-degree, head-up angle to permit pericardial fluid to pool on the inferior surface of the heart. Local anesthetic is given at needle puncture site and more is instilled through the pericardial needle as it is advanced perpendicularly to the skin initially, then at a sharp, low angle (near parallel with the horizontal plane) under the xiphoid process toward the left shoulder. If the patient is obese a larger needle and some force may be required to tip the syringe under the subxiphoid process toward the heart.

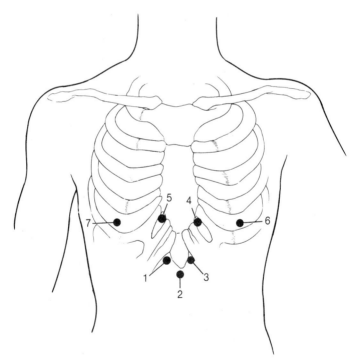

Fig. 7-11 Locations for pericardiocentesis. *1* to *3*, Xiphoid approaches. *4*, Fifth left intercostal space at sternal border. *5*, Fifth right intercostal space at the sternal border. *6*, Apical approach. *7*, Approach for major fluid accumulation on the right side. (Modified from Spodick DH: *Acute pericarditis*, New York, 1959, Grune & Stratton.)

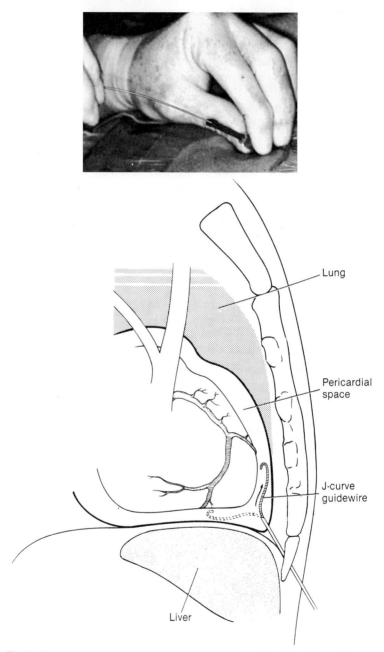

Fig. 7-12 Passing a flexible J tip of guidewire through pericardial needle into the pericardial space. (From Tilkian AG, Daily EK: *Cardiovascular procedures: diagnostic techniques and therapeutic procedures,* St Louis, 1986, Mosby.)

For elective procedures a balloon-tipped catheter is positioned in the pulmonary artery (PA) to assess equalization of diastolic right-sided pressures (and to document the change with intervention), then withdrawn into the right atrium for continuous monitoring of RA pressure during pericardial puncture and effusion drainage. Often, a 5 F sheath placed in a femoral artery is useful for monitoring arterial pressure.

Puncture of the Pericardium. Aspiration during passage of the needle through the skin may block the needle with subcutaneous tissue. Any tissue that may have accumulated in the needle during passage is flushed before the pericardium, a rigid fibrous membrane, is punctured. The pericardial puncture feels similar to a lumbar puncture to the operator. The operator should exercise care when advancing the needle through the diaphragm. Excessive forward pressure may result in crossing suddenly through the pericardium and into a cardiac chamber. Chronic effusions are often clear yellow, occasionally serosanguineous, or, less commonly, dark brown. Acute effusions resulting from trauma, cancer, or artery perforation are frankly bloody.

If hemodynamic monitoring is used, after fluid is aspirated through the needle, the operator can immediately confirm that the needle tip has entered the pericardial space by turning the stopcock and observing the pressure. In this manner inadvertent RV puncture can be recognized at once. In cases of tamponade, pericardial pressure resembles RA pressure.

Alternatively, if echocardiographic guidance is used, injection of 5 to 10 ml of agitated saline through the needle appears as microbubbles in the pericardial space to confirm position. If the needle tip is in a cardiac chamber (e.g., RV), the bubbles will be seen in the RV cavity and can be dispersed rapidly by RV ejection.

If electrocardiographic guidance is used, a current of injury is seen on contact with the epicardium (Fig. 7-13). Of these methods, we favor hemodynamic monitoring for its ease of application in the catheterization laboratory.

When the needle is in the pericardial space, a guidewire is passed, under fluoroscopy, high into the pericardial space and the needle is exchanged for a multiple side–hole plastic catheter (or sheath) over the guidewire. Pericardial and RA pressures are measured (Figs. 7-14 and 7-15), the effusion is aspirated,

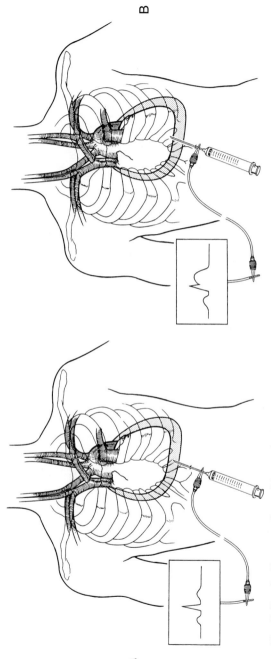

Fig. 7-13   A, Electrocardiographic monitoring of pericardial needle tip. Note normal ST segment while tip is not touching the epicardium. **B,** When needle tip touches epicardium, current of injury ("contact" current) with elevated ST segment is seen. (From Tilkian AG, Daily EK: *Cardiovascular procedures: diagnostic techniques and therapeutic procedures,* St Louis, 1986, Mosby.)

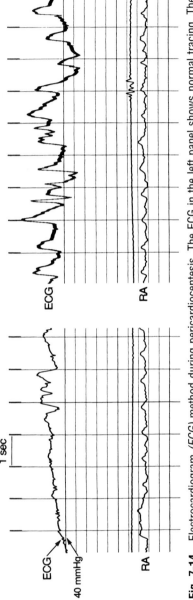

Fig. 7-14 Electrocardiogram (*ECG*) method during pericardiocentesis. The ECG in the left panel shows normal tracing. The ECG clip is attached to the pericardial needle. On advancement of the needle through the pericardium, contact is made with the heart, as shown by the ECG injury current in the right panel. *RA*, Right atrial pressure. (From Kern MJ, Aguirre FV: *Cathet Cardiovasc Diagn* 26:152-158, 1992.)

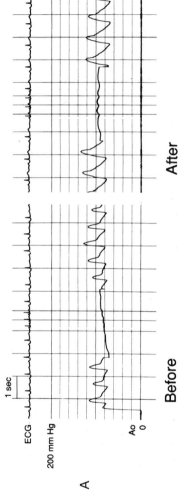

Fig. 7-15 Hemodynamic results of pericardiocentesis. **A,** Aortic *(Ao)* pressure and **B,** right atrial (RA) pressure before and after withdrawal of pericardial fluid. Note the elimination of pulsus paradoxus of aortic pressure and return of Y descent of right atrial waveform after pericardiocentesis (see also Chapter 3).

Continued

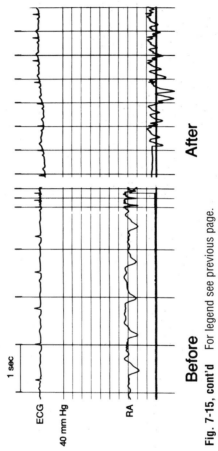

Fig. 7-15, cont'd For legend see previous page.

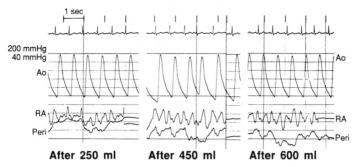

Fig. 7-16 Hemodynamic results of pericardiocentesis after withdrawal of 600 ml of pericardial fluid. This patient did not have tamponade. *Ao,* Aortic pressure (0 to 200 mm Hg scale); *RA,* right atrial pressure; *Peri,* pericardial pressure (0 to 40 mm Hg scale).

and pressures are measured after the pericardial space is empty (Fig. 7-16). If the exact position of the needle or catheter is uncertain, even after measurement of the pressure, a small amount of radiographic contrast medium may be injected. Agitated saline injection under echocardiographic guidance may also be performed. Contrast medium pools in the dependent portion of the pericardial space but rapidly washes out of a vascular space if a cardiac chamber has been entered inadvertently. Bloody pericardial fluid has a lower hematocrit value than intravascular blood and will not clot rapidly when placed in a red-top tube. Balloon pericardiotomy has been used as a therapeutic approach to chronic pericardial effusions.

INTRAVASCULAR FOREIGN BODY RETRIEVAL

Several catheter systems have been designed to retrieve foreign bodies, which are usually fragments of previous catheters or guidewires. Most catheter fragments result from injudicious insertion or removal of catheters from the subclavian, jugular, or, rarely, inferior vena caval approaches. Refined techniques are required for removal of fragments of angioplasty guidewires in coronary arteries. A catheter-housed wire loop or snare is commonly available (Fig. 7-17). An intracoronary guidewire fragment can be retrieved from the coronary artery with the use of a loop passed through a small intracoronary guiding catheter. The snare and loop technique has been used success-

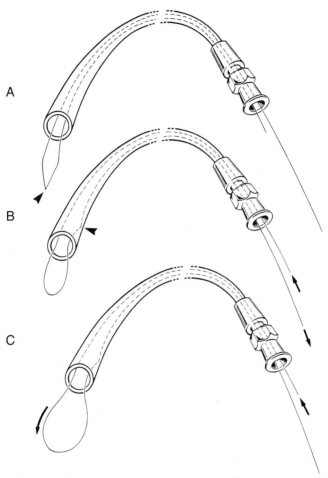

Fig. 7-17 Making a loop snare. **A,** Guidewire with a tight fold (arrow) beyond the catheter tip. **B,** Tight fold is withdrawn into the catheter by withdrawing one free end of the guidewire while advancing the other end, forming a nontraumatic, blunt-tip loop snare. **C,** The size of loop snare is enlarged by further advancement of the guidewire end not containing the initial tight fold. *Continued*

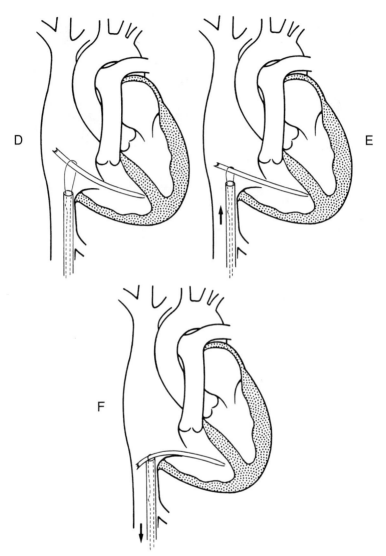

Fig. 7-17, cont'd   **D,** The catheter fragment is snared. **E,** The catheter is advanced while the wire is held so that the catheter rests gently on the fragment, confirming encirclement and securing of the fragment. **F,** The loop is closed down tightly, and the fragment is pulled out with the catheter.

Continued

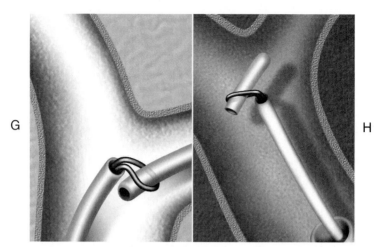

Fig. 7-17, *cont'd* **G,** Loop snare is used to capture a catheter end. **H,** Loop snare can be used to capture catheter fragment. (**A** through **F,** from Tilkian AG, Daily EK: *Cardiovascular procedures: diagnostic techniques and therapeutic procedures,* St Louis, 1986, Mosby. **G** and **H,** courtesy of Microvena Company, Minneapolis, Minn.)

fully in venous and arterial applications. Extra care must be exercised with any snare that has a rigid tip that may damage surrounding structures as the catheter fragment is retrieved. The catheter fragment or guidewire material that is being retrieved may scratch or tear the cardiac chamber unless it is captured at a distal end with the free, sharp edge of the fragment contained.

TRANSLUMINAL ALCOHOL SEPTAL ABLATION FOR HYPERTROPHIC OBSTRUCTIVE CARDIOMYOPATHY

Some patients with hypertrophic obstructive cardiomyopathy (HOCM) have refractory symptoms resulting from outflow obstruction produced by hyperdynamic LV contraction with a hypertrophied septum. A controlled septal infarction can be produced with a new method of nonsurgical septal mass reduction that uses alcohol. In brief, a small balloon catheter is inserted into the septal artery with angioplasty technique and alcohol is instilled. This causes the septal muscle to infarct, become noncontractile, and scar, which eliminates the LV outflow tract gradient.

Criteria for alcohol septal ablation for HOCM include (1) refractory symptoms on maximal medical therapy, (2) a septal thickness of 1.8 cm or more, (3) an outflow tract gradient greater than 40 mm Hg at rest and greater than 60 mm Hg with provocation (e.g., PVC or Valsalva's maneuver, dobutamine challenge), and (4) the gradient localized to the septal obstruction. Other considerations should be moderate or mild mitral regurgitation with no organic abnormalities of the mitral valve and minimal coronary artery disease responsible for the symptoms.

Technique of Alcohol Septal Ablation

Complete hemodynamic and angiographic study should precede alcohol-induced septal ablation. The right and left femoral arteries and veins are cannulated. A 5 F pigtail or Halo ventriculography catheter is positioned in the left ventricle. Arterial pressures are measured through the sidearm of a 6 F arterial sheath. A 6 F left Judkins 4-cm guide catheter is inserted into the left coronary ostium from the contralateral artery. A 5 F balloon-tip pacemaker is positioned in the right ventricle for prophylactic pacing if complete heart block is induced. In some patients an internal jugular vein is selected for pacer insertion in case more than 48 hours of temporary pacing is needed. In some patients a pulmonary artery catheter is positioned to provide more data and cardiac output. After the catheters are positioned, coronary arteriography identifies the large septal artery originating in the proximal left anterior descending artery. The echocardiography technician performs imaging of the LV septum and LV outflow tract gradient. Heparin, 40 U/kg as a bolus, is administered because manipulations of guidewires and catheters may induce thrombus. Heparin is not continued after the procedure. Demerol, 50 mg intravenously, is given before septal cannulation and occlusion.

A 0.014-inch angioplasty guidewire is used to cannulate the large, first septal artery. A large double 45-degree bend on the angioplasty guidewire facilitates entry into the 90-degree origin of the septal branch. A 2-mm × 10-mm balloon catheter is advanced over the guidewire into the septal artery. The balloon is inflated. Angiography is performed to show that the balloon is located properly within the septum and that the balloon occludes antegrade septal flow. The guidewire is removed when the balloon occludes the septal artery. A small amount of contrast material is injected into the septal balloon to (1) ensure no reflux of contrast material or, later, alcohol and (2) opacify the septal artery and subbranch distribution. Subselective septal artery branch ablation may render hemodynamic results equivalent to those with complete septal artery ablation, as well as a lower rate of heart block. After septal contrast opacification, echocardiographic contrast material, such as Optison, is diluted and 0.5 to 1 ml is injected into the septal artery, which allows echocardiographic visualization of the distribution of blood to the septum. This is best seen on the four-chamber, long-axis and two-chamber echocardiographic views.

After echocardiographic confirmation of correct septal branch occlusion, 1 to 2 ml of 98% denatured alcohol is delivered slowly over 3 minutes into the septal artery followed by a 5-minute observation period. Complete heart block may occur with the need for temporary pacing. Chest pain with alcohol instillation is a common occurrence and a sign of septal infarction. Hemodynamic values are obtained continuously before, during, and after alcohol septal ablation. The LV out-flow tract gradient is frequently abolished immediately with the septal infarction. After the observation period the balloon catheter is aspirated and then deflated. Suction is kept on the catheter lumen, the catheter is withdrawn from the LAD and angiography is repeated. Final hemodynamic values are again measured. In most cases the LV outflow gradient is abolished; 10% to 20% of patients may need permanent ventricular pacing. A modest myocardial infarction occurs with creatine phosphokinase elevation of 500 to 2000 U. Patients are monitored in the hospital for 4 to 5 days after the procedure to ensure absence of late heart block. (Examples are shown in Figs. 7-18 to 7-20.)

SPECIAL CONDITIONS
Cardiac Catheterization in the Heart Transplant Recipient

Cardiac transplantation is now a common procedure in most tertiary care centers. Routine yearly follow-up of the patient after transplantation includes cardiac catheterization, coronary angiography, and assessment of LV function, PA pressures, and endomyocardial biopsy. Patients who have undergone cardiac transplant have unique problems that may include altered anatomic relationships, absence of anginal pain, contrast allergic reactions, and high sensitivity to infection, all of which must be considered in the approach to this unusual patient population. Routine left- and right-sided heart catheterization is usually performed from the femoral approach in the patient

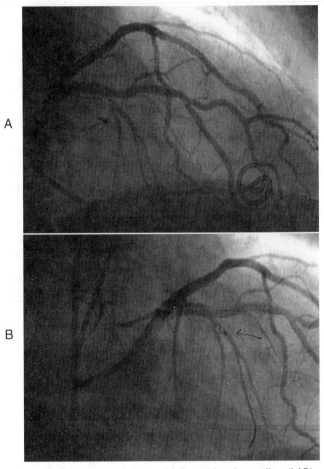

Fig. 7-18   A, Coronary angiogram of left anterior descending (LAD) and first and second septal arteries. **B,** A small angioplasty balloon is placed in *(arrow)* and position verified by echocardiographic and radiographic contrast imaging.   *Continued*

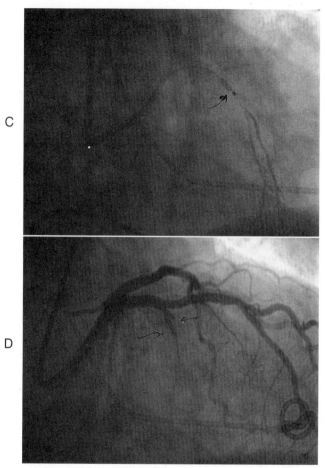

Fig. 7-18, cont'd   C, Selective x-ray contrast injection into septal artery through occlusion balloon *(arrow).* **D,** After alcohol (1 to 2 ml) is instilled, balloon is deflated and removed. Angiogram shows cutoff of thrombosed first septal artery.

after heart transplantation. If femoral scar tissue is excessive on one side, approach from the opposite groin or arm may be necessary. If endomyocardial biopsy is considered, the internal jugular or femoral venous approach may be suitable with the use of fluoroscopy or echocardiographically guided biopsy (see Endomyocardial Biopsy earlier).

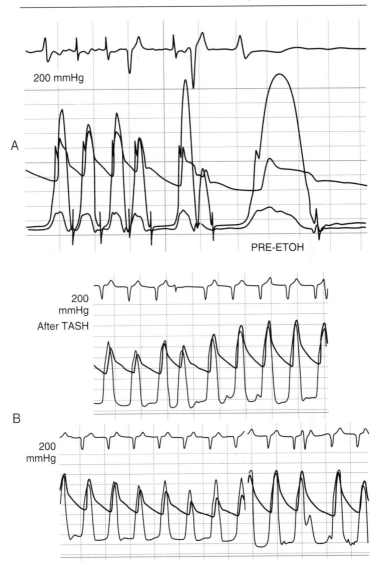

Fig. 7-19 Hemodynamics of left ventricular and aortic pressures, **A,** before transluminal alcohol septal ablation for hypertrophic cardiomyopathy (TASH), and, **B,** after TASH during Valsalva maneuver.

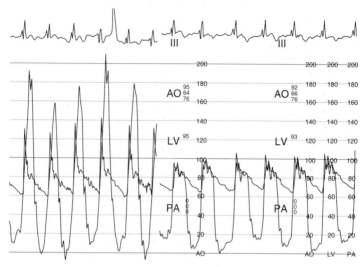

Fig. 7-20   Hemodynamics of hypertrophic cardiomyopathy before *(left)* and after *(right)* transluminal alcohol septal ablation for hypertrophic cardiomyopathy.

Angiographic Notes for the Heart Transplant Recipient. The transplanted heart is rotated clockwise compared with a normal heart. The right coronary ostium is anterior and the left coronary ostium is located in a more posterior plane than in the normal heart. A suture ridge in the lower ascending aorta at the site of the aortic anastomosis may cause the Judkins catheter to snag or bend as it is advanced. A guidewire may be needed to move the left Judkins catheter across this ridge. A left Judkins 5-cm curved catheter may be useful to reach the posterior position of the left coronary orifice. The anterior position of the right coronary ostia may be better engaged with the use of an anteroposterior or slightly rightward oblique view. The multipurpose angiographic catheter may be required for unusual positions of the coronary ostia.

Adherence to sterile techniques cannot be overemphasized. An anaphylactoid reaction to contrast media for multiple post-transplant studies must be considered and pretreated. These patients are generally preload dependent, and recommended administration of intracoronary nitroglycerin for angiographic studies may result in a significant decrease in the patient's blood pressure.

Adult Complex Congenital Heart Disease

Adults who have corrected congenital heart disease are encountered with increasing frequency by nonpediatric cardiac catheterization physicians. Detailed knowledge of previous cardiac surgery and catheterization and echocardiographic findings is necessary for the performance of a complete and efficient catheterization. Residual hemodynamic and electrophysiologic abnormalities must be identified in these patients to maintain their long-term survival.

Ventricular septal defects may occur at the muscular septum or at the site of an old patch in hearts that have been corrected. Great vessel shunts may occur from collateral supply, especially in patients with repaired cyanotic heart disease or incompletely occluded shunts. Cyanosis in these individuals may be the result of the following:

1. Persistent left SVC–to–left atrium shunting with or without CS or septal defect
2. Right pulmonary arteriovenous fistula (Glenn anastomosis)
3. Acquired lung disease
4. A combination of the above

Careful hemodynamic and oximetric measurements are important for identification of shunts in adult patients. Right and left pulmonary arteries must be sampled for oxygen saturations during the oximetry run. For the most accurate results the entire oximetry run should be performed in less than 10 minutes (see Chapter 3). Patients with cyanosis are given 100% oxygen so that cardiac causes of cyanosis can be differentiated from noncardiac causes.

Large-flow (8 F) pigtail catheters with a high-contrast volume load (50 ml at 25 ml/sec) may be required for optimal ventriculographic results. Large-format image intensifiers (9-inch screen) are needed for simultaneous display of both ventricles. Coronary artery abnormalities may be present in adults with congenital heart disease and can contribute to ventricular dysfunction. The late natural history of coronary atherosclerosis in corrected forms of congenital heart disease is unknown. It is recommended that any patient older than age 35 with evidence of ventricular dysfunction undergo coronary arteriography.

Patients with complex congenital heart disease, such as tetralogy of Fallot with an overriding aorta, ventricular septal defect, and pulmonary stenosis or truncus arteriosus (common arterial trunk with ventricular septal defect), may have abnormally large aortic roots, and modified coronary catheters must be used in arteriography in these patients. Single coronary arteries or anomalous origins of the left coronary artery from the right coronary artery may be part of the truncus arteriosus (a common pulmonary and aortic outflow tube) and transposition of the great vessels (switching of the PA and the aorta).

Simultaneous RV and PA pressure recordings are frequently required when patients have residual RV outflow tract obstruction or PA stenosis. The measurements can be accomplished by use of a combination of a long 7 F sheath and an extra-long coronary catheter, such as a multipurpose catheter. After the guidewire has been positioned in the PA, the sheath-catheter combination can be advanced into the PA. The operator can perform stepwire withdrawal of the sheath and maintain the position of the multipurpose catheter in the PA. The simultaneous recording and detection of pressure gradients across the chambers of the right side of the heart and localization of areas of stenosis can be determined.

Catheter Therapy. Balloon dilation or occluder catheter therapy may be performed to dilate narrowed heart valves or to close atrial or ventricular septal defects in children and adults with congenital heart disease. Special devices are available to close patent ductus arteriosus (fetal communication between the aorta and the PA that normally closes at birth). These lesions should be 10 mm in diameter or smaller for catheter therapy. Balloon catheter valvulotomy can be performed for aortic and mitral stenosis. Pulmonic valvuloplasty is commonly performed in children with congenital heart disease and may be practical in adults (see Chapter 9).

Suggested Readings

Bell CA, Kern MJ, Aguirre FV, et al: Superior accuracy of anatomic positioning with echocardiographic over fluoroscopic-guided endomyocardial biopsy, *Cathet Cardiovasc Diagn* 28:291-294, 1993.

Croft CH, Lipscomb K: Modified technique of transseptal left heart catheterization, *J Am Coll Cardiol* 5:904-910, 1985.

Kern MJ, Deligonul U, editors: *The interventional cardiac catheterization handbook*, St Louis, 1996, Mosby.

Mason JW, O'Connell JB: Clinical method of endomyocardial biopsy, *Circulation* 79:971-979, 1989.

Miller LW, Labovitz AJ, McBride LA, et al: Echocardiography-guided endomyocardial biopsy: a 5-year experience, *Circulation* 78(suppl 3):99-102, 1988.

8

HIGH-RISK CARDIAC CATHETERIZATION

Kevin Lisman, Glenn Levine, Hassan Rajjoub, Steve Herrmann, Saad Bitar, and Morton J. Kern

HIGH-RISK PATIENT
Definition

Patients classified as high risk are more likely to die or have myocardial infarction or ventricular fibrillation during cardiac catheterization than are other patients. Numerous studies have summarized the clinical and anatomic characteristics of patients at high risk: patients with known significant three-vessel or left main coronary artery disease, severe left ventricular (LV) dysfunction, diabetes, or poorly controlled hypertension (Box 8-1). Markedly abnormal exercise treadmill test results suggesting severe coronary artery disease are also an indication of potential high-risk status. Patients with congestive heart failure, recent acute myocardial infarction, unstable angina, and severe valvular heart disease (especially critical aortic stenosis) have a high incidence of morbidity and mortality during and after cardiac catheterization. The occurrence of major complications in the cardiac catheterization laboratory has increased markedly with the development of increasingly complex interventional procedures.

INCIDENCE OF COMPLICATIONS IN THE HIGH-RISK PATIENT

The risk of major complications during a diagnostic cardiac catheterization in a patient who is not at high risk is low. In an initial report of 53,581 patients from 1979 through 1982, the Society for Cardiac Angiography reported a 2% risk of major complications (0.14% risk of death, 0.07% myocardial

450

Box 8-1

Patient and Clinical Characteristics Associated with Increased Mortality from Cardiac Catheterization

Age
Infants (<1 year old) and the elderly (>65 years old)
Elderly women seem to be at higher risk than elderly men

Functional Class
Mortality in class IV patients is more than 10 times greater than in class I and II patients

Severity of Coronary Obstruction
Mortality for patients with left main coronary artery disease is more than 10 times greater than for patients with one- or two-vessel disease

Valvular Heart Disease
Severe valvular heart disease, especially severe aortic stenosis, is associated with increased risk of cardiac death

Left Ventricular Dysfunction
Mortality for patients with left ventricular ejection fraction <30% is more than 10 times greater than in patients with ejection fraction ≥50%

Severe Noncardiac Disease
Increased risk of adverse events associated with the following comorbid conditions:
Diabetes
Severe pulmonary disease
Advanced cerebrovascular or peripheral vascular disease
Renal insufficiency

Modified from Grossman W: *Complications of cardiac catheterization: incidence, causes and prevention.* In Grossman W, editor: *Cardiac catheterization and angiography,* ed 3, Philadelphia, 1986, Lea & Febiger.

infarction, and 0.07% cerebrovascular accident). Several clinical variables are associated with an increased risk of death. Age, New York Heart Association functional class, ejection fraction, and extent of coronary heart disease are the most powerful predictors of mortality during cardiac catheterization. An ejection fraction of less than 30% and left main coronary artery stenosis are associated with a 10-fold increase in risk of death. The incidence of major complications for important clinical and angiographic variables is given in Table 8-1.

Prevention of Complications

Meticulous attention to the precatheterization patient assessment and recognition of potential risks decreases procedure-related complications.

Patient Medications. Patients taking warfarin generally do not take it for 48 to 72 hours before the procedure. Elective procedures should be performed only when the patient's international normalized ratio is less than 1.5.

Table 8-1

Incidence of Complications During Diagnostic Cardiac Catheterization for Various Clinical and Angiographic Variables

	Death (%)	MI (%)	CVA (%)	Arrhythmia (%)
Age				
<60	0.07	0.07	0.05	0.43
>60	0.12	0.06	0.09	0.51
NYHA Class				
I	0.02	0.02	0.12	0.53
II	0.02	0.03	0.05	0.32
III	0.05	0.07	0.05	0.43
IV	0.29	0.12	0.08	0.65
Ejection Fraction				
>50%	0.03	0.04	0.05	0.35
30%-49%	0.12	0.06	0.08	0.55
<30%	0.30	0.12	0.09	0.94
Extent of CHD				
1 vessel	0.05	0.06	0.04	0.42
2 vessels	0.07	0.08	0.08	0.45
3 vessels	0.12	0.08	0.09	0.53
LM	0.55	0.17	0.13	0.66

Modified from Johnson LW, et al: *Cathet Cardiovasc Diagn* 17:5-10, 1989.
CHD, Coronary heart disease; *CVA,* cerebrovascular accident; *LM,* left main disease; *MI,* myocardial infarction; *NYHA,* New York Heart Association.

Diuretics should generally not be taken the morning of the procedure. Dehydration may decrease renal flow and increase the risk of contrast nephropathy and hypotension.

Regular morning insulin should not be taken, and the morning dose of long-acting insulin should be halved. Patients who take insulin should receive dextrose in intravenous fluids.

Patients taking metformin (Glucophage) should not take this medication the morning of the procedure (or for 48 hours before the procedure in patients at high risk of contrast nephropathy), and the medication should be resumed 48 hours later only when it has been verified that renal function has not been compromised.

The use of sildenafil (Viagra) within the 48 hours before the procedure is a contraindication to elective catheterization in which nitrates may be used.

Contrast Allergy. Patients who have had previous allergic reactions to contrast media should be pretreated with prednisone (60 mg the night before and morning of the procedure) and diphenhydramine (50 mg intravenously [IV] the morning of the procedure). For patients who have had severe allergic reactions (bronchospasm, laryngospasm, hypotension) additional pretreatment with an H_2 blocker (cimetidine, 300 mg IV, or ranitidine, 50 mg IV) should be considered.

Renal Insufficiency. Contrast nephropathy, defined as a rise in serum creatinine level of 1 mg/dl, occurs in 5% of patients who undergo cardiac catheterization and in 20% to 30% of patients with baseline renal insufficiency, diabetes, or both. Patient hydration before and after the procedure (0.45% saline at 1 mg/kg/hr for 12 hours before and 12 hours after the procedure) decreases the risk of contrast nephropathy and should be used. Data supporting the use of acetylcysteine (600 mg orally twice daily the day before and day of the procedure) or the selective dopamine-1 receptor agonist fenoldopam to reduce risk of contrast nephropathy, although modest, suggest that these agents can be considered for patients at high risk of contrast nephropathy.

Contrast Media Selection. Procedures in which low osmolar and nonionic contrast agents are used are associated with a lower incidence of bradycardia, hypotension, and myocardial ischemia developing in the patient, and these agents are routinely used during cardiac catheterizations. All cardiac catheterizations performed on patients with indications that put them in the high-risk category (including acute myocardial infarction, congestive heart failure, depressed ejection fraction, suspected left main or three-vessel coronary artery disease, and severe aortic stenosis) should preferentially be performed with nonionic, low-osmolality agents. Conditions in which nonionic, low-osmolality agents should be used are listed in Box 8-2.

Vasovagal Reactions

Vasovagal reactions occur more commonly during the painful period in which arterial access is obtained, but may also occur during or after the procedure (particularly during arterial sheath removal and application of pressure to the groin area). In addition to bradycardia and hypotension patients often have pallor, nausea, or diaphoresis. Vasovagal reactions are treated with administration of atropine, 0.5 to 1 mg IV. The dose may be repeated quickly if necessary up to a total dose of 3 mg. Doses of less than 0.5 mg have been associated with paradoxical responses and should not be used. Because in most patients the hypotension is due to a combination of

---

Box 8-2

Conditions in Which Nonionic, Low-Osmolality Contrast Agents Should Be Used Preferentially During High-Risk Cardiac Catheterization

Acute myocardial infarction
Congestive heart failure
Ejection fraction ≤30%
Suspected left main or three-vessel coronary artery disease
Severe aortic stenosis
Complex or multiple ventricular arrhythmias
Acute or chronic renal insufficiency
Anticipated use of large contrast agent volume

Adapted from Hildner FJ: Complications of cardiac catheterization and strategies to reduce risks. In Pepine CJ, editor: *Diagnostic and therapeutic cardiac catheterization*, ed 2, Philadelphia, 1994, Lippincott Williams & Wilkins.

bradycardia and peripheral vasodilation, administration of fluids, as discussed later, can be initiated in patients before the response to atropine occurs.

Fluids

Hypotension resulting from volume depletion and most other causes should be treated with aggressive fluid resuscitation with normal saline (which is preferable to the use of half-normal saline solutions). Rapid administration of at least several hundred milliliters of fluid is usually necessary. Elevation of the patient's legs (to approximately 30 degrees) increases blood return to the heart and increases effective ventricular filling, which improves cardiac output. Placement of a Swan-Ganz catheter helps guide fluid administration in patients with depressed ejection fraction, recent congestive heart failure, severe aortic stenosis, critical illness, or unknown fluid status.

Management of Complications During Cardiac Catheterization

Complications of coronary arteriography in high-risk patients must be managed at once (Table 8-2). If myocardial ischemia develops, the location and cause (thrombus, dissection, spasm) by coronary arteriography should be rapidly assessed, and reperfusion should be attempted with intracoronary nitroglycerin (spasm), thrombolytic agents or thrombectomy (if a thrombus is identified), or emergency revascularization with angioplasty or bypass surgery.

Causes of peripheral arterial complications should be identified early. If a large dissection or thrombotic occlusion occurs, a vascular surgeon should be consulted immediately. Enlarging hematomas should be drained if they compromise circulation to the legs.

Arterial thromboembolism to other areas, such as the brain, may not be immediately treatable but requires close observation or prolonged heparin, depending on neurologic findings. Occipital blindness, a rare event that is caused by hyperosmolarity of the contrast agent, is usually transient and requires no definitive treatment except for hydration and maintenance of blood pressure. Steroids have also been used to

Table 8-2

Management of Complications During Cardiac Catheterization

Complications and Precautions	Treatment
Myocardial Infarction (0.2%)	Intracoronary nitroglycerin (rule out spasm) Consider intracoronary thrombectomy or aspiration, coronary angioplasty, or emergency aortocoronary bypass
Cerebrovascular Accident (0.1%) Systemic heparinization Cleaning of guidewires before use Limit guidewire-blood exposure (<2 min) Use guidewire to cross aortic arch (especially in atherosclerotic aortas, and especially for Amplatz or bypass graft catheter) Aspirate and flush catheters frequently Remove air bubbles in any of the tubing, solutions, or injection syringe Ensure all tubing and catheter connections are tight	
Dissection (0.1%) Never advance guidewire or catheter against resistance; catheter tip location confirmed by gentle contrast injection Do not manipulate catheter in coronary ostium, monitoring pressure of catheter tip Do not inject with damped pressure	No further coronary injections If ischemia produced, stent or emergency aortocoronary bypass If dissection associated with thrombus but no ischemia, use heparin (controversial) and consider coronary stenting

Table 8-2

Management of Complications During Cardiac Catheterization— cont'd

Complications and Precautions	Treatment
Acute Pulmonary Edema	
Treat preexisting CHF optimally	Elevate patient's trunk 30 to 45 degrees
Limit contrast medium in high risk; avoid LV angiography in severe aortic stenosis, marked CHF, or pulmonary hypertension	Oxygen, morphine (2 to 5 mg IV), nitrates (100 to 200 µg IC), furosemide (20 to 100 mg IV); nitroprusside for afterload reduction; inotropic support with dopamine or dobutamine
Use nonionic or low-osmolar contrast media agents	
Avoid hypotension	
Limit flush solution volume	Intraaortic balloon pumping
Monitor LV filling pressure (PCW)	
Cardiogenic Shock	
Careful patient selection: (1) left main coronary artery stenosis, (2) aortic stenosis at high risk, and (3) acute infarction	If shock caused by coronary occlusion, treat with emergency PTCA or CABG surgery
Prophylactic IABP for high-risk left main coronary artery angiography; minimize number of injections; treat hypotension	Vasopressor support IABP
Stop procedure if hypotension persists	Intubation and mechanical ventilation
Atropine, adequate volume expansion, Aramine ([metaraminol] intraaortic injection of 0.125 to 0.250 mg), IABP	Pacemaker as needed
Rule out pericardial tamponade with RA and RV pressures; consider urgent echocardiogram	
Monitor filling pressures	

CABG, Coronary bypass graft; *CHF,* congestive heart failure; *IABP,* intraaortic balloon pump; *IC,* intracoronary; *IV,* intravenous; *LV,* left ventricular; *PCW,* pulmonary capillary wedge; *PTCA,* percutaneous transluminal coronary angioplasty; *RA,* right atrial; *RV,* right ventricular.

Continued

Table 8-2

Management of Complications During Cardiac Catheterization—cont'd

Complications and Precautions	Treatment
Ventricular Tachycardia, Asystole, or Fibrillations (0.6%)	
Use nonionic contrast agents in high-risk patients	Cough for temporary increase in BP
Do not wedge coronary artery catheter; contrast material washout should be brisk; ECG and BP should be normal before next injection	Remove catheter from RV, LV, or coronary ostium
	CPR followed by prompt defibrillation
Do not inject when catheter tip pressure is damped	Defibrillation (200 J)
	Lidocaine (50 mg bolus, 2 to 4 mg/min IV)
Use atropine, volume expansion, or metaraminol (Aramine) for hypotension	Amiodarone (300 mg bolus) then infusion
Limit contrast medium injected into coronary arteries; avoid prolonged injections	Refractory VF usually as a result of extensive CAD; emergency percutaneous cardiopulmonary bypass should be considered
Air Embolism	
For prevention and treatment see p. 454	Same as cerebrovascular accident
Hematoma in Femoral Artery (0.1% Major, 1% to 2% Minor)	
Puncture below inguinal ligament	Evacuation rarely required
Attention to compression	Surgical consult for enlarging hematoma, compartment syndrome, or cool extremity
Prolonged compression if patient coughing, aortic insufficiency, hypertension, or heparin not reversed	
Vascular closure device	
Retroperitoneal Bleeding	
Avoid high (above inguinal ligament) femoral artery puncture	Reverse anticoagulants
	Volume replacement
Watch for hypotension, low abdominal or flank pain within 2-12 hours of procedure	Transfusion if hematocrit <25
	Surgical consultation
Low hematocrit, tachycardia (if not receiving β-blockers)	CT scan

BP, Blood pressure; *CAD,* coronary artery disease; *CPR,* cardiopulmonary resuscitation; *CT,* computed tomography *ECG,* electrocardiogram; *VF,* ventricular fibrillation.

Table 8-2

Management of Complications During Cardiac Catheterization—cont'd

Complications and Precautions	Treatment
Cardiac Tamponade	
Avoid stiff catheters in RA or RV; pacing catheters handled gently	Prompt pericardiocentesis with catheter drainage
Avoid posterior LA wall during transseptal catheterization	Cardiovascular surgery consultation
	Surgical exploration and closure for persistent bleeding
Contrast Agent Nephrotoxicity	
Hydration and nonionic contrast agents	Generally self-limited; dialysis rarely needed
Contrast agent reaction	
Vasovagal reaction	

Modified from Tilkian AG, Daily EK: *Cardiovascular procedures: diagnostic techniques and therapeutic procedures*, St Louis, 1986, Mosby.

treat this condition. An air embolus to the central nervous system may cause the patient to show features of acute stroke such as agitation, confusion, or aphasia. A small air embolus usually resolves and does not often result in permanent damage. Although hyperbaric oxygen chambers have been used successfully for treatment, these are not widely available.

Hypotension

Hypotension may occur before, during, and after cardiac catheterization from a variety of conditions. Before cardiac catheterization hypotension may be caused by hypovolemia induced by fasting before the procedure (water intake should be allowed) or diuretics. During the cardiac catheterization procedure hypotension may be due to vasovagal reaction. Untreated vasovagal reactions with hypotension can lead to irreversible shock. Vasovagal reactions are frequently elicited by pain at the site of vascular access. In some elderly patients a vagal reaction may occur without bradycardia and appear as unexplained hypotension. Hypotension that develops after coronary arteriography or left ventriculography is generally transient and self-limited and responds to IV fluids. Aggressive treatment is occasionally required.

After the cardiac catheterization procedure hypotension is often caused by hypovolemia resulting from excessive contrast-induced diuresis, myocardial ischemia, unsuspected bleeding from the puncture site, or anticoagulation-related retroperitoneal hematoma. Other causes of hypotension include occult cardiac tamponade and hemorrhage from arterial access bleeding.

Acute myocardial ischemia may cause hypotension at any time. If hypotension caused by myocardial ischemia occurs, the operator may need to insert an intraaortic balloon pump (IABP) before the procedure can be safely completed.

Management of Hypotension. Hypotension resulting from hypovolemia is treated with IV saline infusion. Patients often respond acutely to elevation (>30 degrees) of the lower extremities (increased venous inflow, "internal transfusion"). Generally, several hundred milliliters of saline is required to restore adequate blood pressure in patients who have hypotension caused by hypovolemia. Hypovolemia in patients undergoing catheterization can be avoided by the infusion of IV saline (more than 500 ml for 4 to 6 hours) before the start of the procedure (particularly in patients who will be fasting for more than 12 hours) and more than 1000 ml for 4 to 6 hours after the procedure. Administration of blood products is necessary for patients who have hypovolemia caused by hemorrhage. Hemostasis must be achieved at once in such patients. Care should be taken to prevent volume overload in patients with congestive heart failure. Generally, careful measurement of fluid intake and urine output helps the laboratory staff to monitor such patients. If a patient's volume status cannot be determined clinically, a pulmonary artery catheter and pulmonary capillary wedge pressure measurement may be needed.

For patients with hypotension resulting from vasovagal or ischemia reaction, pharmacologic therapy may be necessary to restore adequate blood pressure. Atropine for vasovagal hypotension (0.6 to 1.2 mg IV) is used first. IV (not coronary) aramine (1 mg) or epinephrine bolus (1 ml of 1:10,000 U dilution) temporarily increases blood pressure to normal range while the staff member continues to assess the patient and other vasopressors are prepared. For patients with prolonged hypotension or patients who have hypotension without hypovolemia, pharmacotherapy may be initiated and can be titrated up as needed. A higher initial infusion rate of dopamine at 10 μg/kg/min should be considered for patients with profound hypotension. A second therapy is bolus norepinephrine (Levophed) administration. Intermittent bolus administration of norepinephrine is extremely effective because bolus administration of this agent leads to rapid (within 3 to 5 minutes) improvement in blood pressure, is easily titratable, and has a relatively short half-life. Doses of 5 μg should be administered as indicated. The premixing regimen for norepinephrine is given in Box 8-3.

Drug-induced hypotension should be addressed with agents that antagonize, ameliorate, or minimize the actions of the offending agent. Narcotic-induced hypotension can be treated with administration of naloxone (Narcan). The dose is 0.4 mg (1-ml ampule), which may be repeated every 2 to 3 minutes as needed. Hypotension (or hypoventilation) resulting from benzodiazepam administration can be treated with flumazenil (Romazicon). The initial dose is 0.2 mg (2 ml) administered over 30 seconds; additional doses of 0.3 to 0.5 mg (3 to 5 ml) can be administered as indicated up to a total maximum dose of 3 mg.

Box 8-3

Premixing Regimen Used in the Preparation of Norepinephrine (Levophed) for Bolus Therapy for Blood Pressure Support

1. Dilute 1 mg norepinephrine in 9 ml normal saline
   = 1000 μg/10 ml
   = 100 μg/ml
2. Take 1 ml of above mixture and further dilute in another 9 ml normal saline
   = 100 μg/10 ml
   = 10 μg/ml
3. Administer bolus doses of 5 μg (0.5 ml) approximately every 5 minutes as needed. Blood pressure usually responds within 3 to 5 minutes

Hypotension resulting from negative inotropic, negative chronotropic, and vasodilatory actions may be caused by calcium channel blockers. The vasodilatory actions can be at least partially reversed by administration of calcium chloride (1 ampule, 13.6 mEq). Administration of glucagon (1 mg) may partially ameliorate the effects of β-blockers.

If nitroglycerin-induced hypotension develops, the IV infusion should be stopped or the nitropaste wiped off. Hypotension resulting from cardiac tamponade is an emergency condition that requires immediate pericardiocentesis.

Allergic Reactions. Hypotension caused by anaphylactoid reaction usually occurs within 20 minutes of exposure to contrast media. Patients at highest risk for anaphylactoid reactions are those with prior anaphylaxis (recurrence in 16% to 44% of patients) and those with atopy or asthma (who are twice as likely as other patients to have reactions to contrast agents). Recommendations by the Society for Cardiac Angiography and Intervention for treatment of severe anaphylactoid reactions include IV epinephrine with large volumes of normal saline, diphenhydramine, and hydrocortisone. If the patient does not respond to this therapy, an H_2 blocker and dopamine may be administered. Specific dosage regimens are given in Box 8-4. Patients with bronchospasm should be treated with supplemental oxygen and inhaled β-agonists such as albuterol. If laryngeal edema develops, the anesthesia service should be called at once, and an intubation tray and a tracheostomy tray should be prepared. IV bolus of epinephrine is most commonly used to treat laryngeal edema.

Management of Refractory Myocardial Ischemia and Hemodynamic Instability. Transient ischemia and coronary artery occlusion can be caused by catheter-induced spasm, cannulation of a severely diseased coronary artery, or a severe ostial lesion. Initial intervention is removal of the catheter from the coronary ostium. Continued myocardial ischemia should initially be treated with pharmacologic therapy. Initial pharmacologic therapy begins with nitrates, either sublingual nitroglycerin (0.4 mg every 5 minutes) or IV or intracoronary nitroglycerin (100-μg boluses repeated every 5 minutes as necessary). Nitroglycerin can be used, provided that the patient

Box 8-4

Treatment of Severe Anaphylactoid Reactions: Recommendations from the Society of Cardiac Angiography and Interventions

Initial Pharmacological Therapy
Epinephrine 10 µg/min IV until desired blood pressure response, then 1 to
   4 µg/min to maintain desired blood pressure, given simultaneously with large
   volumes of normal saline
Diphenhydramine (Benadryl) 50 to 100 mg IV
Hydrocortisone 400 mg IV

If Unresponsive to Initial Therapy
H_2 blocker therapy
   Cimetidine 300 mg in 20 ml normal saline administered IV over 15 minutes
   Ranitidine 50 mg in 20 ml normal saline administered IV over 15 minutes
Dopamine 2 to 15 µg/kg/min IV infusion

does not have hypotension. For patients with tachycardia, negative inotropic therapy with a β-blocker, such as metoprolol (5 mg IV every 5 minutes), or a calcium channel blocker, such as verapamil (2.5 to 5 mg IV every 5 minutes), should be considered if the patient is otherwise hemodynamically stable.

When ischemia persists after optimal medical treatment, or when it is associated with significant hemodynamic instability, including pulmonary edema or hypotension or both, mechanical assistance should be considered, usually IABP counterpulsation.

MANAGEMENT OF ARRHYTHMIAS IN HIGH-RISK PATIENTS

Serious arrhythmias (including ventricular fibrillation, ventricular tachycardia, supraventricular tachycardia, asystole, and heart block) occur in approximately 1% of either right-sided or left-sided heart catheterizations. In almost all instances the arrhythmia can be managed successfully by prompt recognition and treatment. Arrhythmias may result from intracardiac catheter manipulation or contrast-induced myocardial ischemia during angioplasty.

For malignant ventricular arrhythmias with hypotension the most important determinant of short- and long-term (neurologically intact) survival of the patient is the interval from the onset of hemodynamic collapse to the restoration of effective, spontaneous circulatory and respiratory function. The following section provides suggestions for optimal treatment. These suggestions do not preclude other measures that may be indicated on the basis of the specific clinical circumstances of the individual patient.

Primary Prevention of Arrhythmias

Electrocardiographic Monitoring. Continuous electrocardiographic (ECG) monitoring is essential for the performance of a safe cardiac catheterization. If a problem develops with the ECG leads or equipment during the procedure, the operator must remedy it before the procedure continues.

Intravenous Access. Before the procedure is begun, a functioning 18-gauge peripheral IV line should be established in the patient. If peripheral venous access cannot be obtained, the operator should place a femoral venous sheath large enough to accommodate a pacing wire and allow rapid saline infusion. A 6 F or larger femoral venous sheath should be placed in potentially unstable or acutely ill patients.

Standby Transvenous Pacing. The need for a prophylactic temporary transvenous pacemaker is determined by the patient's risk of bradyarrhythmia or heart block and the patient's ability to tolerate these arrhythmias should they occur. The use of flexible, balloon-tipped, flow-directed pacemaker wires provides the lowest risk for cardiac perforation. Risk factors for bradyarrhythmia include the following:

1. Preexisting right bundle-branch block during left-sided heart catheterization
2. Preexisting left bundle-branch block during right-sided heart catheterization, particularly when stiff catheters (e.g., Cournand) are used
3. Heart block greater than first degree
4. Marked sinus bradycardia
5. Coronary artery angioplasty involving the (dominant) artery supplying the atrioventricular (AV) node, especially when rotational atherectomy or thrombus extraction devices are used.

Box 8-5

Conditions in Which Venous Femoral Access Should Be Obtained and a Transvenous Pacemaker Considered
Poor peripheral access
Hemodynamic instability
Suspected left main coronary artery disease
Active arrhythmia

Conditions for which femoral venous access and transvenous pacing should be considered are summarized in Box 8-5.

Limitation of Cardiac Catheter Manipulations. Catheter passage through the heart should be performed with caution and a smooth motion. Particular note should be made of ventricular ectopy during catheter manipulation. Atrial arrhythmias (atrial fibrillation, supraventricular tachycardia) may be caused by vigorous stretching of the right atrium. Ventricular arrhythmias are associated with stimulation of the right ventricular outflow tract or papillary muscles by catheter contact. Removal of stimulating catheters usually terminates the arrhythmia.

Limitation of Occlusive Engagement of Coronary Arteries. The engaged coronary catheter pressure should always be checked before contrast medium is injected. Occlusion of flow through the coronary artery (or vein graft) by the catheter is reflected by a damped pressure wave. Ostial occlusion in combination with contrast dye injection can lead to the development of ventricular fibrillation, particularly during right coronary artery angiography.

Limitation of Coronary Artery Contrast. Injections of contrast medium should be sufficient to opacify the arterial tree without excessive volume or rates of injection. Ionic contrast media predispose a patient to bradycardia and ventricular fibrillation, especially during injection of the right coronary artery. The operator should ask the patient to cough when sustained hypotension is recognized before loss of consciousness (and cardiac arrest). Forceful coughing can generate sufficient blood flow to the brain to maintain consciousness until definitive treatment can be initiated.

Atropine Administration. Atropine, 0.6 to 1 mg IV, may be administered before coronary angiography when ionic contrast media is utilized or in patients with baseline heart rates of less than 60 beats/min.

Defibrillation and Cardioversion. Definitive electrical treatment has the highest priority of any modality. A defibrillator should be located near the patient in each cardiac catheterization laboratory suite. Before the procedure is begun, the defibrillator should be turned on and conductive jelly should be ready to apply to the defibrillator paddles to avoid delay in defibrillation. The time to successful defibrillation is the major determinant of the patient's survival. If pulseless ventricular tachycardia or ventricular fibrillation is present, defibrillation should be performed at once. An algorithm for treatment of ventricular fibrillation with cardiopulmonary resuscitation (CPR) is provided in Figure 8-1.

Proper paddle placement (Fig. 8-2) and the use of conducting gel are essential to successful defibrillation. One paddle should be placed along the upper right sternal border, below the clavicle, and the other paddle should be placed lateral to the patient's nipple with the center of the electrode in the midaxillary line. The paddles should be applied with firm pressure (about 25 lb). The person who performs the defibrillation must ensure that no one is touching the bed or the patient during defibrillation. Large defibrillation patches used with automatic external defibrillators are also highly effective. These patches may be put on the high-risk patient who has had prior ventricular tachycardia episodes in anticipation of an arrhythmia.

Continuing Modalities

Securing of Adequate Routes for Drug Administration. A central venous (internal jugular or femoral) line should be used for drug administration. If an antecubital vein is used, rapid entry of drugs into the central circulation can be facilitated by use of large volumes of flush solutions (50 ml) after bolus medication injection and elevation of the arm.

The distal wrist, hand, and saphenous veins provide poor access to the central circulation and are not useful or appropriate for rapid drug administration. A long catheter that

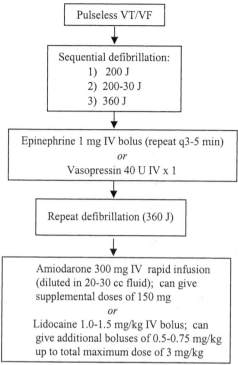

Fig. 8-1 Advanced cardiac life support algorithm for pulseless ventricular tachycardia or ventricular fibrillation. *IV,* Intravenous; *J,* joule; *VF,* ventricular fibrillation; *VT,* ventricular tachycardia.

reaches above the diaphragm via the femoral venous route provides prompt access to the central circulation. Direct intracardiac injections are not indicated.

Cardiopulmonary Resuscitation. Chest compressions (1.5- to 2-inch depression; 5:1 compression-to-breath ratio) should be performed if no blood pressure is present (Fig. 8-3). The catheterization laboratory table is moved over the support base to accommodate chest compression (Fig. 8-4).

Intravenous Fluids. Rapid volume expansion is not necessary in most patients with cardiac arrest unless an indication of preexisting volume depletion is present. Volume expansion may diminish blood flow to the cerebral and coronary circulations.

Sodium bicarbonate should be used when a clearly defined metabolic derangement (e.g., hyperkalemia or preexisting acidosis) exists. These conditions are not present in most patients with cardiac arrest in the catheterization laboratory. Adequate ventilation of the patient corrects acidosis better than sodium bicarbonate. Sodium bicarbonate should be administered only after rhythm-stabilizing and contractility-stabilizing interventions have been used and acidosis is likely to develop in the patient. The initial dose is 1 mEq/kg followed by

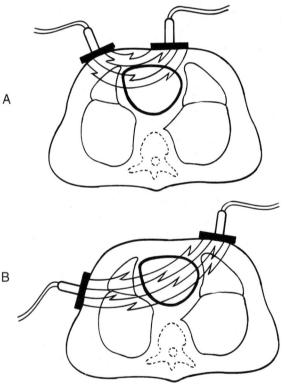

Fig. 8-2 Cardioversion paddle positions. **A,** Avoid too close positioning of electrode paddles (a substantial amount of current shunts between them and an insufficient amount reaches the heart). **B,** Space paddles widely, allowing a sufficient amount of current to reach the left ventricle. (**A** and **B** modified from Ewy GA: *J Cardiovasc Med* 7:44, 1982.) *Continued*

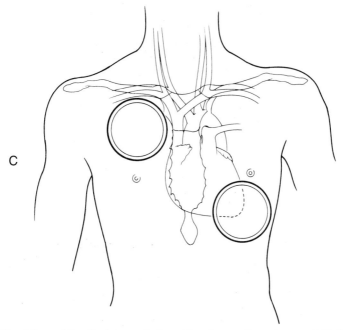

Fig. 8-2, cont'd   C, Anteroapical position for cardioversion or defibrillation. See text for details. (**C** from Tilkian AG, Daily EK: *Cardiovascular procedures: diagnostic techniques and therapeutic procedures,* St Louis, 1986, Mosby.)

0.5 mEq/kg every 10 minutes. Sodium bicarbonate should not be given in the same IV line as catecholamines (inactivation) or calcium (formation of precipitates). Postresuscitation sodium bicarbonate administration should be guided by the physician's knowledge of acid-base status from arterial blood gases.

Administration of calcium does not improve the patient's chances of survival from cardiac arrest. High serum calcium levels induced by calcium administration may be detrimental, especially when reperfusion occurs. The patient should not be given calcium unless hyperkalemia, hypocalcemia (e.g., after multiple blood transfusions), or calcium channel blocker toxicity is present. When calcium administration is indicated, 10% calcium chloride administered IV is the preferred preparation.

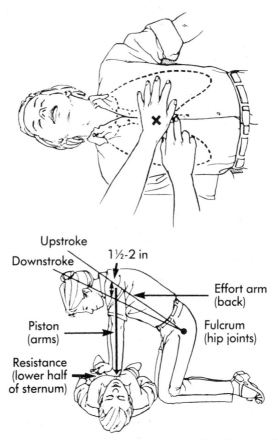

Fig. 8-3 Techniques for external chest compression. *Top,* Locating the correct hand position on the lower half of the sternum. *Bottom,* Proper position with shoulders directly over the sternum and elbows locked. (From Standards and guidelines for cardiopulmonary resuscitation [CPR] and emergency cardiac care [ECC], *Cardiopulmonary Resuscitation,* Washington, DC, 1981, American National Red Cross.)

Treatment of Specific Arrhythmias

The following sequences are useful to treat a broad range of patients with arrhythmias in the catheterization laboratory, but the sequences should be modified as the clinical situation warrants.

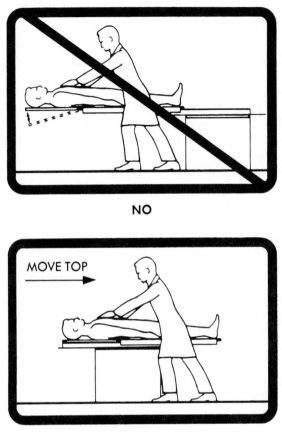

Fig. 8-4 Emergency cardiopulmonary resuscitation (CPR) procedures on the cardiac catheterization table. CPR may not be effective with the table top extended. Position the top caudally to the end of travel to provide additional support and minimize the possibility of table damage or failure. The patient load capacity of this carbon fiber top is 350 lb (159 kg). (Courtesy of Phillips Radiographic, Inc, Shelton, Conn.)

Vasovagal Reactions. Vasovagal reactions, which are often preceded by a slowing of heart rate before a decrease in blood pressure occurs, respond dramatically to IV atropine (0.6 to 1 mg). Elevation of the patient's legs and infusion of saline may increase blood pressure transiently. Early signs of vasovagal reaction include pallor, nausea, yawning, sneezing, or coughing.

Bradycardia. Bradycardia (ventricular heart rate <60 beats/min) may be caused by autonomic influences (vagal) or intrinsic disease of the cardiac conducting system (ischemia). Atropine sulfate is the treatment of choice for symptomatic bradycardia, a heart rate inappropriate for the hemodynamic state (e.g., a heart rate of <80 beats/min with hypotension). The initial dose to treat symptoms of bradycardia is 0.6 to 1 mg IV, to be repeated every 5 minutes as needed to a maximum dose of 3 mg. Doses of less than 0.5 mg may induce vagotonic effects. A pacemaker is rarely needed to treat bradycardia. Isoproterenol, a pure β-adrenergic agonist with positive chronotropic (heart rate) and inotropic (contractility) properties, is contraindicated in cardiac arrest.

Sinus or junctional rhythms and second-degree AV block (type I) often do not require specific treatment. In patients with symptoms of these conditions, these rhythms usually respond to atropine. Atropine should be given as needed, up to 3 mg in divided doses (0.5 mg). If symptoms of bradycardia persist after the maximal dose of atropine, the operator should place a transvenous pacemaker in the patient. An external pacemaker can be used to maintain the patient until a transvenous pacemaker can be inserted (Box 8-6).

Second-degree AV block (type II) and third-degree AV block are treated with a temporary transvenous pacemaker even in the absence of symptoms. If bradycardia is associated with hypotension, congestive heart failure, ischemia, or infarction, atropine (doses of ≤3 mg) should be administered until a pacemaker can be inserted.

Box 8-6

Conditions in Which a Temporary Transvenous Pacemaker Should Be Placed
Severe bradycardia
High-degree atrioventricular block
Pre-existing left bundle-branch block if right-sided heart catheterization is to be performed

Ventricular Fibrillation. If ventricular fibrillation is present, the operator should quickly remove intracardiac catheters and perform defibrillation at once (Fig. 8-5). Thereafter, guidelines are as follows (see Fig. 8-1):

1. Three consecutive unsynchronized defibrillations in rapid sequence are recommended for adults as necessary. The first defibrillation is performed at unsynchronized 200 J, the second at 300 J, and the third at 360 J. For children, 2.5 to 50 J (2 J/kg) is used.

2. If the defibrillations are unsuccessful, the operator should begin CPR. Epinephrine, 1 mg IV, or vasopressin, 40 U IV, is given. The patient is intubated if possible and ventilated manually. A mouthpiece should be inserted and the patient ventilated with a facemask if intubation is not possible. Vasopressin should be administered and CPR continued until a pulse is established. The success of treatment at this point depends in large part on the adequacy of CPR. CPR should not be stopped for more than 5 seconds except to defibrillate or intubate the patient. Treatment of underlying abnormalities (e.g., hypokalemia, hypomagnesemia, ischemia, infarction,

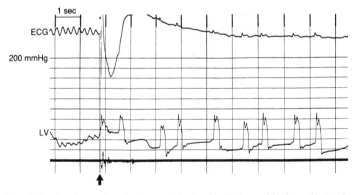

Fig. 8-5 Cardioversion during ventricular fibrillation with the catheter in the left ventricle. The electrocardiogram *(ECG)* shows coarse ventricular fibrillation with left ventricular *(LV)* pressure between 30 and 40 mm Hg. Arrow shows when cardioversion with 200 J is performed. The normal rhythm then returns with generation of LV pressure (70 to 80 mm Hg systolic). (From Kern MJ: *Hemodynamic rounds: interpretation of cardiac pathophysiology from pressure waveform analysis,* New York, 1993, Wiley-Liss.)

airway obstruction, or hypoxia) that may be causing the arrhythmia is crucial.

3. Defibrillation is repeated again at 360 J.
4. If defibrillation is unsuccessful, lidocaine (1 mg/kg bolus) or amiodarone (300 mg bolus) is administered, and defibrillation is repeated at 360 J.
5. Defibrillation is repeated at 360 J after each dose of antiarrhythmic agent.
6. If ventricular fibrillation does not respond to the above-listed measures, repeat amiodarone dose or emergency cardiopulmonary bypass should be considered.
7. If ventricular fibrillation recurs during the arrest sequence, defibrillation should be reinitiated at the energy level that had previously resulted in successful defibrillation.

Sustained Ventricular Tachycardia. If sustained ventricular tachycardia persists after removal of intracardiac catheters, management proceeds according to the stability of the patient. In patients who are hemodynamically unstable (e.g., hypotension [systolic blood pressure <90 mm Hg], pulmonary edema, or unconsciousness), synchronized cardioversion at 200 J is performed.

Synchronized cardioversion uses the largest R wave. If the QRS cannot be distinguished, the unsynchronized mode is used:

1. Paddles are lubricated with conduction gel
2. Excessive gel, which may conduct energy to the operator or bystanders, is avoided
3. All personnel are cleared before the paddles are discharged
4. Paddles are positioned properly (see Fig. 8-2)

In patients who are hemodynamically stable, the first approach to sustained ventricular tachycardia is antiarrhythmic therapy. Lidocaine and amiodarone are the drugs of first choice. If still this approach is unsuccessful, synchronized cardioversion, beginning with 100 to 200 J, is indicated. The patient should be sedated and given analgesics.

Nonsustained Ventricular Tachycardia. Nonsustained ventricular tachycardia usually can be eliminated by repositioning of or withdrawal of intracardiac or coronary catheters. Frequent nonsustained ventricular tachycardia caused by acute myocardial ischemia rather than catheter irritation should be treated with lidocaine.

Antiarrhythmic Agents for Ventricular Tachycardia. Amiodarone is the drug of choice for the management of ventricular ectopy, including ventricular tachycardia and ventricular fibrillation. Amiodarone is given to stable patients as a 150-mg infusion over 10 minutes, then 1 mg/min every 6 hours and 0.5 mg/min every 18 hours. An initial dose of 300 mg is given to unstable or pulseless patients.

Alternatively, lidocaine should initially be given as a bolus of 1.0–1.5 mg/kg. Additional boluses of 0.5 mg/kg can be given subsequently (every 8 to 10 minutes) to a total dose of 3 mg/kg in the arrest setting. In the nonarrest setting, the initial bolus should be reduced by half if any of the following conditions are present: congestive heart failure, shock, hepatic dysfunction, or age greater than 70 years. After a successful resuscitation a constant infusion of lidocaine at a rate of 2 to 4 mg/min should be initiated if lidocaine has been used successfully during the resuscitation.

Procainamide administration requires a relatively long time to achieve therapeutic levels. In urgent situations, 1 g of procainamide HCl can be administered over 30 minutes. A constant infusion rate (1 to 4 mg/min) is then administered and later titrated to serum drug levels. In situations that are not urgent, 1 g should be given over at least 1 hour. The rate of drug administration should be reduced or discontinued if hypotension is induced or if a greater than 50% prolongation of the QRS complex or Q-T interval occurs. Procainamide is contraindicated in Wolff-Parkinson-White syndrome.

Note: Wide-complex tachycardia of uncertain cause (i.e., ventricular tachycardia versus paroxysmal supraventricular tachycardia [PSVT] with aberrancy) should be treated as ventricular tachycardia until proved otherwise. Verapamil is contraindicated.

Sustained ventricular tachycardia in the patient who remains hemodynamically stable can first be treated with antiarrhythmic therapy. Amiodarone and lidocaine are reasonable choices. The dosages of these medications are given in Box 8-7.

Box 8-7

Medications and Dosage Regimens for Arrhythmias That Develop During the High-Risk Cardiac Catheterization

Stable Ventricular Tachycardia
Amiodarone: Can administer in one of two regimens, as dictated by clinical setting
Regimen 1: 150 mg over 10 minutes, followed by infusion rate of 1 mg/min
Regimen 2: 300 mg IV rapid infusion after dilution in 20 to 30 ml fluid; can give additional 150 mg rapid infusions in similar manner as indicated
Lidocaine 1-1.5 mg/kg IV bolus; can give additional boluses of 0.5 to 0.75 mg/kg IV as indicated, up to 3 mg/kg

Pulseless Ventricular Tachycardia or Ventricular Fibrillation
Epinephrine 1 mg IV bolus; can repeat every 3 to 5 minutes
Vasopressin 40 U IV bolus × 1 (either epinephrine or vasopressin can be given after three unsuccessful defibrillation attempts)
Amiodarone 300 mg IV rapid infusion after dilution in 20 to 30 ml fluid; can give additional 150-mg rapid infusions in similar manner as indicated
Lidocaine 1-1.5 mg/kg IV bolus; can give additional boluses of 0.5 to 0.75 mg/kg IV as indicated, up to 3 mg/kg

Patients who are hemodynamically stable but do not respond to antiarrhythmic therapy or patients who become mildly symptomatic can be treated with synchronized cardioversion (beginning at 100 J and increasing stepwise to 360 J as necessary).

Patients in whom pulseless ventricular tachycardia or ventricular fibrillation develops should initially be treated with a precordial thump. After this, immediate defibrillation is indicated (beginning at 200 J and increasing stepwise to 360 J). *No other intervention should interfere with the immediate and rapid first three sequential attempts at defibrillation.* Patients who do not convert after these three initial attempts at defibrillation should be treated with epinephrine (1 mg IV, repeated every 3 to 5 minutes) or vasopressin (40 U IV × 1), with defibrillation repeated afterward. Patients who still do not respond can be treated with amiodarone (300 mg IV bolus after dilution in 20 ml of fluid) or lidocaine (1 to 1.5 mg/kg IV bolus), with repeated attempts at defibrillation afterward. Simultaneous with these interventions should be the initiation of CPR. The advanced cardiac life support algorithm for the treatment of pulseless ventricular tachycardia or ventricular fibrillation is presented in Figure 8-1.

Asystole. Asystole is usually the result of extensive myocardial ischemia. Pacing of the right ventricle should be instituted as quickly as possible. Atropine (1 mg) should be given and can be repeated in 5 minutes if necessary. Because it may be difficult to distinguish fine ventricular fibrillation from asystole, asystole should be confirmed in two leads. If the diagnosis is unclear, the physician should assume that fine ventricular fibrillation is present and treat the patient accordingly. External pacing can be used if right ventricular pacing cannot be established immediately. Metabolic abnormalities, including hyperkalemia or severe preexisting acidosis, may cause the arrhythmia and may respond to bicarbonate.

Epinephrine has vasoconstrictor α-adrenergic properties, which makes it superior to other α-adrenergic agents (methoxamine and phenylephrine). The dose of epinephrine is 1 mg and may be given at least every 5 minutes. If asystole does not respond to the aforementioned measures, emergency cardiopulmonary bypass should be considered.

Pulseless Electrical Activity. Pulseless electrical activity is a heart rhythm disturbance that is fatal unless the underlying cause can be identified and treated at once. Causes of pulseless electrical activity include the following:

1. Hypovolemia, especially if it is a result of bleeding. Treatment is aggressive volume repletion and transfusions. Hemostasis is obtained by reversing anticoagulation.
2. Pericardial tamponade, especially in patients with acute infarction, recent cardiac biopsy, recent endocardial pacer insertion, or uremia. If tamponade is suspected, blind pericardiocentesis is warranted (see Chapter 7).
3. Massive pulmonary embolism may precipitate pulseless electrical activity. On rare occasions the embolus may break up during prolonged resuscitative efforts. Some patients may survive long enough for the operator to use thrombus aspiration catheters to treat this condition.
4. Tension pneumothorax may occur in patients after internal jugular or subclavian venous access is obtained.

Fluoroscopy may visualize air in the patient's chest. If the operator suspects that tension pneumothorax is present, he or she should carefully insert a small-bore needle attached to a syringe into the pleural space. If a tension pneumothorax is present, air under pressure is expelled.

Supraventricular Arrhythmias. The hemodynamic stability of the patient determines how PSVT and atrial fibrillation should be treated.

1. In patients who are unstable (e.g., with hypotension, chest pain, congestive heart failure, acute ischemia, or infarction), synchronized cardioversion is used at once. Sedation with a rapidly acting intravenous agent (e.g., diazepam [Valium] or midazolam [Versed]) can be used for patients who are conscious and do not have hypotension as long as it does not delay the procedure. The initial discharge is 75 to 100 J. If conversion occurs but PSVT or atrial fibrillation recurs, repeated electrical cardioversion is *not* indicated. If conversion does not occur, energy levels are increased (e.g., 200 J, 360 J) and cardioversion is repeated. If these maneuvers fail, IV amiodarone is used, after which cardioversion is repeated. Digitalis toxicity is a relative contraindication to cardioversion because severe bradycardia or asystole may occur after cardioversion. The ventricular response can be controlled with β-blockers or intravenous diltiazem in patients who have atrial fibrillation and are hemodynamically stable. The irregular heart rhythm can be abolished with use of procainamide or elective cardioversion.

2. PSVT without atrial fibrillation should initially be treated with vagal maneuvers. The Valsalva maneuver is usually successful. If carotid disease or a carotid bruit is not present, carotid sinus massage can be used. If unsuccessful, diltiazem or adenosine (6 to 12 mg IV bolus) may be used. Patients who fail to respond to diltiazem or adenosine may respond to amiodarone, overdrive pacing, elective cardioversion, or β-blockers.

Verapamil (for reentrant supraventricular tachycardia) is a calcium channel blocker with electrophysiologic effects on the

AV node and, to a lesser extent, the sinoatrial node. It also has negative inotropic properties. It is commonly used for the rate control of narrow QRS complex paroxysmal supraventricular tachycardia in patients who are hemodynamically stable if maneuvers that increase vagal tone are unsuccessful. Verapamil is also useful for rate control in patients with atrial fibrillation and a rapid ventricular response. Initially a 5-mg dose should be given IV over 1 minute and additional doses of 2.5 to 5 mg given in 5- to 10-minute intervals up to a maximum dose of 20 mg if PSVT persists without an adverse response to the initial dose. Contraindications to verapamil include history or presence of bradycardia, hypotension, or decompensated congestive heart failure or concomitant use of an IV β-blocker. Adverse reactions to verapamil include severe bradycardia, hypotension, congestive heart failure, and rapid accessory conduction in patients with Wolff-Parkinson-White syndrome. Hypotension may often be reversed with IV calcium chloride (0.5 to 1.0 g).

Adenosine is a naturally occurring agent that produces AV nodal blockade and increases coronary blood flow. It is 90% to 100% effective in terminating reentrant supraventricular or AV nodal tachycardia in 6- to 12-mg IV bolus doses. It has a 30-second onset of action and a 60-second offset of action. Transient flushing is the only major side effect.

Digitalis is useful for the control of a rapid ventricular response in patients with atrial fibrillation, atrial flutter, or PSVT. The toxic-to-therapeutic ratio is narrow, and the onset of action is slower than that of verapamil (i.e., digitalis is not useful for acute situations).

β-Blockers (including metoprolol, 5 mg IV push) can be used to control recurring episodes of PSVT. The use of β-blockers may be hazardous when cardiac dysfunction is present. The dosage for propranolol is 1 mg every 5 minutes IV up to a total of 0.1 mg/kg. Short-acting β-blockers (esmolol) are administered in 5- to 15-mg boluses and have 5- to 10-minute half-lives.

CARDIAC SUPPORT DEVICES
Intraaortic Balloon Pump

IABP counterpulsation increases diastolic pressure and coronary blood flow and decreases myocardial oxygen demand (i.e., reduces afterload). Balloon inflation in diastole (at the dicrotic notch on the central arterial pressure tracing) increases diastolic pressure, which increases coronary artery pressure and coronary flow. Deflation of the balloon just before systole (at end diastole, the upstroke of arterial pressure tracing) results in decreased ventricular afterload, which decreases myocardial oxygen consumption and increases the cardiac output (Fig. 8-6).

In high-risk patients or patients who are unstable, an IABP may be inserted before catheterization. During catheterization or interventional procedures hypotension (not responding to volume loading or IV vasopressors) and refractory angina are indications for IABP placement. Indications and contra-indications for IABP use are summarized in Box 8-8.

Technique.   Before the percutaneous insertion of an intraaortic balloon, the operator assesses the iliofemoral arteries and aorta for vascular disease. Significant peripheral vascular disease is a relative contraindication. An abdominal aortogram helps identify the course and disease of iliac and femoral vessels before IABP insertion.

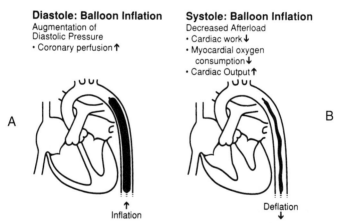

Diastole: Balloon Inflation
Augmentation of
Diastolic Pressure
• Coronary perfusion ↑

Systole: Balloon Inflation
Decreased Afterload
• Cardiac work ↓
• Myocardial oxygen
  consumption ↓
• Cardiac Output ↑

A

B

↑
Inflation

Deflation
↓

Fig. 8-6   A schematic representation of, **A,** balloon inflation during diastole and, **B,** deflation just before the onset of systole. Diastolic augmentation increases coronary artery perfusion, whereas deflation of the balloon just before the onset of systole decreases afterload, which results in decreased myocardial oxygen demand, decreased cardiac workload, and increased cardiac output.

Box 8-8

Indications and Contraindications for Intraaortic Balloon Counterpulsation

Indications
Refractory unstable angina
Cardiogenic shock
Postoperative hemodynamic compromise
Acute myocardial infarction with mechanical impairment as a result of mitral regurgitation or ventricular septal defect
Intractable ventricular tachycardia as a result of myocardial ischemia
Patients with left main coronary stenosis or severe three-vessel disease undergoing anesthesia for cardiac surgery
High-risk PTCA
Maintenance of vessel patency after PTCA with slow flow

Contraindications
Anatomic abnormality of femoroiliac artery
Iliac or aortic atherosclerotic disease impairing blood flow runoff
Moderate or severe aortic regurgitation
Aortic dissection or aneurysm
Patent ductus (counterpulsation may augment the abnormal pathway of aortic to pulmonary artery shunting)
Bypass grafting to femoral artery
Bleeding diathesis
Sepsis

PTCA, Percutaneous transluminal coronary angioplasty.

Complications of intraaortic balloon placement most commonly result from a puncture site that is too low, perforation of the superficial femoral artery, or forceful artery dissection caused by advancement of the guidewire. The puncture site should be located similar to or slightly more cranial than a standard femoral puncture for diagnostic catheterization. A puncture lower than the prescribed site may involve the superficial femoral artery, which is too small to accept the IABP, and leg ischemia can result.

The 8 F IABP balloon sheath (or sheathless IABP catheter) is inserted into either groin using standard Seldinger technique. Before IABP catheter insertion a negative vacuum to the balloon is applied using a large syringe and the one-way valve provided in the IABP insertion kit. The catheter is loaded with the 0.018-inch or 0.025-inch guidewire provided in the IABP kit. The assembly is inserted through the sheath with the guidewire leading. The marker at the tip of the IABP catheter should be 1 to 2 cm below the top of the aortic arch. The guidewire is removed. The central lumen is carefully flushed and connected to a pressure transducer. Fluoroscopic observation of the balloon inflation above the renal arteries confirms optimal placement.

After the catheter is positioned, the IABP tubing is connected to the IABP console. Counterpulsation is initiated. In short patients pumping may not begin if the distal end of the balloon catheter remains in the sheath. Partial withdrawal of the sheath from the femoral artery may remedy this problem. The balloon catheter is secured with sutures. The position of the balloon is rechecked before the patient is moved. After the patient has been returned to the intensive care unit, the position of the IABP is checked again with a chest radiograph.

The timing cycle of the IABP inflation should begin at 1:2 pumping (one inflation for every two beats). The balloon inflation timing is adjusted to optimize augmented diastolic pressure waveform (Fig. 8-7). The central aortic pressure through the IABP lumen is used to assess hemodynamic effects (Fig. 8-8).

Optimal balloon timing is guided by direct pressure readings. If no pressure wave is available, the ECG may be used for timing the balloon; however, this practice is not recommended. The ECG is used to trigger the balloon. IABP inflation should occur at the aortic dicrotic notch (T wave on ECG), and deflation should occur immediately before systole (at or before the R wave) to provide maximal diastolic flow and maximal reduction of "presystolic" pressure (Fig. 8-9). After proper adjustment of balloon inflation and deflation, the timing cycle is set at 1:1 pumping. Factors that affect diastolic pressure augmentation are listed in Box 8-9.

The effects of the IABP on coronary blood flow depend on the degree of coronary arterial obstruction that is present. In patients who undergo coronary angioplasty, flow distal to severe stenoses showed no effect of IABP. After coronary angioplasty, flow was increased markedly and augmented further with IABP (Fig. 8-10).

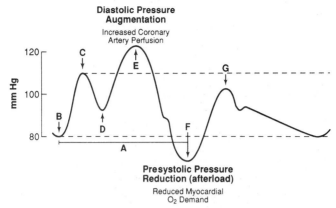

Fig. 8-7 Arterial waveforms during 2:1 intraaortic balloon pump counter-pulsation. *A*, One complete cardiac cycle. *B*, Unassisted aortic end-diastolic pressure. *C*, Unassisted aortic systolic pressure. *D*, Dicrotic notch (balloon inflation). *E*, Diastolic augmentation. *F*, Assisted aortic end-diastolic pressure. *G*, Assisted systole. Diastolic augmentation occurs during balloon inflation, which results in increased coronary artery perfusion. Reduction in the presystolic pressure (afterload) occurs with balloon deflation and re-duces myocardial oxygen demand. The assisted systolic pressure, *G*, should be lower than the unassisted aortic systolic pressure, *C*, because of a reduction in the aortic end-diastolic pressure, *F*.

Assessment of the patient after IABP placement includes evaluation for infection, thrombocytopenia, hemorrhage, hemolysis, and vascular obstruction with limb ischemia. Thrombus or dissection may be present at or proximal to the puncture site. Heparin administration (5000 U bolus with 1000 U/hr) is standard practice in most institutions. Aortic dissection may occur if the balloon has not been advanced and positioned carefully over a guidewire. *Blind insertion of a counterpulsation balloon without a leading guidewire is not recommended under any circumstances.* The patient must remain comfortable and relatively supine while the IABP is in place, although 30 degrees of hip flexion may be permitted. When angiography is performed from the contralateral femoral artery, the IABP is placed on standby while the J-guidewire and catheter pass the deflated balloon so that the potential for balloon puncture is minimized. Causes of poor IABP augmentation are summarized in Boxes 8-10 to 8-13.

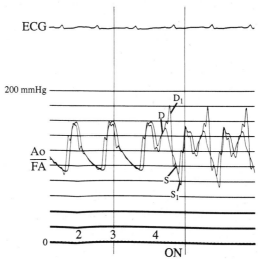

Fig. 8-8 Hemodynamic tracings of femoral artery *(FA)* and central aortic *(Ao)* pressure during intraaortic balloon pumping shows the augmentation in diastole in the central position *(D)* and femoral artery position *(D₁)* and reduction in systolic load in the central position *(S)* and the femoral artery position *(S₁)*. Moving the timing of inflation toward the dicrotic notch and the timing of deflation away from systolic upstroke augments the diastolic pressure and optimally reduces systolic load. *ON,* The point at which the balloon pump is turned on.

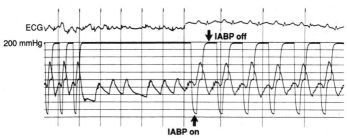

Fig. 8-9 Arterial pressure wave and influence of intraaortic balloon pumping *(IABP)*. A timing signal from the balloon pump shows effective diastolic pressure augmentation and systolic pressure reduction.

Box 8-9

Factors Affecting Diastolic Augmentation

Patient Hemodynamics
Heart rate
Stroke volume
Mean arterial pressure
Systemic vascular resistance

IAB Mechanical Factors
IAB in sheath
IAB not unfolded
IAB position
Kink in IAB catheter
IAB leak
Low helium concentration

IABP Console Factors
Timing
Position of IAB augmentation dial

IAB, Intraaortic balloon; *IABP,* intraaortic balloon pump.

Prophylactic Intraaortic Balloon Pump. In current practice an IABP is rarely placed prophylactically before diagnostic cardiac catheterization. Prophylactic placement should be considered for patients with known severe left main coronary artery disease, recalcitrant pulmonary edema, or hemodynamic instability. In patients in whom prophylactic IABP insertion is considered but not implemented and in patients who undergo high-risk cardiac catheterization in which the risk of the patient becoming hemodynamically compromised is high, arterial access in the contralateral femoral artery should be obtained with placement of a 4 F or 5 F sheath.

Intraaortic Balloon Pump Removal. When clinically indicated, the balloon is removed first by aspiration of negative pressure on the balloon lumen and then joint withdrawal of the sheath and balloon assembly while compression is applied to the puncture site. The deflated IABP catheter profile is larger than the 8 F sheath lumen, and therefore the catheter cannot be

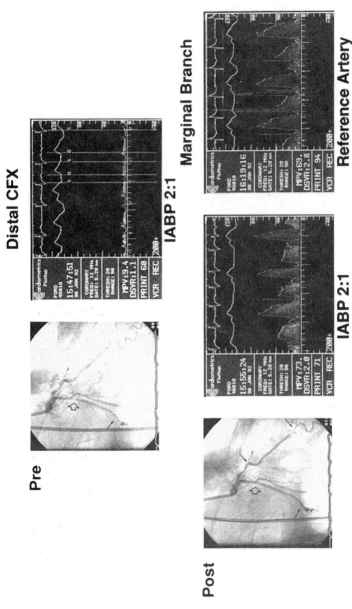

Fig. 8-10   For legend see opposite page.

Fig. 8-10   Effects of intraaortic balloon pumping *(IABP)* on distal coronary flow (velocity) before and after angioplasty. *Top panels, Pre,* Before angioplasty, severe narrowing in the circumflex coronary artery *(open arrow)* is associated with minimal flow velocity (by Doppler guidewire) and no effect of intraaortic balloon pumping. *Bottom panels, Post,* After angioplasty *(open arrow),* distal coronary flow velocity is increased markedly and augmented further by intraaortic balloon pumping; these findings are nearly identical to flow patterns in a normal adjacent reference artery. *CFX,* Circumflex artery. (From Kern MJ, Aguirre F, Bach R, et al: *Circulation* 87:500-511, 1993.)

withdrawn completely into the sheath before removal. Pressure on the puncture site must be maintained for 30 to 60 minutes with frequent assessment of distal pulses. Anticoagulant medication should be discontinued 4 hours before removal of the balloon catheter. The activated clotting time should be less than 150 seconds before the IABP is removed.

Complications of Intraaortic Balloon Pump. Complications of IABP most commonly result from a low puncture site, insertion perforation of the superficial femoral artery, or damage to the arterial entry site from forceful advancement of the catheter. The most common serious complication of IABP is ischemia of the lower extremity, which occurs in 2% to 10% of patients. Prolonged IABP use is also associated with hemolysis and platelet destruction. Blood counts of patients with an IABP should be monitored.

Percutaneous Cardiopulmonary Support. Cardiopulmonary support is rarely used in the catheterization laboratory as an adjunct to high-risk angioplasty for maintenance of adequate perfusion in hemodynamic catastrophes instead of, or in conjunction with, an IABP, and for rescue of an unexpected catastrophe during diagnostic and interventional procedures. The CPS system uses one of several types of pumps. A flow probe, heat exchanger, and membrane oxygenator are often in series in the circuit. Two large cannulae, venous and arterial, are inserted percutaneously or by the cutdown method. The

---

Box 8-10

Poor Intraaortic Balloon Pump Augmentation Because of Catheter Problems

IABP membrane not fully exited from the sheath. Pull the sheath back until the membrane fully exits the sheath.

IAB membrane has not fully opened. Inject and immediately evacuate 60 cm^3 of air or helium into the balloon (using a syringe and a stopcock). Do not inject through any extender tubing that may be attached. *Warning:* Never inject air into the central lumen (female Luer-Lok fitting).

Augmentation-volume knob on IABP console set inappropriately. Check that augmentation-volume knob on IABP console is set appropriately.

IAB is positioned in the subclavian artery or malpositioned. Ensure that the balloon position is appropriate, under fluoroscopy; if balloon position is poor, loosen the sheath seal and reposition IABP.

IAB is in a false lumen. Use fluoroscopy to check intraluminal position of the balloon tip.

— Aspirate a 3-ml volume of blood from the central lumen of the balloon (female Luer-Lok).

— Inject 10 to 20 ml of contrast medium through the central lumen of the balloon while the balloon is pumping.

If the balloon tip is within the aortic lumen, contrast medium will wash away in the next two or three heartbeats.

If the balloon tip is in a false lumen, contrast medium remains around the balloon. In this case, the balloon should be removed and replacement should be considered.

Avoid excessive pressure when injecting contrast medium through the central lumen.

Avoid use of a syringe smaller than 20 ml to inject through the central lumen. If resistance is met, consider the lumen obstructed and permanently seal off the lumen.

Do not use an angiographic flow rate injector; the high pressure generated by the injector may damage the central lumen.

IAB, Intraaortic balloon; *IABP,* intraaortic balloon pump.

large venous cannula (16 F to 20 F and 75 cm in length) is inserted over a tapered dilator. It is positioned with the distal end in the right atrium for venous blood withdrawal. The arterial cannula (16 F to 20 F and 32 cm in length) is inserted into the femoral artery for retrograde aortic perfusion.

An experienced invasive cardiologist can insert the cannulae relatively easily with the percutaneous technique. If a cutdown

Box 8-11

Poor Intraaortic Balloon Pump Augmentation Because of Physiologic Problems

Low mean arterial blood pressure
Low systemic vascular resistance
Tachycardia (compromises ventricular filling and ejection)
If after a review of all the above, the reason for poor augmentation cannot be
    determined, remove the intraaortic balloon

Box 8-12

Poor Intraaortic Balloon Pump Augmentation Caused By Poor Inflation-Deflation Timing

Early Inflation: Inflation of the IAB Before Aortic Valve Closure
Waveform characteristics
Inflation before the dicrotic notch
Diastolic augmentation encroaches onto systole

Physiologic effects
Potential premature closure of the aortic valve
Potential increase in left ventricular end-diastolic volume and left ventricular end-
    diastolic pressure
Increased left ventricular wall stress (afterload)
Aortic regurgitation
Increased myocardial oxygen demand

Late Inflation: Inflation of the IAB Some Time After Closure of the Aortic Valve
Waveform characteristics
Inflation of the IAB after the dicrotic notch
Absence of sharp v wave
Suboptimal diastolic augmentation

Physiologic effects
Suboptimal coronary artery perfusion

IAB, Intraaortic balloon.   *Continued*

Box 8-12

Poor Intraaortic Balloon Pump Augmentation Caused By Poor Inflation-Deflation Timing—cont'd

Early Deflation: Premature Deflation of the IAB During Diastole
Waveform characteristics
Deflation of the IAB seen as a sharp drop after diastolic augmentation
Suboptimal diastolic augmentation
Assisted aortic end-diastolic pressure may be less than or equal to unassisted aortic end-diastolic pressure
Assisted systolic pressure may rise

Physiologic effects
Suboptimal coronary perfusion
Potential for retrograde coronary and carotid blood flow
Angina may occur as a result of retrograde coronary blood flow
Suboptimal afterload reduction
Increased myocardial oxygen demand

Late Deflation
Waveform characteristics
Assisted aortic end-diastolic pressure may be less than or equal to unassisted aortic end-diastolic pressure
Rate of rise of assisted systole prolonged
Diastolic augmentation may appear widened

Physiologic effects
Afterload reduction essentially absent
Increased myocardial oxygen consumption caused by the left ventricle ejecting against greater resistance
Prolonged isovolumic contraction phase
IAB may impede left ventricular ejection and increase afterload

---

is used, a surgeon or a cardiologist proficient with this technique should insert the cannulae.

A separate arterial access is necessary for the monitoring of blood pressure. During an operator's early experience, the procedure should be performed with a perfusionist and cardiac anesthesiologist in attendance.

An alternative technique for in-laboratory CPS is a left atrium–aorta bypass in which a transseptal puncture is used to

---

Box 8-13

Poor Intraaortic Balloon Pump Augmentation Caused by Arrhythmias

Atrial Fibrillation
Use auto timing and ECG trigger

Ectopics
To ensure triggering, select the lead that minimizes the amplitude difference between the normal QRS and the ectopic

Cardiac Arrest or Defibrillation
Use ECG or pressure trigger during cardiopulmonary support
If ECG or pressure trigger cannot be used, internal trigger may be used
The operator must be sure to stand clear of the IABP during defibrillation
The intraaortic balloon should not remain immobile for more than 30 minutes in situ

ECG, Electrocardiogram, *IABP*, intraaortic balloon pump.

place a long cannula in the left atrium, and returning left atrial blood is pumped into the aorta via a large femoral artery cannula. The patient's lungs are used as the oxygenator with this method. The limitations of large cannulae and the need for anticoagulant medication are the same as for other types of CPS.

Percutaneous femoral CPS can be lifesaving in refractory cardiac arrest when it is initiated within 30 minutes in a patient with surgically- or angioplasty-remediable disease or in a candidate for cardiac transplantation. CPS should *not* be considered for a patient who does not fulfill these criteria. Safe and effective application of CPS in the catheterization laboratory requires teamwork among the cardiologist, the cardiac surgeon, and the perfusionist. When initial attempts to resuscitate the patient fail, the patient's eligibility for CPS and further treatment should be determined, and CPS should be initiated without delay if appropriate.

Cautionary Notes

CPS cannulae are large-bore catheters. When CPS is used, the likelihood of vascular problems is high, especially in the elderly or in patients with peripheral vascular disease. In an emergency situation a quick evaluation of the extremity circulation is performed, and the artery and vein are approached as described. While the cannulae are inserted, the external circuit is prepared, primed, and purged of all air. When adequate flow is established, the resuscitation can be stopped. Arrhythmias are treated by standard methods. Ventricular fibrillation is defibrillated by direct current shock. Further treatment (e.g., bypass surgery or percutaneous transluminal coronary angioplasty [PTCA]) is planned at once.

The elective use of CPS in high-risk patients undergoing PTCA may help such patients remain hemodynamically stable during the procedure. Class 1 indications for elective use of CPS are undefined. For some high-risk patients undergoing PTCA (e.g., patients with poor LV function, dilation of only remaining vessel, dilation of a territory supplying ≥50% of the myocardium), standby CPS seems reasonable. In this method, 5 F sheaths are placed into the contralateral femoral artery and vein. These small sheaths allow rapid placement of the cannula, which saves valuable time in the event of hemodynamic collapse. Angiography should always be performed to document the accuracy of the iliac femoral system. In patients with obstructive disease in the iliofemoral system, CPS should not be attempted. Because CPS will not increase regional myocardial blood flow or alleviate myocardial ischemia, acute coronary dissection or occlusion should be treated immediately with stenting or emergency coronary artery bypass graft surgery (if possible).

The complications of percutaneous CPS are primarily vascular in nature: bleeding, thromboembolism, and pseudoaneurysm formation. Complications specific to CPS (e.g., thrombocytopenia, disseminated intravascular coagulation) develop especially in patients in whom long-term support (>6 hours) was necessary.

Suggested Readings

Boehrer JD, Lange RA, Willard JE, et al: Markedly increased periprocedure mortality of cardiac catheterization in patients with severe narrowing of the left main coronary artery, *Am J Cardiol* 70:1388-1390, 1992.

Colyer WR Jr, Moore JA, Burket MW, Cooper CJ: Intraaortic balloon pump insertion after percutaneous revascularization in patients with severe peripheral vascular disease, *Cathet Cardiovasc Diagn* 42:1-6, 1997.

Ferguson JJ, Cohen M, Freedman RJ, et al: The current practice of intra-aortic balloon counterpulsation: results from the Benchmark Registry, *J Am Coll Cardiol* 38:1456-1462, 2001.

Folland ED, Oprian C, Giacomini J, et al: Complications of cardiac catheterization and angiography in patients with valvular heart disease, *Cathet Cardiovasc Diagn* 17:15-21, 1989.

Heupler FA: Guidelines for performing angiography in patients taking metformin, *Cathet Cardiovasc Diagn* 43:121-123, 1998.

International Consensus on Science: Guidelines 2000 for cardio-pulmonary resuscitation and emergency cardiovascular care, *Circulation* 102(suppl I):1-370, 2001.

Kern MJ, Aguirre F, Bach R, et al: Augmentation of coronary blood flow by intra-aortic balloon pumping in patients after coronary angioplasty, *Circulation* 87:500-511, 1993.

Kern MJ, Aguirre FV, Tatineni S, et al: Enhanced coronary blood flow velocity during intraaortic balloon counterpulsation in critically ill patients, *J Am Coll Cardiol* 21:359-368, 1993.

Kini AS, Mitre CA, Kim M, et al: A protocol for prevention of radiographic contrast nephropathy during percutaneous coronary intervention: effect of selective dopamine receptor against fenoldopam, *Cathet Cardiovasc Interv* 55:169-173, 2002.

Landau C, Lange RA, Glamann DB, et al: Vasovagal reactions in the cardiac catheterization laboratory, *Am J Cardiol* 73:95-97, 1994.

Laskey W, Boyle J, Johnson LW: Multivariable model for prediction of risk of significant complication during diagnostic cardiac catheterization, *Cathet Cardiovasc Diagn* 30:185-190, 1993.

Millereau M: Dilution of potent drugs, *Am J Cardiol* 68:418, 1991.

Solomon R, Werner C, Mann D, et al: Effects of saline, mannitol, and furosemide to prevent acute decreases in renal function induced by radiocontrast agents, *N Engl J Med* 331:1416-1420, 1994.

Tepel M, van der Giet M, Schwarzfeld C, et al: Prevention of radiographic-contrast-agent-induced reductions in renal function by acetylcysteine, *N Engl J Med* 343:180-184, 2000.

Tommaso CL: Contrast-induced nephrotoxicity in patients under-going cardiac catheterization, *Cathet Cardiovasc Diagn* 31:316-321, 1994.

Tommaso CL, Johnson RA, Stafford JL, et al: Supported coronary angioplasty and standby coronary angioplasty for high-risk coronary artery disease, *Am J Cardiol* 66:1255-1257, 1990.

Vignola PA, Swaye PS, Gosselin AJ: Guidelines for effect and safe percutaneous intra-aortic balloon pump insertion and removal, *Am J Cardiol* 48:660-664, 1981.

Vogel RA, Shawl F, Tommaso C, et al: Initial report of the National Registry of Elective Cardiopulmonary Bypass Supported Coronary Angioplasty, *J Am Coll Cardiol* 15:23-29, 1990.

Welton DE, Young JB, Raizner AE, et al: Value and safety of cardiac catheterization during active infective endocarditis, *Am J Cardiol* 44:1306-1310, 1979.

Wyman RM, Safian RD, Portway V, et al: Current complications of diagnostic and therapeutic cardiac catheterization, *J Am Coll Cardiol* 12:1400-1406, 1988.

9

INTERVENTIONAL TECHNIQUES

Morton J. Kern, Saad Bitar, Sanjeev Puri, Hassan Rajjoub, and Steve Herrmann

The widespread use of interventional techniques after diagnostic angiography for patients with ischemic and valvular heart disease is now commonplace. The expansion of this field has prompted a separate handbook dedicated to this area. *The Interventional Cardiac Catheterization Handbook* expands on the materials and concepts presented in this chapter and provides a more detailed foundation at the basic level for indications, techniques, contraindications, and complications of interventional cardiology approaches.

PERCUTANEOUS CORONARY INTERVENTIONS

Until 1977 coronary artery bypass graft surgery was the only alternative to medicine for the treatment of coronary artery disease. Coronary artery bypass graft surgery attaches a segment of leg vein (or chest wall artery) to the heart to detour blood around the narrowed portion (i.e., stenosis) of a coronary artery. Percutaneous transluminal coronary angioplasty provides an alternative to bypass graft surgery in which the narrowed portion of the artery can be enlarged selectively without surgery by the insertion of a long thin balloon to open the blocked artery. In addition to balloons, interventional cardiologists may use metallic stents, cutters, grinders, and aspiration catheters to treat a wide variety of artery problems. These methods are collectively referred to as PCI:

Percutaneous—refers to the insertion of a catheter into the body through a small puncture site in the skin, usually into an artery.

Coronary—identifies the specific artery to be dilated.

*I*ntervention—a technique for remodeling a blood vessel through the introduction of an expandable stent, balloon catheter, or other specialized tool for treating a diseased artery.

Figure 9-1 shows how to perform PCI. A guiding catheter is seated in the coronary ostium. A thin, steerable guidewire is introduced into the coronary artery and positioned across the stenosis into the distal aspect of the artery. An angioplasty catheter, which is considerably smaller than the guiding catheter, is inserted through the guiding catheter and positioned (in the artery) across the stenotic area by tracking it over the guidewire. The balloon or stent is on the PCI catheter. When the balloon or stent is placed correctly within the area to be treated, the balloon on the PCI catheter is inflated several times for periods ranging from 10 seconds to several minutes. The inflation and deflation of the balloon-stent in the blocked artery restores blood flow to an area of the heart previously deprived by the stenosed artery. If no complications occur, only one day more in the hospital is required. Patients can usually resume their normal routine within several days.

How Balloon Angioplasty Works

Several theories regarding the mechanisms of angioplasty have been proposed.

Disruption of Plaque and Arterial Wall. The inflated balloon exerts pressure against the plaque and arterial wall, causing fracturing and splitting of the plaque. The concentric lesion fractures and splits at its thinnest and weakest point. Eccentric lesions split at the junction of the plaque and the arterial wall. Dissection or separation of the plaque from the medial wall releases the "splinting" effect that is caused by the lesion and results in a larger lumen. This is the major effective mechanism of balloon angioplasty.

Loss of Elastic Recoil. Balloon dilation causes stretching and thinning of the medial wall. Stretching causes the medial wall to lose its elastic properties. The degree of elastic recoil loss is affected by the balloon-to-artery size ratio. Over time (1 to 6 weeks), there may be renarrowing of the artery as a result of

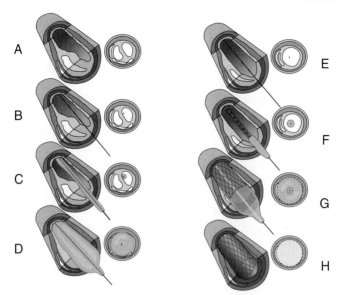

Fig. 9-1   How angioplasty and stenting works. **A,** The artery is filled with atherosclerotic material compromising the lumen. A cross section of the artery is shown on the right. **B,** A guidewire is positioned past the stenoses through the lumen. **C,** A balloon catheter is advanced over the guidewire. **D,** The balloon is inflated. **E,** The balloon is deflated and withdrawn. **F,** The balloon catheter is exchanged for a stent (on a balloon). **G,** The stent is expanded. **H,** The expanded stent remains in place after the deflated balloon is withdrawn. (Reproduced with permission from the American Heart Association.)

elastic recoil, which is prevented by placement of a stent in the artery.

Redistribution and Compression of Plaque Components. Shear pressures cause denudation or stripping of endothelial cells and the extrusion or pushing out of plaque components. There may be some molding of the softer lipid material, but this effect accounts for a small part of the overall effect of angioplasty.

Mechanism of Stents. Stents scaffold the lumen and plaque open, holding back dissection flaps and stopping recoiling and renarrowing of the lumen.

Indications

Indications for PCI are as follows:
1. Angina pectoris causing sufficient symptoms despite optimal medical therapy
2. Mild angina pectoris with objective evidence of ischemia (abnormal stress testing or physiology) and high-grade lesion (>70% diameter narrowing) of a vessel supplying a large area of myocardium
3. Unstable angina
4. Acute myocardial infarction (MI) as primary therapy or in patients who have persistent or recurrent ischemia after failed thrombolytic therapy
5. Angina pectoris after coronary artery bypass graft surgery
6. Restenosis after successful PCI

Contraindications

Contraindications for PCI are as follows:
1. Unsuitable coronary anatomy
2. Extremely high-risk coronary anatomy in which closure of vessel would result in patient death
3. Contraindication to coronary artery bypass graft surgery (however, some patients have PCI as their only alternative to revascularization)
4. Bleeding diathesis
5. Patient noncompliance with procedure and post-PCI instructions
6. Multiple PCI restenosis
7. Patients who cannot give informed consent

Complications

Complications associated with PCI include the following:
1. Death (<1%)
2. MI (<3% to 5%)
3. Emergency coronary artery bypass graft surgery (<3%) and abrupt vessel closure (0.8%)
4. All the complications that can occur during cardiac catheterization; access site bleeding is more common

Although not a true complication, restenosis, intimal hyperplasia at the site of PCI, occurs in approximately 10% to 30% of patients after placement of a stent, leading to recurrence of anginal symptoms. Typically, restenosis occurs in the initial 6 months after PCI. In-stent restenosis is expected to be <10% with drug-eluting stents.

Equipment

PCI equipment consists of three basic elements: the guiding catheter; the balloon, stent, or atherectomy catheter; and the coronary guidewire (Fig. 9-2).

Guiding Catheter. A special large-lumen catheter is used to guide the coronary balloon catheter to the vessel that has the lesion to be dilated. Compared with diagnostic catheters, guiding catheters have thinner walls and larger lumens, which allows contrast injections to be done while the balloon catheter is in place. The guiding catheters are stiffer than diagnostic catheters to provide support for advancing the balloon catheter into the coronary artery and they respond differently to manipulation than diagnostic catheters. The guiding catheter tip is not tapered, occasionally causing pressure dampening on engaging the coronary ostium. 6 F guiding catheters are generally used. Some catheters have relatively shorter and more flexible tips than other catheters, theoretically to decrease catheter-induced trauma. Others may have side holes to help maintain blood flow during PCI. Larger lumens (>0.70 inch) may be needed for kissing balloons, rotoblator burrs larger than 2 mm, and some cutting balloons.

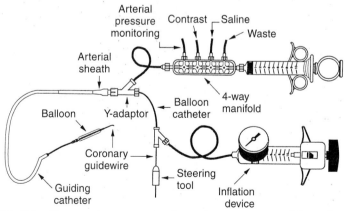

Fig. 9-2 Diagram of components of percutaneous coronary intervention equipment. (From Freed M, Grines C, Safian RD: *The new manual of interventional cardiology*, Birmingham, Mich., 1996, Physicians' Press.)

There are many different shapes of guiding catheters for different anatomic variations.

Functions of the Guiding Catheter. There are three major functions of a guiding catheter during PCI (Fig. 9-3):

1. *Balloon-stent catheter delivery.* The guiding catheter is the delivery device of the balloon catheter to the coronary artery. If the guiding catheter is not seated properly in a coaxial manner, it may not be possible to advance the balloon across the stenotic area. After seating the guide catheter in the coronary artery (cannulation), the guiding catheter provides the necessary backup support or "platform" to push the balloon catheter across the stenosis.

Several terms that are commonly used when referring to guiding catheters are important:

Backing out: The guiding catheter is being ejected from the coronary ostium into the aortic root when pressure is applied to the balloon in an attempt to cross the lesion. This is caused by an insufficient support position or a tight stenosis.

Backup: A stable support position of the guiding catheter at the orifice of the coronary ostium provides the necessary platform to advance the balloon across the lesion.

Deep seat: This refers to the process of manipulating the guide over the balloon catheter shaft past the ostium and

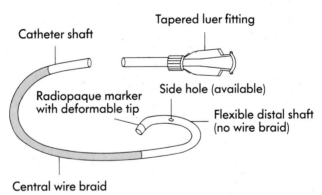

Fig. 9-3 Illustration of a guiding catheter shows variable position of central wire braid, optional distal side hole, deformable tip, and radiopaque marker. (From Avedissian MG, Killeavy ES, Garcia JM, et al: *Cathet Cardiovasc Diagn* 18:263, 1989.)

further into the vessel to obtain increased backup support for crossing difficult lesions. This maneuver is typically used as a last resort because of the increased chance of guide catheter–induced dissection of the proximal vessel.

2. *Contrast injection.* The guiding catheter permits visualization of the target by contrast administration with or without the balloon catheter in place. Some large PCI devices may block good contrast injection, which makes the procedure more difficult.

3. *Pressure monitoring.* The guiding catheter lumen measures aortic pressure for determination of the transstenotic pressure gradient for physiologic lesion assessment, ostial lesions (pressure wave damping), and hypotension during prolonged ischemia.

Balloon Catheters

Development of Coronary Angioplasty Balloon Catheters. Technologic refinements of balloon catheter equipment and increased operator experience have dramatically improved the primary success rate of PCI.

Over-the-Wire Angioplasty Percutaneous Coronary Intervention Systems. A standard over-the-wire PCI catheter (Fig. 9-4) has a central lumen throughout the length of the catheter for the guidewire and a separate lumen for the balloon inflation. These catheters are approximately 145 to 155 cm long and can be used with long or short guidewires, usually 0.014 inch.

The advantages and limitations of over-the-wire angioplasty balloon catheters are listed in Table 9-1. These catheters accept multiple guidewires, which allows for the exchanging of additional devices that may require stronger, stiffer guidewires. Maintenance of distal wire position beyond the target stenosis is paramount in coronary angioplasty. For over-the-wire balloon catheters the guidewire can be extended to help maintain distal position while the balloon catheter is withdrawn completely over the guidewire to permit another balloon catheter to be exchanged and introduced over the same guidewire for additional dilations. A 300-cm exchange wire is also commonly used.

Over-the-wire angioplasty balloon catheters have few limitations. A primary operator and experienced personnel are

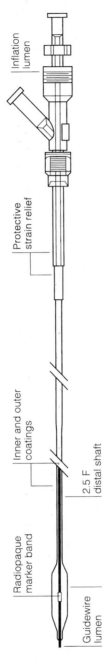

Fig. 9-4   Schematic design of a typical over-the-wire angioplasty balloon catheter. The guidewire extends the entire length of the catheter. (From Talley JD, Joseph A, Kupersmith J: *Cathet Cardiovasc Diagn* 20:108-113, 1990.)

Table 9-1

Advantages and Limitations of Angioplasty Balloon Types

Advantages	Limitations
Over the Wire	
Distal wire position	Two experienced personnel required for exchanges
Distal port available for pressure measurement or contrast media injection	
Accepts multiple guidewires	
Rapid Exchange (monorail)	
Distal wire position	Excellent guiding catheter support
Enhanced visualization	Exchanging balloons at hemostatic valve can be demanding
Single-operator system	Poor balloon tracking if wire lumen not flushed
Fixed Wire	
Enhanced visualization	Lack of through lumen
Single-operator system	Exchanging balloon requires complete removal of percutaneous coronary intervention catheter
Access to distal lesions	
Use with small guiding catheters	
Very low-profile balloons	

required to perform catheter exchanges. Several different types of devices can be used to fix a 155-cm guidewire in place to permit over-the-wire catheters to be exchanged without using a 300-cm guidewire. These devices include a wire entangler, a balloon trapper, and a magnet fixation system (see later).

Rapid-Exchange (Monorail) Percutaneous Coronary Intervention Catheters. Rapid-exchange balloon catheters were developed to allow the operator to exchange over-the-wire PCI catheters unassisted. This catheter differs from other PCI catheters in that only a variable length of the shaft has two lumens (Fig. 9-5, *A*). One lumen is for balloon inflation and the other, which extends through only a portion of the catheter shaft, houses the guidewire. Because only a limited portion of the balloon requires dual lumens, the catheter shafts can be made smaller.

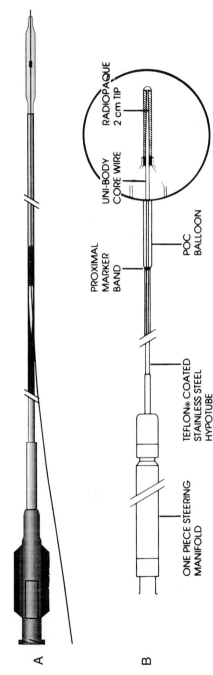

Fig. 9-5 A, Schematic design of a typical rapid-exchange angioplasty balloon catheter. The guidewire extends on "through" the distal part of the catheter allowing for single-operator use. (Courtesy of SciMed Life Systems, Maple Grove, Minn.) **B,** Schematic design of a standard fixed-wire angioplasty balloon catheter. This design has only one "through" lumen for balloon inflation, and the device itself serves as a "steerable guidewire." (From Talley JD, Joseph A, Killeavy ES, et al: *Cathet Cardiovasc Diagn* 22:310-316, 1991.)

Rapid-exchange balloon catheters address certain inherent limitations of over-the-wire systems. First, over-the-wire balloon exchanges requiring extension of the distal wire or a long wire are unnecessary because the rapid-exchange portion of the catheter is short. Second, a single operator can use rapid-exchange balloon catheters without the aid of other assistants to maintain distal guidewire position or facilitate balloon navigation.

Monorail catheters also have limitations, including the need for excellent guiding catheter support and more operator skill for the complexity in manipulation of the guidewire, balloon catheter, and guiding catheter. Blood loss during removal of the monorail balloon catheter at the rotating hemostatic valve can be reduced with better technique and valve connectors.

Fixed-Wire Angioplasty Balloon Catheters. The fixed-wire catheter has the balloon mounted on the wire with a distal flexible steering tip (Fig. 9-5, *B*). The proximal end of the catheter consists of a single, nonremovable port connected to a hollow metal tube (hypotube). A core wire extends from the hypotube to the end of the distal steerable tip. This assembly is coated with a thin plastic shaft that enhances flexibility. Fixed-wire balloons have only one enclosed lumen for balloon inflation.

The advantages and limitations of fixed-wire angioplasty balloon catheters are listed in Table 9-1. The small shaft size of the single-lumen design provides excellent coronary visualization. Because the balloon is mounted on the distal guidewire, the device can easily be used by a single operator. Fixed-wire balloon catheters are particularly useful for distal lesions, subtotal stenoses, and lesions located in tortuous small vasculature.

Fixed-wire catheters have significant limitations. These catheters lack the inherent safety advantage of over-the-wire and rapid-exchange systems because the balloon is mounted on a guidewire. To exchange this catheter for a different balloon size, the catheter is removed completely, and the lesion recrossed with a different size catheter. Alternately, the catheter remains across the lesion, and a second guidewire is advanced to secure access to the lesions. The fixed-wire balloon can be withdrawn and the procedure completed with standard techniques. A narrowed or dissected lesion may not permit balloon advancement or even may close the vessel. The lack of a distal lumen prevents measurement of distal pressure or injection of contrast media to evaluate distal vessel runoff.

Procedure Notes for Percutaneous Coronary Intervention. The balloon is inflated and deflated using a hand-held syringe device with a pressure gauge. Balloon catheters come in different sizes (1.5 to 5 mm for coronary arteries), which refer to the inflated diameter of the balloon. The balloon diameter is selected according to the angiographic size of the vessel to be dilated. Coronary balloon catheters are made of plastic materials that determine the flexibility of the catheter shaft and the balloon characteristics (e.g., burst pressure and actual diameter under different pressure levels). There are special-purpose coronary balloon catheters (e.g., catheters with side holes in the shaft, permitting distal autoperfusion during prolonged balloon inflations).

Angioplasty Guidewires. Coronary angioplasty guidewires are small-caliber (0.014- to 0.018-inch) steerable wires. They are advanced into the coronary artery or branches beyond the lesion that is to be dilated. A J tip of varying degree may be shaped by the operator to negotiate side branches and tortuous artery curves. The balloon-stent catheter is advanced over the wire and, after artery dilation, removed from the artery with the wire remaining in place beyond the dilated lesion. Extra-long guidewires (300 cm) are used to exchange over-the-wire balloon catheters. The tip flexibility and torque control characteristics of these coronary guidewires vary. Generally the softer wires are safer and easier to advance into tortuous branches, whereas the stiffer wires give better torque control and may be useful for crossing difficult or total occlusions. Some guidewires have special coatings to cross totally occluded stenoses better. These hydrophilic wires generally carry a small risk of perforation if the tip position is not kept in the major vessel lumen.

Exchange and Extension Guidewires and Wire Fixation Devices. An exchange guidewire is similar to guidewires mentioned previously except that its length is 280 to 300 cm.

This long wire replaces the initial wire when the exchange of an over-the-wire balloon catheter is necessary. Alternatively a 120- to 145-cm extension wire can be connected to the end of the initial guidewire to allow balloon catheter exchanges.

Several guidewire fixation or exchange systems are available. One uses a special short balloon on a wire that is not long enough to leave the guide. When inflated, the balloon traps the guidewire inside the guide catheter, permitting the balloon catheter to be pulled off without moving the guidewire. A different-size balloon catheter can be advanced over the wire, the trapper balloon deflated, and the balloon catheter readvanced into the artery. This system usually requires a catheter caliber of 7 F or larger.

Another wire fixation device has a twisting wire that entraps the guidewire and fixes it while the balloon is removed and replaced with another. When the new balloon catheter is inserted with the end of the guidewire sticking out of the catheter end for manual fixation, the tangling wire is retracted into its holder and removed from the guide catheter.

A third system has a magnet and special guidewire, and can be used with any guide catheter and balloon system. The magnet fixes the guidewire in place while the balloon catheter is exchanged.

Other Equipment

Y Connector (Adjustable Hemostasis Device). The Y connector is an accessory device that minimizes back-bleeding while the balloon catheter is inserted into the guiding catheter. This device allows the injection of contrast media and pressure monitoring through the guiding catheter, regardless of balloon catheter position.

Inflation Device. A disposable syringe device is used to inflate the balloon on the balloon catheter with precise measurement of the inflation pressure in atmospheres (atm). Balloons are generally inflated at pressures of 4 to 12 atm. Although stents may be inflated at 10 to 18 atm, the balloon is typically inflated with sufficient pressure to compress the plaque and fully expand the "dumbbell," or indentation, at the waist of the partially inflated balloon caused by the undilated stenosis. Occasionally, hard lesions (calcium or fibrosis) may require high pressures (>14 atm) to remove the dumbbell. Needless overinflation of the balloon increases the risk of dissection and balloon rupture.

Torque (Tool) Device. A small cylindrical pin vise clamp slides over the proximal end of the angioplasty guidewire, permitting the operator to perform fine manipulations of the guidewire by turning the torque tool (i.e., pin vise on the guidewire). Fig. 9-6 shows examples of the inflation device, Y' connectors, guidewire introducers, and torque tool.

Clinical Procedure

   A. Noninvasive testing for ischemia
      1. Electrocardiogram (ECG) (evidence of resting ischemia or recent infarction)
      2. Exercise stress with or without perfusion imaging or echocardiography for left ventricular (LV) wall motion as indicated; pharmacologic stress study (e.g.,

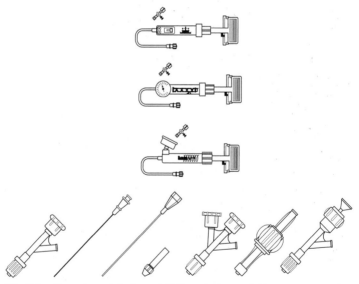

Fig. 9-6 Examples of balloon inflation device and Y connectors, wire introducer needles, and torque tool. (Courtesy of Meritt Medical, Inc., Salt Lake City, Utah.)

dipyridamole); two-dimensional echocardiography (as indicated for assessment of LV function or valvular heart disease)

   3. Coronary angiography evaluation (may require in-laboratory translesional physiology assessment of flow or pressure for objective evidence of ischemia before intervention)

Note: Order of tests depends on clinical presentation

B. Pre-PCI preparation

   1. Patient preparation (intravenous [IV] line, medications, consent)

   2. Patient and family teaching (procedure, results, complications)

   3. Cardiothoracic surgeon consultation, particularly for high-risk patients and patients with multivessel disease or decreased LV function

   4. Appropriate laboratory work (type and crossmatch blood, complete blood cell and platelet counts, prothrombin time, partial thromboplastin time, electrolytes, blood urea nitrogen, creatinine)

C. Patient preparation in catheterization suite

   1. ECG (inferior and anterior wall leads): 12-lead (radiolucent) ECG

   2. Skin preparation; inguinal area for femoral artery or wrist for radial artery

   3. Venous access for temporary pacing is no longer routine; venous access should be considered for high-risk patients, acute MI, left bundle-branch block needing right coronary artery PCI or rotoblator or thrombus aspiration device

   4. Aspirin (325 mg orally); failure to administer aspirin before PCI is associated with a two to three times higher acute complication rate

   5. Administration of calcium antagonists is no longer routine unless for hypertension or known coronary spasm.

   6. Benadryl (25 mg IV or orally)

   7. Heparin, 40-70 µg/kg bolus (or smaller bolus if glycoprotein IIb/IIIa blocker used); target activated coagulation time is greater than 200 seconds

   8. Glycoprotein IIb/IIIa blockers should be considered

9. Meperidine (Demerol) (25 to 50 mg IV) or fentanyl (50 to 100 μg IV)

D. Guiding coronary arteriograms (perform after administration of 100 to 200 μg of nitroglycerin by the intracoronary route)
   1. Definition of coronary anatomy and collateral supply (if any)
   2. Storage of guiding shots to use as reference map for balloon-stent positioning
   3. Selection of device size; known guide catheter diameter is used to select the balloon-stent diameter

Note: 8 F = 2.87 mm, 6 F = 2 mm. (Size of PCI device based on distal artery normal reference segment; balloon/artery ratio <1:1.2)

E. PCI procedure
   1. Guiding catheter selected for angle of vessel takeoff and optimal backup
   2. Guiding catheter is seated; coaxial alignment is best
   3. Guidewire is advanced beyond target vessel stenosis to distal position
   4. Balloon-stent is inserted through hemostasis valve on guide catheter
   5. Balloon-stent is advanced into center of lesion
   6. Centering of the balloon is maintained with the use of radiopaque markers on balloon)
   7. Balloon-stent is inflated; adequate inflation pressure (to remove dumbbell indentation of lesion on partially inflated balloon) must be used; a balloon may be inflated for 60 to 120 seconds as tolerated; stents may be inflated for 10 to 20 seconds

F. Assessment of the dilation result
   1. Enlarged artery lumen (≤20% residual lesion)
   2. Good angiographic flow (TIMI [Thrombolysis in Myocardial Infarction] grade 3)
   3. Observe for adverse angiographic markers (thrombus or dissection)
   4. No residual ischemia (ECG changes with or without chest pain)

G. Considerations for additional stenting
   1. Target segment recoil
   2. Large dissection

3. Slow flow (may require fractional flow reserve [FFR] or intravascular ultrasound to establish presence of dissection)
4. Ischemia

H. Postprocedure angiograms and sheath care
   1. Removal of guidewire for final images after additional intracoronary nitroglycerin
   2. Femoral angiography before vascular closure device selection (right anterior oblique view is obtained for right femoral artery)
   3. Vascular closure device is chosen
   4. Alternatively, suture arterial and venous sheaths in place; they are removed in 4 hours; no prolonged (>6 hours) heparin infusions are indicated unless special circumstances

I. Postprocedure outside laboratory
   1. Teaching about hospital course and bleeding problems, late complications, and restenosis
   2. Notification of departments, intensive care (or other appropriate patient care area), operating room, and surgical team stand-down
   3. Laboratory and ECG

J. Post-PCI medications
   1. Aspirin (325 mg orally daily)
   2. Clopidogrel (325 mg loading dose and 75 mg/day orally, at least 2 to 4 weeks after stenting); initiation of statin drugs should be considered; antihypertensive or antianginal medications are restarted depending on the patient's clinical needs

K. Follow-up schedule
   1. Exercise treadmill test (≥6 weeks after PCI)
   2. If symptoms or signs of ischemia are present, coronary angiography is repeated
   3. The patient returns to activities of daily living

Stenosis Assessment With Use of Fractional Flow Reserve With a Pressure Guidewire

Pressure transmitted from an angioplasty guidewire and the guiding catheter can be used to determine the hemodynamic significance of additional lesions or the end point of PCI. To measure translesional pressure, the operator matches the pressures of the guidewire and guide catheter before the stenosis is crossed. Pressures are normalized (matched) to eliminate any intrinsic gradient. Figure 9-7 shows the translesional gradient at rest and during hyperemia. The gradient measured during adenosine-induced hyperemia reflects the blood flow through the artery. The distal pressure/proximal pressure ratio during hyperemia is called the fractional flow reserve (FFR) and is a more accurate indication of the narrowing artery than the resting gradient. Before PCI in the patient example (Fig. 9-7, *top right*), the proximal aortic pressure is obtained through the guiding catheter. The proximal pressure (Pa) is 145/68 mm Hg. The distal pressure (Pd) is measured from the sensor angioplasty guidewire at 110/50 mm Hg. During intracoronary administration of adenosine, the hyperemic mean pressures used to compute FFR (at peak hyperemia, Pd/Pa = FFR) show FFR = 0.72 (FFR <0.75 is associated with inducible ischemia). The resting gradient was insignificant and does not correlate to inducible ischemia.

After PCI the gradient between the proximal and distal artery pressures decreases. An FFR of >0.9 is considered a successful result. Normal arteries have FFR greater than 0.94. In this patient after PCI the FFR = 0.98 (Fig. 9-7, *bottom*).

A persistently low FFR (<0.75), especially if the angiographic result is suboptimal, is an indication for further inflations (either prolonged inflations or upsizing of the balloon) or stenting. FFR and distal coronary flow velocity data (see Chapter 6) have important value when questionable angiographic results are obtained. The use of adjunctive imaging and diagnostic techniques during PCI is presented in Table 9-2. Intravascular ultrasound imaging measures anatomy, not flow, and is primarily used to confirm optimal stent implantation in artery stenosis.

Stent Implantation

Elective stent placement is performed as part of a planned revascularization strategy and can be performed with or without prior balloon inflation of the target lesion. Elective stent implantation improves long-term results compared with balloon angioplasty as reflected by the reduced restenosis rates in the BENESTENT and STRESS trials and in specific subsets,

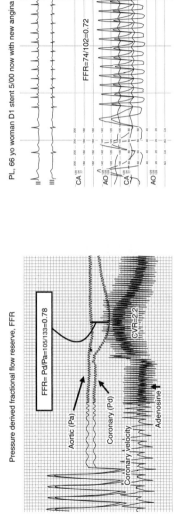

PL, 66 yo woman D1 stent 5/00 now with new angina

FFR=74/102=0.72

PL, 66 yo woman, post PTCA of LAD

Pressure derived fractional flow reserve, FFR

FFR= Pd/Pa=105/133=0.78

Aortic (Pa)

Coronary (Pd)

Coronary velocity

CVR=2.2

Adenosine

Fig. 9-7 Calculation of fractional flow reserve *(FFR)*. *Top left*, Proximal guide catheter pressure *(Aortic, Pa)* and distal coronary pressure *(Pd)* and coronary flow velocity at rest and after intracoronary adenosine *(arrow)*. Hyperemia widens gradient and decreases Pd when velocity is maximal (coronary vasodilatory reserve [CVR] = 2.2), FFR = Pd/Pa = 105/133 = 0.78, above the ischemic threshold value (0.75). *Top right*, Patient example: before percutaneous coronary intervention, FFR = 0.72. *Bottom*, After percutaneous coronary intervention, FFR = 0.98.

Table 9-2

Diagnostic and Imaging Adjuncts to Endovascular Intervention

Advantages	Disadvantages
Intravascular Ultrasound Imaging (IVUS)	
1. Quantifies wall thickness	1. Requires iterative IVUS catheter-balloon exchanges
2. Qualitative tissue characterization	2. Remote potential for vascular damage
3. Provides a 360-degree tomographic view	3. Spasm
4. Helpful for vessel sizing and stenting	
Intravascular Pressure Wire (FFR)	
1. Ease of signal interpretation	1. IC or IV adenosine and heparin
2. Easily combined with stents	2. IC nitroglycerin
3. FFR is lesion specific	3. Spasm
4. FFR is independent of hemodynamics	
Doppler FloWire (CFR)	
1. On-line assessment of coronary flow before, during, and after intervention	1. Complexity in interpretation of microcirculation
2. Easily combined with PCI	2. Signal is operator dependant
3. Assesses CFR and relative CFR	3. IV, IC adenosine, heparin, spasm
Angioscopy	
1. Best method to see thrombus-plaque surface	1. Requires blood displacement by constant flushing
2. Forward viewing	2. Limited image acquisition time ($\leq$60 seconds)
	3. Potential for vascular damage
	4. Does not provide quantitative data
	5. No longer available in United States

Modified from Siegel RJ, Forrester JS: *ACC Curr J Rev* 2:77, 1993.
CFR, Coronary flow reserve; *FFR,* fractional flow reserve; *IC,* intracoronary; *IV,* intravenous; *IVUS,* intravascular ultrasound imaging; *PCI,* percutaneous coronary intervention.

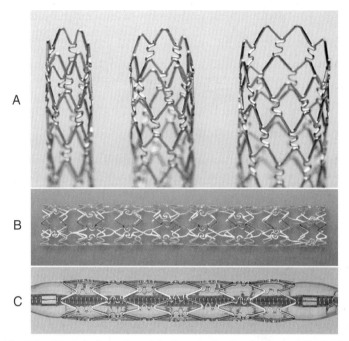

Fig. 9-8   Stent designs. **A** and **C,** Bx velocity, Cordis Corp., Miami, Fla. **B,** Jostent, Jomed, Rancho Cordova, Calif.

such as saphenous vein grafts, total occlusions, and restenotic lesions. Several different kinds of stents are used (Fig. 9-8).

Stenting of angioplasty-induced dissection decreases the need for emergency bypass surgery and the risk of MI. Emergency stent implantation is performed for acute or threatened vessel closure. Emergency stent implantation may need to be performed during periods of significant ischemia, which may limit optimization of stent expansion or precipitate subtle changes in technique, such as incomplete stent coverage of the entire lesion or a willingness to accept a less than optimal angiographic result. These features may make the difference between a successful and an unsuccessful long-term outcome.

Indications

Elective stenting is indicated in the following patients:
1. Those eligible for balloon angioplasty
2. Those with symptomatic ischemic heart disease caused by discrete stenosis (length <20 mm)

3. Those with de novo or restenostic coronary artery lesions with a vessel diameter ≥2.5 mm (preferably >3 mm)

Compared with percutaneous transluminal coronary angioplasty, stenting produces a larger minimal luminal diameter, maintains arterial patency, and reduces restenosis at 6 months. Follow-up for stenting at 1 and 5 years is highly favorable.

Contraindications

Contraindications are classified based on patient and anatomic factors. Relative contraindications based on patient factors are similar to those for balloon angioplasty and include the following:
1. Inability to take antiplatelet therapy
2. History of bleeding or other conditions that preclude anticoagulation during the stent procedure
3. Noncardiac surgery required within 2 weeks

Figures 9-9 to 9-11 are case examples of PCI.

Coronary Atherectomy

Because atherosclerotic plaque remains in the artery after balloon dilation, physical removal of the plaque from inside the coronary artery may improve procedural and clinical results. Three devices developed for this purpose are approved for coronary intervention: the high-speed rotablator, directional atherectomy catheter (DCA), and transluminal extraction catheter.

Rotational Atherectomy (Rotablator)

The rotablator is made of an olive-shaped steel burr (1.25 to 2.5 mm in diameter, Fig. 9-12) that is embedded with microscopic diamond particles in the front half and is rotated with a torque wire at up to 200,000 rpm by an external air turbine. The device is inserted through 6 F to 9 F guide catheters over a special 0.009-inch guidewire. A continuous pressurized heparin saline infusion is administered through the device to aid lubrication and heat dissipation. After the burr is placed just proximal to the lesion, the system is activated, and the burr is advanced through the lesion in a slow, steady manner. The abrasive surface of the burr selectively ablates (pulverizes) the hard plaque while sparing the softer normal wall. Several burr passes are performed before removal

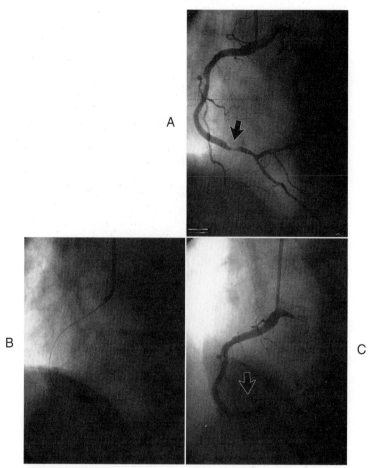

Fig. 9-9 Single-vessel stenting. **A,** Right coronary artery with lesion proximal to posterior descending artery *(arrow).* **B,** Direct stenting was performed. **C,** Final result with 0% residual narrowing *(arrow).*

of the burr and a decision for a larger burr or complementary balloon inflation is made. Additional angioplasty balloon inflations are needed to decrease the residual stenosis. The maximum burr diameter should be no larger than 70% to 80% of the normal arterial luminal diameter.

The rotablator is most suitable for rigid calcified and long lesions in which balloon angioplasty success is likely to be low. The complication and restenosis rates are similar to balloon

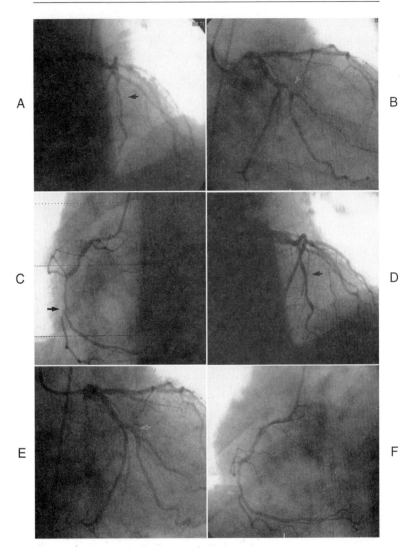

Fig. 9-10 Multivessel stenting. **A,** Before percutaneous coronary intervention, significant stenoses are present in left anterior descending (LAD) artery *(arrow)*. **B,** Circumflex (CFX) artery. **C,** Right coronary artery (RCA) *(arrow)*. **D,** After stenting LAD artery. **E,** CFX artery. **F,** RCA.

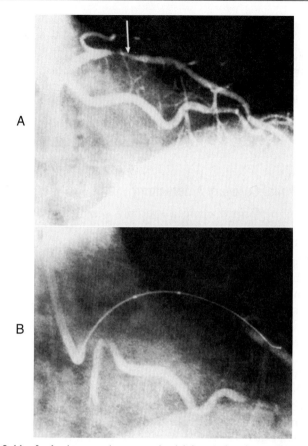

Fig. 9-11 A, Angiogram shows proximal left anterior descending artery stenosis *(arrow).* **B,** A guidewire across the stenosis with balloon markers in place. Note persistent stain of contrast material in the circumflex artery consistent with left main coronary artery dissection. This complication required emergency bypass surgery in 1989. Today, left main stenting would be considered.

angioplasty. Randomized comparisons indicate no restenosis advantage, but procedure success is higher in the calcified small vessel or long lesion subset. A specific complication of the rotablator is temporary no-reflow phenomenon with creatine kinase enzyme increase in some patients. This problem may necessitate insertion of a prophylactic pacemaker wire, especially for right coronary lesions.

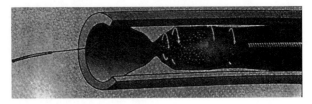

Fig. 9-12 Rotoblator burr.

Directional Coronary Atherectomy

DCA is performed using a specially designed catheter with a metal cutting chamber that contains a cylindrical cutter (Fig. 9-13). The operator uses a posteriorly located supporting balloon to push the cutting chamber against the lesion. The cutter is rotated by a hand-held motor at 2000 rpm and is advanced within the cutting chamber to shave the plaque and deposit it to the nose cone of the catheter. DCA works via three interactive mechanisms: "Dotter" technique or pushing effect created by the bulk of the catheter (5 F to 7 F), balloon dilation effect caused by inflation of supporting balloon, and actual cutting and removal of the plaque. The last-mentioned is usually the dominant mechanism.

Because of the large size of the DCA catheter and rigid cutter housing, large-lumen guide catheters with specially designed curves are needed. An appropriately sized long sheath and a large-bore rotating hemostatic adapter are required. The large size of the sheaths has been a significant source of morbidity and mortality, especially in elderly patients.

Randomized studies suggest a small restenosis benefit with DCA compared with balloon angioplasty only in patients with proximal left anterior descending artery lesions in large arteries. Some studies indicate increased complications with DCA. The risk/benefit ratio should be carefully evaluated for each patient. Patients with large vessels (>3 mm) and ostial or eccentric lesions, which decrease the success with balloon dilation, seem to be the most suitable candidates for DCA. Patients with calcified, angulated, long (<20 mm) narrowings, spiral dissections, and friable graft lesions are not suitable candidates for DCA. Stenting has largely replaced DCA.

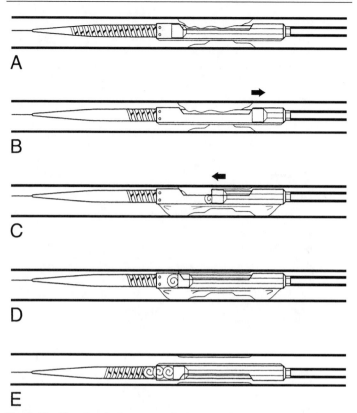

Fig. 9-13 Directional atherectomy catheter cutting sequence. **A,** Catheter housing is positioned in the coronary lesion. Cutter is forward. **B,** Cutter is retracted. **C,** Balloon is inflated, cutter motor is turned on, and cutter is advanced slowly, shaving tissue. **D,** Cutter is advanced to deposit the specimen into the nose cone chamber. **E,** Balloon is deflated. Keep the cutter forward until after the catheter is rotated to the next position. Repeat steps **A** to **E**. (From Simpson JB, Selmon MR, Robertson GC, et al: *Am J Cardiol* 61:96G-101G, 1988.)

Thrombus Aspiration System

The AngioJet Rheolytic Thrombectomy System opens an artery by aspirating clot. High-pressure water jets directed backward into the catheter create a strong suction at the space near the tip and effective thrombus evacuation occurs (Fig. 9-14). Conventional treatment for thrombus in the past involved mostly a "lyse and wait" procedure that used thrombolytic

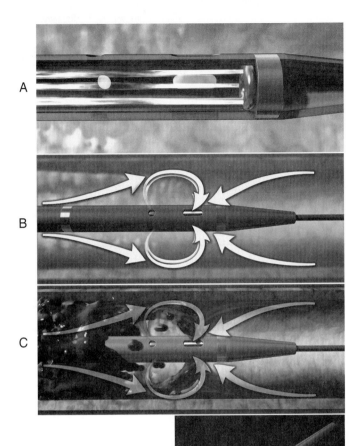

Fig. 9-14 *Top,* Thrombus aspiration catheter (Angiojet) from Possis Medical Inc., Minneapolis, Minn. **A,** A high-pressure water jet is direct from the tip back into the catheter lumen. **B,** This jet creates a Venturi suction at the top and, **C,** aspirates materials. **D,** Several different designs are available.

therapy to dissolve thrombus. The AngioJet System removes thrombus from the artery as safely as thrombolytic therapy and, in some lesions, with less risk of breaking up thrombus with the distal thromboembolism.

In the VeGAS 2 trial of thrombectomy in saphenous vein graft thrombosis, procedural success (i.e., achievement of a final residual diameter stenosis of <50% and TIMI 3 flow post procedure, in the absence of death, emergent bypass surgery, or Q-wave MI) was high (>90%). Success was significantly higher with the AngioJet System regardless of the age of the thrombus. Procedural success was also achieved in 81.3% of interventions with chronic (>2 weeks old) thrombus. The incidence of major adverse events was 52% less with the AngioJet System. MI (Q wave or large non–Q wave) was reduced with the AngioJet System, an effect that was sustained for 1 year after the procedure. Procedures with the AngioJet often require temporary pacing and may be less effective in large-diameter conduits. A full discussion of these devices can be found elsewhere (see the Suggested Readings section).

Peripheral Arterial Balloon Angioplasty

Peripheral arterial disease is a common manifestation of atherosclerosis and is often present in patients who undergo cardiac catheterization for coronary artery disease. Generally, peripheral arterial disease can be managed conservatively, although some patients require revascularization therapy (either via surgery or peripheral arterial balloon angioplasty). Certain anatomic considerations often make a patient a better candidate for one procedure as opposed to the other. In coronary artery disease discrete localized lesions are usually treated best by balloon angioplasty, whereas diffuse disease and long total occlusions can often be treated better with bypass surgery. A team approach involving input from the vascular interventionalist and vascular surgeon results in optimal treatment for the patient. The nomenclature for the peripheral vessels below the diaphragm is shown in Fig. 9-15.

Indications. Indications for peripheral arterial balloon angioplasty are as follows:

1. Intermittent (lifestyle-limiting) claudication for more than 6 months
2. Severe limb ischemia

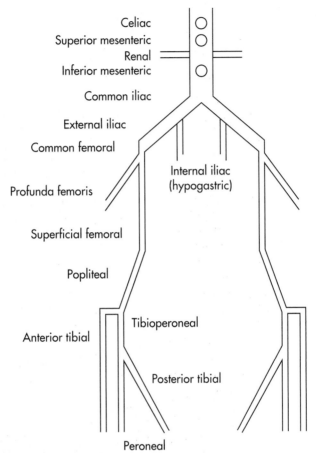

Fig. 9-15 Peripheral vascular interventional sites of the lower extremities. (Courtesy of CJ White, SR Ramee, and TJ Collins, Ochsner Medical Institutes, New Orleans, La.)

3. Pain while resting
4. Nonhealing ulcer
5. Diabetes mellitus

Revascularization is elective in nondiabetic patients and in patients who smoke with intermittent claudication because (1) it does not affect long-term survival and (2) the incidence of severe limb-threatening ischemia is low because of distal vessel patency.

Indications for peripheral arterial thrombolysis therapy are as follows:

1. Native arterial thrombosis
2. Graft thrombosis
3. Acute emboli
4. Thrombosis from popliteal artery aneurysms. Peripheral arterial thrombolysis therapy is used with caution before surgery. Chronic thrombosis is better treated with surgery.

Contraindications. Contraindications for peripheral arterial thrombolysis include the following:

1. Nonsignificant arterial disease based on Doppler studies and ankle-brachial flow index
2. Medically unstable patient
3. Long (>15 cm) arterial occlusion
4. Lesion that jeopardizes supply of critically dependent collaterals

Technique
Vascular Access

1. Antegrade, common femoral

   The common femoral artery is entered above the midpoint of femoral head

   Most superficial femoral artery (SFA)–profunda bifurcations below this point

   Access to ipsilateral SFA, profunda, popliteal, and below-knee vessels

2. Retrograde, common femoral

   Access to ipsilateral iliac artery

   Renal angioplasty

   Contralateral approach to iliac lesions, SFA

3. Brachial-axillary

   Requires extra-long catheters and balloons (120 to 145 cm)

   Access when bilateral iliofemoral vessels are occluded

4. Popliteal

   Retrograde access for SFA occlusions

   Minimizes likelihood of entering side branches in total occlusions

   Risk of joint space (knee) injury

Angiography

1. Cardiac catheterization laboratory equipment; digital subtraction angiography should be considered

   Image intensifier, 9-inch mode

   Digital imaging subtraction to reduce radiation exposure

   Cine film shows flow dynamics (helpful in assessing collaterals)

   Speed of 15 frames/sec is adequate

2. Abdominal aortogram

   Catheter is positioned above or at the level of renal arteries (L1 or L2 disk space)

   Contrast medium injection, 15 ml/sec × 3 seconds or 20 ml/sec × 2 seconds

   Pan to iliofemoral vessels

   Lateral plane for celiac, superior mesenteric, or inferior mesenteric origins

3. Selective iliofemoral angiography with runoff to feet

   Catheter is positioned in proximal common iliac artery

   Simmons, Cobra, internal mammary, NIH, or pigtail catheters are used (Fig. 9-16)

   Contrast medium injection, 6 to 8 ml/sec × 4 to 6 seconds

   Lateral angulation of image intensifier at 30 degrees (SFA-profunda bifurcation)

   Pan from common iliac artery to foot vessels

   Figure 9-17 illustrates a common peripheral vascular intervention.

Complications. Complications of angiography include the following:

1. Vasospasm—200 to 600 mg of intraarterial nitroglycerin should be administered (2 to 10 mg of papaverine intraarterially or 50 mg of lidocaine may also be administered)
2. Thrombus—heparin should be increased; thrombolytics or thrombectomy catheter aspiration can be considered
3. Arterial dissection
4. Vessel perforation (1%)
5. Death (<0.5%)

Devices

Balloons. Long shaft coronary balloons are used for below-knee angioplasty. Approximate vessel sizes are as follows:

Common iliac, 8 to 10 mm diameter

Simmons   Internal mammary   Cobra

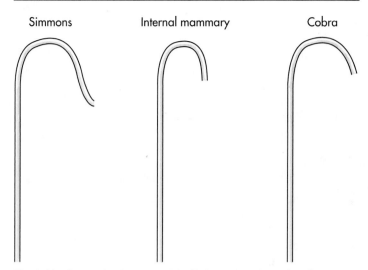

Fig. 9-16   Types of catheters used for iliofemoral angiography. (Courtesy of CJ White, SR Ramee, and TJ Collins, Ochsner Medical Institutes, New Orleans, La.)

Common femoral, 6 to 8 mm
Superficial femoral artery (SFA), 4 to 6 mm
Tibial artery, 2 to 4 mm

Stents
1. Approved for peripheral vascular interventions, including renal, iliac, and SFA
2. For SFA, useful for suboptimal balloon results
3. Good long-term patency in large vessels
4. Abrupt occlusion or thrombosis not generally a problem in large (iliac) vessels

Note: In contrast to coronary stenting, adjunctive thieno-pyridine (clopidogrel) therapy is not mandatory because of low incidence of thrombotic occlusion.

Anticipated Results of Peripheral Arterial Balloon Angioplasty.
Anticipated results can be summarized as follows:
1. Iliac
   85% to 90% 5-year patency
   Combine with peripheral bypass, provide inflow without abdominal surgery

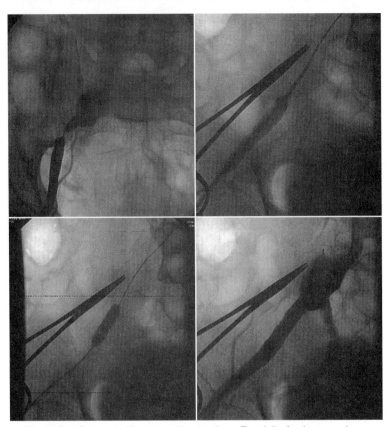

Fig. 9-17 Common iliac stenosis stenting. *Top left,* Angiogram shows severe stenosis and proximal ectatic region. *Top right,* A hemostat is used to mark location, and self-expanding stent is released in lesion. *Bottom left,* A balloon is expanded in stent to ensure complete apposition. *Bottom right,* Final angiogram with 0% residual narrowing.

2. Femoropopliteal
   Stenoses: 3-year patency, 70%
   Occlusions: 3-year patency, 55%
   Poorer results with longer lesions, diabetes, poor runoff, and tobacco use
3. Infrapopliteal
   Smaller vessels, poorer results
   Reserved for limb salvage procedures
   May provide runoff to aid bypass graft patency

Methods of Clinical Assessment for Peripheral Vascular Insufficiency. Peripheral vascular insufficiency can be assessed by the following methods:

1. Ankle-brachial index (ratio of upper-extremity blood pressure to lower-extremity blood pressure)
2. Color flow Doppler
3. Magnetic resonance imaging
4. Angiography

Renal Balloon Angioplasty and Stenting

Nonsurgical opening of the narrowed renal artery may alleviate renovascular hypertension or improve renal function and permit use of angiotensin-converting enzyme inhibitors in patients with congestive heart failure.

Indications. Indications for renal balloon angioplasty and stenting include the following:

1. Renovascular hypertension caused by atherosclerotic or fibromuscular narrowing of the renal artery (approximately 1 in 50 hypertensive patients) after failed medical therapy with three antihypertensive medications, including a diuretic
2. Increased renal vein renin on side of arterial disease
3. Renal transplant artery stenosis
4. Renal artery or vein bypass graft stenosis
5. Renal insufficiency with greater than 50% artery stenosis or 10 to 20 mm Hg translesional gradient
6. Renal artery stenosis in patients with a single kidney

Contraindications. Contraindications for renal balloon angioplasty include the following:

1. Unstable medical condition
2. Borderline lesion (<50% diameter or no translesional pressure gradient, no lateralized elevated renin)

Technique

1. Femoral approach
   a. The operator obtains femoral arterial access, inserts sheath and guiding catheter (renal artery guide), and performs initial angiograms
   b. IV heparin, 5000 U, and intraarterial nitroglycerin, 100 to 200 µg is administered

   c. Gradient is assessed
   d. The operator advances the guidewire across lesion and watches for small-vessel spasm
   e. The balloon-stent system is advanced across the lesion; primary stenting may also be performed (4- to 8-mm diameter stents are commonly used)
   f. Balloon-stent inflated at 4 to 10 atm
   g. Balloon is deflated and withdrawn
   h. Pressure gradient is assessed
   i. Angiography is performed
   j. Renal stenting: *Technical note*: After step *f*, the operator deflates the balloon and slides the guide catheter into the renal artery; the operator crosses the lesion with the renal stent, withdraws the guide, checks the position, and deploys the stent
   k. Vascular closure device or manual compression of puncture is used
2. Radial-brachial arterial approach for downward origin of renal arteries
   a. The radial-brachial artery is accessed by percutaneous technique
   b. Above-listed steps *c* through *g* are performed

Figure 9-18 shows an example of renal artery stenting.

Postprocedural Care
1. Blood pressure is monitored for 24 hours
2. Poststent care regimen (see coronary stenting).

Complications. Complications resulting from renal balloon angioplasty are as follows:
1. Death (1%)
2. Thrombus (1%)
3. Nonocclusive dissection (2% to 4%)
4. Worsening renal failure (1.5% to 6%)
5. Embolus to peripheral artery (1.5% to 2%)
6. Embolus to distal renal artery (2%)
7. Rupture of artery (1%)

Thrombolysis for Peripheral Vascular Interventions

Indications. Indications for thrombolysis for peripheral vascular interventions are as follows:
1. Acute occlusion

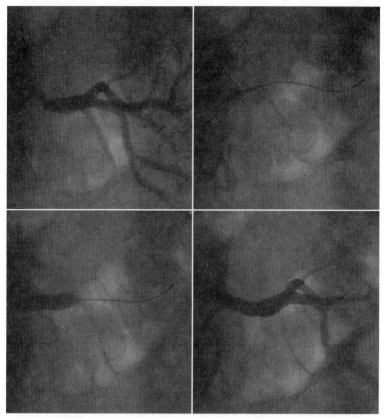

Fig. 9-18 Renal artery stenting. *Top left,* Ostial left renal artery stenosis. *Top right,* Stent is advanced into stenosis. *Bottom left,* Stent is deployed. *Bottom right,* Final angiogram with 0 mm Hg gradient and 0% residual narrowing.

   2. Chronic occlusion
   3. Distal embolization

Contraindications. No absolute contraindications for this procedure exist. Relative contraindications are as follows:
   1. Recent surgery
   2. Bleeding tendency
   3. Trauma
   4. Stroke

Therapeutic Principles. Therapeutic principles include the following:

1. Low systemic dose, high local concentration of agent
2. Pharmacologic lysis atraumatic to vessels and grafts versus Fogarty embolectomy
3. Lysis improves distal runoff
4. Maximize drug delivery to thrombus
   Coaxial delivery systems
   Sos wire (hollow 0.035 wire)
   Craig wire (hollow 0.025 wire)
   Katzen wire (multiholed 0.035 wire)
   EDM (multiholed catheter)
   Tracker catheter (0.018, 0.025, and 0.035 plastic catheter)
   Lacing: hand injection of lytic agent along length of thrombus (Fig. 9-19)

Thrombolytic Agents. Thrombolytic agents include the following:

1. Streptokinase
   Inexpensive
   Associated with lower success rate
   Associated with higher systemic complication rate
2. Urokinase (removed from market by the Food and Drug Administration in 1998; reintroduced in 2002)
3. Recombinant tissue plasminogen activator (rtPA)
   Rapid lysis
   Modest systemic effects
   High success rates
4. Retavase (rtPA)

rtPA is the most commonly used thrombolytic agent. A dosage of 0.001 to 0.02 mg/kg/hr and a non–weight-based dosage at 0.12 to 2.0 mg/hr are recommended. Retavase has been used at a dosage of 0.5 µg/hr. Local infusion of thrombolytic agent is the preferred method. Different techniques, such as pulse spray pharmacomechanics, thrombolysis, lacing, or infusion catheters, can also be used to infuse thrombolytic agents.

VALVULOPLASTY
Percutaneous Balloon Valvuloplasty

Percutaneous techniques as alternatives to surgery for the treatment of valvular and congenital heart disease were

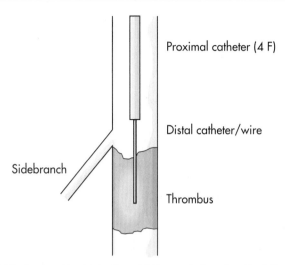

Fig. 9-19 Lacing. Hand injection of lytic agent along length of thrombus. (Courtesy of CJ White, SR Ramee, and TJ Collins, Ochsner Medical Institutes, New Orleans, La.)

introduced in the early 1980s and have undergone sufficient investigation to define their roles in interventional cardiology. In children balloon valvuloplasty is frequently used to relieve selected congenital valvular disorders, especially pulmonic and aortic stenosis. In adults balloon aortic valvuloplasty has been relegated to a palliative role in the management of aortic stenosis in patients who are not surgical candidates, whereas balloon mitral valvuloplasty for mitral stenosis has emerged as an excellent alternative to surgical commissurotomy or valve replacement and, in selected patients, is considered as the initial mechanical treatment of choice.

Percutaneous Balloon Mitral Valvuloplasty. Percutaneous balloon mitral valvuloplasty (PBMV) for the treatment of mitral stenosis has been studied extensively, and when successful has been found to yield marked immediate hemodynamic improvement and sustained clinical benefit. Prospective comparisons of PBMV with surgical commissurotomy in selected patients have shown similar hemodynamic and clinical results in follow-up. Not all patients are optimal candidates for PBMV, however. Echocardiography is essential to evaluate mitral valve structure and to exclude left atrial thrombus.

Indications

SYMPTOMATIC MITRAL STENOSIS. Patients with isolated symptomatic mitral stenosis or stenosis combined with mixed valvular disease with less than moderate mitral regurgitation with suitable valvular characteristics can be offered PBMV because of the comparable risk and the relative ease of the procedure.

Immobile, severely thickened, and fused or calcified valve leaflets may not respond well to balloon valvuloplasty. Patients with symptoms of mitral stenosis with these unfavorable characteristics who are not candidates for surgery may still benefit from the procedure, however. PBMV is contraindicated in the presence of atrial thrombus, which is best detected by transesophageal echocardiography.

Procedure. Antegrade transseptal access to the mitral valve with use of a single, specially designed balloon catheter (Inoue balloon) (Fig. 9-20) is the easiest method of access and is reliable. Clinical success is high, and complication rates are low. Because of its single-balloon design and relative ease in crossing of the mitral valve, use of the Inoue balloon generally requires less fluoroscopic and procedural time than previously used double-balloon techniques.

LEFT ATRIAL ACCESS. After baseline hemodynamic measurements are obtained, transseptal catheterization is performed (see Chapter 7). Care should be exercised not to perform the puncture too high on the septum. This location presents great difficulty in crossing the mitral valve and positioning the balloon catheter. Sometimes it may be necessary to float a balloon catheter through the mitral valve to enter the left ventricle.

DILATING THE INTERATRIAL SEPTUM. After placement of the guidewires, the atrial septum is dilated with a 6- to 8-mm balloon to allow easy passage of the larger dilation catheters. These small atrial septal defects are not generally clinically important.

INOUE BALLOON TECHNIQUE. The Inoue balloon catheter has a unique design that allows inflation of the tip of the balloon to facilitate crossing the mitral valve. A calibrated syringe produces a stepwise incremental valve dilation. Selection of balloon size is based on patient height. After left atrial access is obtained, the interatrial septum is dilated, and the Inoue bal-

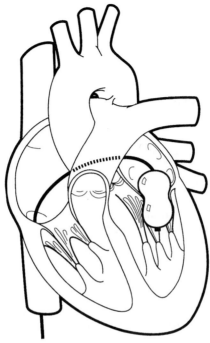

Fig. 9-20 Diagram of Inoue balloon catheter in position across the mitral valve during mitral valvuloplasty.

loon is tracked over the special guidewire into the left atrium. The tip of the balloon is inflated, and the distal balloon tip is floated across the mitral valve, steered with a stylet. Care should be taken that the balloon catheter is free within the ventricular cavity and not entangled in subvalvular chordae tendineae. The partially inflated balloon is withdrawn to engage the mitral valve leaflets and then fully inflated to achieve commissural splitting. The transmitral pressure gradient and an echocardiographic assessment of commissural separation and valvular regurgitation have been recommended after each dilating step to monitor the need for continued large-diameter balloon dilations in an effort to safely obtain the maximum mitral orifice possible without producing mitral regurgitation.

After the last inflation, left atrial-LV pressure and a right-sided oxygen saturation (to detect left-to-right shunting at the atrial septal level) are measured. The average decrease in mitral valve gradient is approximately 50% to 75% of the baseline gradient, and the increase in valve area is usually around 100% (average 2 cm^2). Figs. 9-21 and 9-22 show a case example of PBMV.

Complications. Procedural and hospital mortality is rare (0% to 2%) and usually is the result of ventricular perforation. Complications of transseptal puncture, such as hemopericardium or tamponade, are also rare (<2%), and systemic emboli may occur in 1% to 2% of patients. Mitral regurgitation increases in 20% to 50% of patients but is increased significantly (more than one angiographic grade) in only 8% to 10% of patients. Significant mitral regurgitation may appear late after PBMV. Mitral regurgitation severe enough to require valve replacement occurs in 0.9% to 3% of patients after PBMV and is usually the result of noncommissural tearing of the mitral leaflets or chordal rupture. An atrial septal defect with left-to-right shunting is detectable in 8% to 87% of patients (depending on the sensitivity of the method used for detection); most of these defects have shunt fractions of less than 1.4 to 1, are clinically unimportant, and decrease or disappear during follow-up.

Follow-up. The symptomatic status of the patient generally improves immediately and during follow-up. Short-term symptomatic improvement is present in most patients. Long-term follow-up (≥5 years) remains good in well-selected patients, especially those with less evidence of valve deformity (mobility, thickening, calcification, subvalvular disease) reflected in low preprocedural echocardiographic scores and with low LV end-diastolic pressure. In such patients, event-free 5-year survival is greater than 80%. Patients with more deformed valves and higher echocardiographic scores have a higher rate of restenosis. The incidence of restenosis and long-term outcome after PBMV seem comparable to closed mitral commissurotomy.

Percutaneous Balloon Aortic Valvuloplasty. First introduced in 1985, percutaneous balloon aortic valvuloplasty (PBAV) has been successfully used in the pediatric management of congenital aortic stenosis. PBAV for the treatment of adult

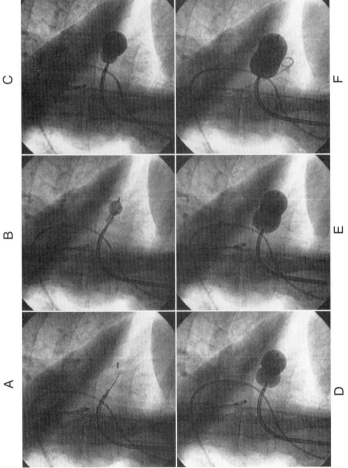

Fig. 9-21 A and **B,** Front half of balloon inflated and passed across the mitral valve orifice. This is analogous to the manner in which a balloon flotation catheter is maneuvered from the right atrium to the right ventricle during right-sided heart catheterization. **C,** The partially inflated balloon is pulled back until it engages the mitral valve. **D,** Front and back portions of balloon inflated, creating a "dogbone" shape that self-positions the balloon in the mitral orifice. **E,** Almost fully inflated balloon opening the commissures. The inferior indentation in the balloon was not as pronounced as the superior, signifying incomplete commissural separation. **F,** Full balloon inflation.

calcific aortic stenosis initially held promise but had disappointingly high restenosis rates (which may approach 50%). PBAV must be considered a short-term palliative procedure to be applied to a select group of patients.

Indications. The indications for PBAV in adults have evolved since its introduction.

1. Symptomatic patients who are not candidates for valve surgery can undergo PBAV. The age of the patient is not itself a contraindication for surgery.
2. In selected patients with poor LV function, PBAV can be used as a bridge to surgery.

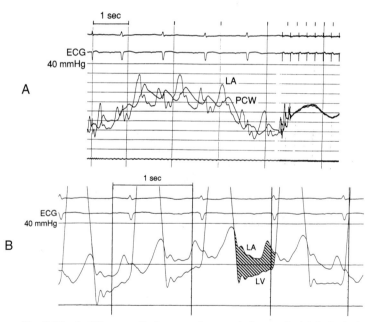

Fig. 9-22 **A,** When monitoring percutaneous balloon mitral valvuloplasty, pulmonary capillary wedge *(PCW)* pressure often is used. Differences between PCW and left atrial *(LA)* pressures may introduce error into final gradient measurements. **B,** Directly measured LA–left ventricular *(LV)* gradient before a percutaneous balloon mitral valvuloplasty shows gradient of 18 mm Hg. *Continued*

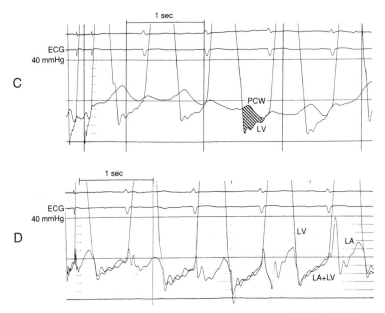

C

D

Fig. 9-22, cont'd C, After a percutaneous balloon mitral valvuloplasty PCW-LV gradient remains greater than 8 to 10 mm Hg. The PCW waveform is damped. **D,** In the same patient as Figure 9-21 and 9-22, LA-LV pressure after a percutaneous balloon mitral valvuloplasty now has no gradient, a highly successful result. (From Kern MJ, Aguirre F: *Cathet Cardiovasc Diagn* 27:52-56, 1992.)

3. Symptomatic aortic stenosis in patients scheduled to undergo major noncardiac surgery or other invasive procedures is another indication for PBAV.

Note: Before PBAV is performed, an evaluation for severe coronary artery disease and peripheral vascular disease is warranted. Significant aortic regurgitation and severe left main coronary artery disease are contraindications to PBAV.

Procedure

1. Arterial access is evaluated. The balloon catheters used for PBAV are large (>10 F), which increases the risk of vascular problems, especially in elderly women with fragile, small arteries. In some patients with peripheral vascular disease, smaller-size balloon catheters can be inserted through the brachial artery.

2. Severe coronary artery disease should be excluded. The possibility of left main coronary artery disease should be excluded by angiograms.

3. Significant aortic insufficiency should be excluded. An aortic regurgitation of more than 2+ is a contra-indication for the procedure because the degree of regurgitation may increase after PBAV.

4. Single or double balloons can be used. The current practice begins with a single balloon (Fig. 9-23). Low-profile balloons allow insertion and removal of 23- to 25-mm balloons with less difficulty. The diameter of the balloons should not be larger than the aortic annulus. There is no generally accepted way of selecting the proper size of balloon. Our practice usually is to start with an 18- to 20-mm balloon, increasing the balloon diameter to 23 mm, or rarely 25 mm, as necessary to reduce the aortic gradient more than 50%.

5. Positioning of the balloon. The patient is given 5000 U of heparin for anticoagulation. After baseline hemo-dynamics are obtained, the aortic valve is crossed, and a stiff (Amplatz 300-cm) guidewire with a large pigtail curve is positioned in the left ventricle. The skin punc-ture site is enlarged. The balloon catheter (prepared by flushing diluted contrast solution, then applying nega-tive pressure) is advanced into the left ventricle over the wire and positioned across the aortic valve. Longer bal-loons (4 to 5 cm) give better stability during inflation. Some operators have used an Inoue balloon in a retrograde fashion.

6. Valve dilation. The balloon catheter is inflated and de-flated by hand with continuous monitoring of arterial pressure and cardiac rhythm. The patient should be observed carefully for syncope and seizures during brief but severe hypotension. Several inflations are performed until disappearance of the balloon indentation or "waist." Before each inflation the arterial pressure and pulmonary artery oxygen saturation (monitored with an oximetric pulmonary catheter) should return to baseline.

Final Result. After a satisfactory reduction in LV-aortic gradient (≤30 mm Hg) and increase in valve area (≥25%

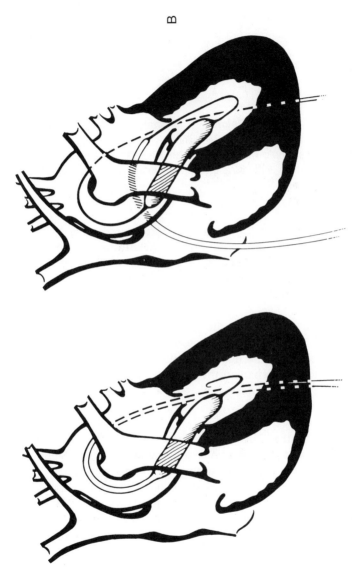

Fig. 9-23 A diagram of two techniques of aortic balloon valvuloplasty. **A,** The retrograde approach. **B,** The antegrade, transseptal approach.

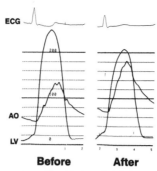

Fig. 9-24 Simultaneous aortic *(Ao)* and left ventricular *(LV)* pressures before and after aortic valvuloplasty in an 86-year-old woman, showing marked reduction in aortic valve gradient and increase in aortic valve area from 0.4 to 0.9 cm^2.

of baseline), the procedure is terminated (Fig. 9-24). Ascending aortography is indicated to determine the presence of postdilation aortic regurgitation. After reversal of anticoagulation with protamine sulfate, the balloon catheter and sheaths are removed, and the site is managed with manual compression.

After the procedure, the patient should be carefully monitored for bleeding, hematoma, pseudoaneurysm, and arteriovenous fistula. If no complications arise, patients can be ambulated and discharged the day after the procedure. *Note:* Significant aortic stenosis, albeit of a lesser severity, is still present after PBAV.

Complications. The most frequent complications of PBAV are vascular and usually involve the arterial entry site. Significant vascular trauma or bleeding occurs in approximately 5% to 20% of patients. Embolic phenomena are infrequent (1% to 2%). Procedural and total in-hospital mortality is low (4% to 7%). LV perforation, cardiac tamponade, and precipitation of severe aortic regurgitation are rare (<2%) but serious complications.

Follow-up. Although the average increase in valve area after PBAV is only approximately 0.5 cm^2, most patients report reduction in dyspnea and angina. In approximately 50% of patients with poor LV function, the ejection fraction improves during follow-up. The reduction in syncope is more difficult to document. The 1-year mortality is up to 25%, especially in the elderly and in patients with New York Heart Association class IV symptoms. Although this mortality figure seems more favorable than the natural history of untreated symptomatic calcific aortic stenosis (1-year mortality of 40% to 50%), a survival benefit with PBAV is not noted. The recurrence of symptoms and renarrowing of the valve are frequent occurrences in the first 6 to 12 months (50% of patients) after PBAV. The follow-up data emphasize the palliative nature of the procedure.

Pulmonary Valvuloplasty

Pulmonary stenosis (pulmonary valve gradient >50 mm Hg) can be easily treated with percutaneous balloon valvuloplasty. The technique is similar to mitral valvuloplasty. Femoral venous access is obtained. Guidewire placement across the pulmonic valve is followed by balloon dilation. Success is determined by the reduction of pulmonary gradient and reduced right ventricular pressure (Fig. 9-25).

Combined Coronary and Valvular Interventional Procedures. In selected patients combined interventional methods have been used successfully in the treatment of coexistent coronary and valvular disease or multivalvular disease. The sequence of the procedures should be determined so as to increase the patient's safety. In combined aortic stenosis and coronary artery disease it may be reasonable to perform PCI several days after PBAV has been performed successfully. In a patient with critical coronary stenosis, PCI may be done first to avoid significant myocardial ischemia in case of profound hypotension, which may occur during PBAV. In combined aortic stenosis and mitral stenosis the aortic stenosis is relieved first to avoid the possibility of increasing diastolic loading with worsened aortic gradient as a result of increased stroke volume.

Fig. 9-26 is a summary of uses of various coronary interventional techniques.

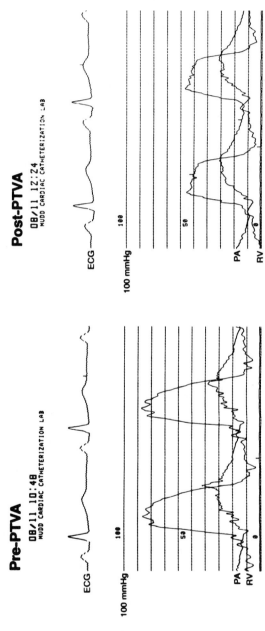

Fig. 9-25 In a patient with pulmonic stenosis, right ventricular *(RV)* pressure is reduced from 80 to 50 mm Hg after a single-balloon technique of pulmonic valvuloplasty. *PA,* Pulmonary artery pressure.

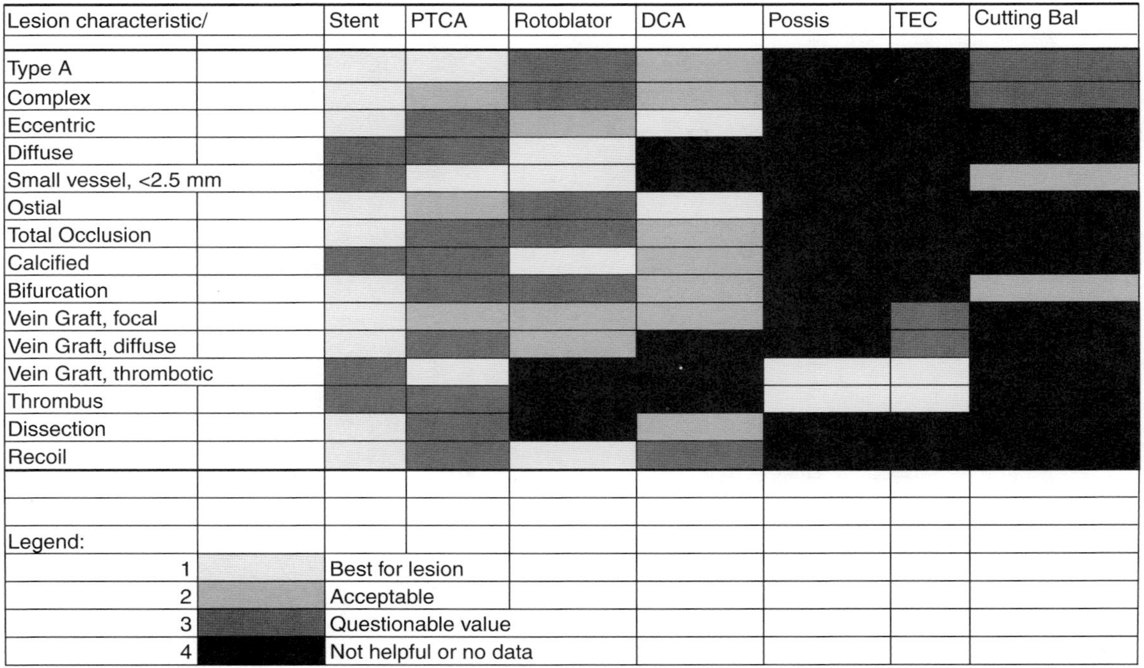

Fig. 9-26 Scheme for niche application of coronary interventional procedures. *DCA,* Directional coronary atherectomy; *Possis,* Anjiojet thrombus aspirator; *PTCA,* percutaneous transluminal coronary angioplasty; *TEC,* transluminal extraction catheter. Shading in boxes denotes best niche uses.

Suggested Readings

Albertal M, Voskuil M, Piek JJ, et al: Coronary flow velocity reserve after percutaneous interventions is predictive of periprocedural outcome, *Circulation* 105:1573-1578, 2002.

Baim DS, Grossman W, editors: *Grossman's cardiac catheterization, angiography, and intervention,* 6th ed, Philadelphia, 2000, Lippincott Williams & Wilkins.

Columbo A: *Techniques in coronary artery stenting,* London, 2000, Martin Dunitz.

Cura FA, Bhatt DL, Lincoff AM, et al: Pronounced benefit of coronary stenting and adjunctive platelet glycoprotein IIb/IIIa inhibition in complex atherosclerotic lesions, *Circulation* 102:28-34, 2000.

Davidson CJ, Laskey WK, Hermiller JB, et al: Randomized trial of contrast media utilization in high-risk PTCA: the COURT trial, *Circulation* 101:2172-2177, 2000.

Grines C, Freed M, Safian RD: *The new manual of interventional cardiology,* Birmingham, Mich., 1996, Physicians' Press.

Gruntzig A, Sennig A, Siegenthaler WE: Nonoperative dilatation of coronary artery stenosis: percutaneous transluminal coronary angioplasty, *N Engl J Med* 301:61-68, 1979.

Kern MJ: Coronary physiology revisited: practical insights from the cardiac catheterization laboratory, *Circulation* 101:1344-1351, 2000.

King SB III, Meier B: Interventional treatment of coronary heart disease and peripheral vascular disease, *Circulation* 102:IV81-IV86, 2000.

Nissen SE, Yock P: Intravascular ultrasound: novel pathophysiological insights and current clinical applications, *Circulation* 103:604-616, 2001.

Smith SC Jr, Dove JT, Jacobs AK, et al: ACC/AHA guidelines for percutaneous coronary intervention (revision of the 1993 PTCA Guidelines)—executive summary: a report of the American College of Cardiology/American Heart Association task force on practice guidelines (committee to revise the 1993 guidelines for percutaneous transluminal coronary angioplasty) endorsed by the Society for Cardiac Angiography and Interventions, *Circulation* 103:3019-3041, 2001.

Teirstein PS, Kuntz RE: New frontiers in interventional cardiology: intravascular radiation to prevent restenosis, *Circulation* 104:2620-2626, 2001.

Williams DO, Holubkov R, Yeh W, et al: Percutaneous coronary intervention in the current era compared with 1985-1986: the National Heart, Lung, and Blood Institute registries, *Circulation* 102:2945-2951, 2000.

10

DOCUMENTATION IN THE CARDIAC CATHETERIZATION LABORATORY

Anne Bradley

HEALTH CARE QUALITY STANDARDS TO REDUCE MEDICAL MALPRACTICE

Medical malpractice actions are frequently initiated as a result of unresolved anger and frustration on the part of the patient. Time and time again, statements such as "no one would answer my questions," "no one took time to explain anything," and "no one returned my calls" are made. At a plaintiff's deposition the defense counsel awaits the disclosure that indicates the underlying motivation that provoked the patient to become a plaintiff. The plaintiff, after the initiation of the lawsuit, sits confident in the expectation that "they'll answer my questions now," "they'll explain it all to me now," or "they'll return this call."

The best approach to avoiding litigation is to always keep the lines of communication open between the provider (physician, nurse, technologist) and the patient. The provider must take the time to let the patient know he or she is important to the provider.

An Institute of Medicine report quoted rates estimating that medical errors kill 44,000 to 98,000 people a year in U.S. hospitals. At 44,000 deaths a year, medical errors would be the eighth leading cause of death in the United States. This loss of lives is staggering. The response from the health care industry has been to improve the quality of health care and patient safety by changing procedural systems. Changing procedures, rather than focusing on human error, helps to ensure that the processes practitioners follow prevent medical errors from continuing to occur. Maintaining the legibility of entries into patient records and the uniformity of the medical care within an institution has proved to prevent errors. The legibility of a health care provider's entry into a patient's record is of paramount importance, which explains the increasing use of electronic medical records, personal data assistants, and medical software that immediately identifies drug interactions. Many medication errors result because a medical record entry is not clear and is misinterpreted. The use of these tools not only affords the patient a better quality of care, but also provides health care professionals safeguards against professional liability lawsuits.

Although written communication in the medical record is important, it is equally important that there is open communication between the health care provider and the patient and the patient's family. Letting the patient know that he or she is important to the health care provider is an integral part of good health care. This chapter assists the health care professional in documenting the health care services that were provided in the patient's medical record.

MEDICAL RECORD: GENERAL POINTS

Despite efforts of health care providers to deliver the highest quality patient care and remain available and approachable to patients, litigation will continue to be initiated. The importance of an accurate and legible medical record in protecting the interests of patients, physicians, and staff cannot be underestimated. The reasons are twofold. First, this record may serve as the basis for determining future medical management of the patient. Illegible, imprecise, or unclear entries may result in medical error and injury to the patient. Second, the medical record forms the basis for either the patient's lawsuit or the medical staff's defense in a professional liability suit.

In most medical malpractice cases the medical record is not only entered into evidence, but is also a determining factor in the outcome of the litigation. Although the parties may introduce many types of evidence to support their respective positions, the medical record is often considered the most reliable, trustworthy, and unbiased piece of evidence because the record was made contemporaneously with the patient's care and before litigation.

The entire medical record, including radiographs, is generally maintained by the medical records department and is the property of the hospital or privately owned cardiac catheterization laboratory. Although the patient or the patient's legal representative or guardian has the legal right to access his or her medical record, each facility has specific policies governing access to medical records.

The information contained within the hospital record, because it was obtained in the course of providing service to a patient, is confidential except as otherwise provided by law. Medical information from the record or a copy of the record may be released only with the written consent of the patient or their legally authorized representative or guardian, court order, or duly executed subpoena.

The Health Insurance Portability and Accountability Act (HIPAA) also has an impact on patient information and how it is to be maintained. The new HIPAA regulations will have an impact on medical records because many medical records are being maintained electronically. Regulations have been passed by the Center for Medical and Medicaid Services to implement these new privacy regulations. Each facility should have policies and procedures in place for complying with these new regulations.

General Guidelines for Documentation

Proper charting in a medical record for the catheterization laboratory generally is no different than charting in all other areas of the hospital.

1. The most important aspect of documentation in the hospital record relates to handwriting and organization. The person making the entry should write legibly and in an organized fashion when making entries in the medical record. The person's signature and professional status (e.g., M.D., R.N., L.V.N., L.P.N., N.A.) should be included. An illegible record can serve as the basis for a lawsuit and result in a settlement or verdict for the plaintiff even though there may be no merit to the claim. An illegible and unorganized medical record has great impact when the attorney projects it on a screen to

the jury, magnified more than 100 times. It is easy for the jury to equate sloppy charting with poor care and side with the plaintiff.

2. Proper spelling, grammar, and punctuation should be used. These errors create an overall negative impression about the quality of care. Whenever in doubt, look it up. The patient's name should be on *every* sheet entered into the record.

3. Only symbols and abbreviations authorized by the facility should be used. The facility maintains and constantly updates its approved abbreviation list, keeping in mind that each symbol or abbreviation should have only *one* meaning.

4. The date, time, method of admission, and transfer or discharge of a patient from the facility should be charted. All valuables that are in the patient's possession and their disposition should be recorded on admission and discharge. The full name of the person receiving the valuables if they are sent home should be recorded.

5. The frequency of chart entries depends on the individual hospital's department policies, acuity of the patient, changes in the patient's condition, national and state standards, standards of the community, and common sense. Charting should occur as soon as possible to the time of the observation or care provided. Routine charting should include a concise and accurate record of the care administered, including pertinent observations, psychosocial and physical manifestations, incidents, unusual occurrences, abnormal behavior, treatments, intake and output, and vital signs.

6. Information in the medical record should reflect only accurate facts regarding the particular patient. Generalizations and speculation can be avoided by the charting of only what is seen, heard, felt, or smelled. Words such as inadvertently, unfortunately, appears, or resembles should not be used. The medical record is a legal document and is not the proper forum for dispute resolution. It is not the appropriate place to settle grudges with other personnel. The chart should not contain flippant or humorous remarks. The professionalism of

the hospital staff should be reflected in the medical record entries.

7. Charting should be done after the delivery of care, not before. Never make an entry in anticipation of something to be done. Only what has taken place, including accurate dates and times, should be charted. It is never appropriate to leave blank spaces on forms designated for chronologic, sequential notes.

8. If it is necessary to add an entry at a later time, the date and time of the entry and the date and time of the occurrence (e.g., 3/10/00 1015 hours charting for 3/8/00 0900 hours) should be clearly identified. For medication charting, hospital policy and procedures as to the method of recording the entry and explanation of why the drug was given late or not given should be followed.

9. All entries in the medical record must be made in permanent ink, and no portion of the medical record is to be obliterated, erased, altered, or destroyed. If a charting error is made, an appropriate way to correct the error is to draw one line through the entry and initial, date, and enter the time at which the correction is made. The reason for the correction should be noted and the correct information charted. *Note:* Most facilities have a policy that addresses the issue of charting errors.

10. At the time of discharge from the cardiac catheterization laboratory, the patient's status, including all teaching efforts and the response from the patient or family, should be noted. All take-home instructions and take-home medications, prescriptions, or equipment should be charted. The patient or their legal representative or guardian should acknowledge the receipt of hand-written or preprinted instructions in writing, and a copy kept in the record.

11. Charting should not be done routinely for another person. *During emergency situations*, such as a cardiac arrest, one person should be designated to be in charge of making a detailed account. The record should document all treatments, medications, responses of the patient, and personnel involved in the emergency

situation. The cosigning of someone else's note generally presumes agreement with the information contained in the note.

MINIMUM DOCUMENTATION IN THE CATHETERIZATION LABORATORY

Minimum documentation includes the following:

1. Patient identifying information
2. Date and time of admission and discharge
3. Vital signs
4. Weight of patient (self-reported generally acceptable)
5. Time of last meal
6. Last menstrual period when applicable
7. Allergy status
8. Current medications, including medications taken in the last 24 hours
9. Previous health history
10. Laboratory and radiology tests
11. All medications and intravenous fluids administered
12. Response to medications
13. Mode of arrival and departure
14. Notification of the physician and the actual time of arrival
15. Discharge assessment
16. Discharge instructions
17. Disposition of patient
18. Registered nurse on duty
19. Patient consent when applicable
20. The use of an interpreter when applicable and the name of that individual

CHARTING RECOMMENDATIONS FOR OUTPATIENT CATHETERIZATION

Charting recommendations for outpatient catheterization include the following:

1. A complete assessment of the patient on admission to the outpatient catheterization unit, including vital signs
2. The identity of anyone who accompanied the patient and the arrangements made to transport the patient home on discharge
3. Allergies

4. Consent forms that have been completed properly; in the event the patient indicates he or she has not been fully informed and has additional questions, the physician should be contacted immediately, and documentation should be made to that effect

5. Information about procedure treatments, preparations, or medications administered and the response of the patient

6. Patient history and physical and preoperative diagnosis data, which must be on the chart before any procedure

7. Completed reports or necessary laboratory tests; notification to the physician of abnormal laboratory values

8. Information about the patient's compliance with preprocedure instructions and details of notification to the physician if the patient states otherwise

9. A completed catheterization laboratory record is required as part of the inpatient medical record

10. Complete postcatheterization assessment and vital signs, plus pertinent observations recorded to indicate that the patient is alert and without postoperative complications before discharge

11. If discharge criteria are used to determine that the patient is stable for discharge, documentation of observations that the criteria have been met

12. Written after-care instructions given to the patient; the patient should sign a written statement that he or she has received a copy of the instructions and understands them

13. The full name of the person who accompanied the patient on discharge and an indication of the method by which the patient departed

14. A discharge note that includes a thorough assessment of the physical and psychosocial status of the patient

15. Any complications that occurred during or after the procedure, documented in a factual, objective manner; an incident report or quality assurance monitoring form should be completed, but no mention should be made of such reports in the medical record

16. Details of any arrangements made for transfer to inpatient status, including the method of transfer plus

the names and titles of the persons accompanying the patient during transfer

17. Documentation of notification to the physician during the recovery period, to include details of the patient's condition as reported and any responsive measures taken

Techniques for Preventing Medication Errors

To prevent medication errors, the following techniques are recommended:

1. Calculate dosages on paper in written form
2. Give what is poured and pour what is given
3. Be alert to drug name similarities (e.g., quinine and quinidine, Maalox and Marax, Dilantin and Dilaudid, meperidine and Methergine)
4. The dosage ranges of the drugs administered should be known
5. When taking telephone orders, drug names should be confirmed by spelling them back to the physician
6. Do not become distracted when preparing medications
7. Listen to the patients; if they question the route, time, or medication being administered to them, double check the physician's order
8. The most recent package insert data for drugs used should be known
9. Medication expiration dates should always be checked
10. "Look-alike" medications should not be stocked on the same shelf (i.e., potassium chloride, sodium chloride)
11. Needles that are the appropriate size for the drug to be administered and for the size of the patient should be used

DOCUMENTATION FOR MEDICAL TREATMENT PROBLEMS OR COMPLICATIONS: EVENTS REQUIRING AN INCIDENT REPORT

Each Joint Commission on Accreditation of Health Care Organizations (JCAHO)–accredited facility should have a policy outlining the requirement of incident and occurrence reporting. Professional health care providers must be aware of their professional liability insurance carrier's reporting requirements and ensure that adverse events, which may give rise to liability, are reported in a timely fashion.

Generally an incident or occurrence is defined as an unanticipated or unexpected event involving a patient that resulted in or may have resulted in an injury to the patient. The JCAHO has identified sentinel events as unexpected occurrences involving death or serious physical or psychological injury or the risk thereof. Serious injury specifically includes loss of limb or function. The event or the risk thereof includes any process variation for which a recurrence would carry a significant chance of a serious adverse outcome. Such events are called sentinel because they signal the need for immediate investigation and response. These events include the following:

1. Suicide of a patient in specified setting
2. Infant abduction or discharge to the wrong family
3. Rape
4. Hemolytic transfusion reaction with major blood group incompatibilities
5. Surgery on the wrong patient or wrong body part
6. Any patient death, paralysis, coma, or other major permanent loss of function associated with a medication error
7. Any suicide of a patient in a setting where the patient is housed around-the-clock, including suicides from elopement
8. Any elopement (i.e., unauthorized departure) of a patient from an around-the-clock care setting resulting in a temporally related death (suicide or homicide) or major permanent loss of function
9. Any procedure on the wrong patient, wrong side of the body, or wrong organ
10. Any intrapartum (related to the birth process) maternal death

"Near miss" is a term used to describe any process variation that did not affect the outcome but for which a recurrence carries a significant chance of a serious adverse outcome. Such a "near miss" falls within the scope of the definition of a sentinel event but outside the scope of sentinel events that are subject to review by the JCAHO under its Sentinel Event Policy. Examples include the following:

1. Medication errors that result in a change in level of care or extended hospital stay

2. Falls that result in an extended hospital stay or rehabilitation
3. Blood transfusion errors that do *not* result in confirmed hemolytic transfusion reactions
4. Restraint injuries that require specific attention outside of the patient's condition or admitting diagnosis
5. Delays in treatment that result in extended hospital stays

The JCAHO has also implemented standards concerning the disclosure of these unanticipated events to patients and "requires that patients, and when appropriate, their families are informed about the outcomes of care, including unanticipated events." The new standards went into effect on July 1, 2001, and require providing patients with information regarding all results and outcomes from diagnostic testing and medical or surgical care as integral components of the treatment process. Although the JCAHO disclosure standards apply to accredited facilities, the accompanying intent provision rests the responsibility for discussions with patients on the professional health care practitioner.

Product Liability Issues in the Cardiac Catheterization Laboratory

In light of publicity surrounding the approval by the Food and Drug Administration (FDA) of newly developed medical devices and generic drugs, discussion of product liability issues in the catheterization laboratory is appropriate. Several areas have serious medicolegal implications, including equipment failure, adverse reactions to contrast media or medication, reuse of equipment, and product recalls.

EQUIPMENT FAILURE

Under ideal conditions equipment can malfunction, devices can fail, and dye or drugs may cause adverse reactions. The result is often immediate or eventual harm to the patient. When such events occur, the first responsibility is appropriate intervention to address the effects of the event on the patient. In the aftermath of the crisis other steps must be taken in the interests of professional responsibility and potential liability. Essential to the entire process is careful and complete documentation of the occurrence, the effect on the patient, the treatment, and the response to treatment.

Hospitals are responsible for reporting adverse incidents caused by or attributed to a medical device's failure or malfunction pursuant to the Safe Medical Devices Act (SMDA) of 1990 (Public Law 101-629, 104 Stat. 4511 [1990]; and 21 U.S.C. 3601 [1990]). The SMDA requires that hospitals report within 30 days certain device-specific and patient-specific information to the manufacturer of a device that caused or contributed to the serious illness, serious injury, or death of a hospital patient. In some situations this information must be reported to the FDA. The SMDA requires that a hospital conduct an investigation of such incidents to determine the cause of the incident (i.e., whether the incident was attributable to device malfunction or failure or some combination of this and user error) and to identify the specific patient and device involved. The hospital is required to establish policies and procedures for implementing the requirements of the SMDA and to identify an individual who will be responsible for coordinating incident investigation, incident reporting, and in-service training and to serve as facility liaison with manufacturers, the FDA, and any other agencies involved in incident reporting. The hospital's risk manager and, in some cases, attorney should be notified and consulted in the event of a device-related incident. Apart from the requirement of the SMDA, it is advisable to record equipment or substance descriptions and such identifiers as serial or lot numbers to facilitate identification of devices or substances that may cause adverse incidents at a later time.

In the case of a device-related incident or equipment failure or malfunction not involving a patient, the equipment must be removed from use at once, sequestered in a safe place, reported to the supervisor, and assessed by a reputable outside specialist as to cause of malfunction or failure. Before or during assessment the device should not be repaired or altered. It is essential that the device is not altered until a full investigation of the incident is conducted and the device manufacturer or the FDA has had an opportunity to conduct an investigation these entities may require. It is advisable not to surrender or release the device to any third party, even an outside specialist or the device manufacturer, without the express agreement that the device will be maintained in the condition in which it was received.

If a piece of equipment has been serviced, maintained, or calibrated to the manufacturer's instructions, and if it was being used properly for the purpose for which it was intended, the liability for the consequences of failure or malfunction is attributable to the manufacturer rather than the health care provider. Records must be maintained to prove this.

Intravascular Device Failure

When problems with catheters and other intravascular devices arise, such as separation or breakage, all portions should be saved in a secure place. When feasible, immediate contact with the manufacturer or distributor should be made to determine whether the device in question was contained in a defective lot or batch, or whether a flaw in design or production may have caused or contributed to the device's failure or malfunction. If time and the situation allow, a different lot of the same make or a different manufacturer's product should be obtained for use until it has been determined that it is safe to use the same type that caused the incident.

Medication Reactions

Reactions to contrast media or medication require notation of lot numbers and other identifying information and contact with the manufacturer or distributor. Similarly, use of another lot or brand should be standard protocol, when possible, until the problem is identified. It is good practice to routinely include the lot numbers of products such as contrast media in the catheterization laboratory record because adverse effects are not always immediate; without that information in the record, it is often impossible to determine the source of the problem. The hospital should also be familiar with and in compliance with any state and federal law that requires the reporting of adverse incidents related to the use of the products.

It is the conscientious reporting of product hazards and deficiencies that enables the FDA and other agencies and services to identify problems and issue warnings and recalls that ultimately protect other patients from injury and death. These agencies have a duty to observe certain standards of confidentiality regarding patient-identifiable information that may be contained in such reports.

Hand in hand with the responsibility for reporting goes the responsibility for responding effectively to reports received regarding product warnings and recalls. In too many organizations such reports are either ignored or erroneously routed, and the information never reaches the areas or individuals affected.

The hospital must establish and follow policies and procedures that designate an individual as responsible for coordinating the investigation and reporting of devices and other products' adverse incidents pursuant to existing law for communicating warning and recall information and for ensuring that appropriate action is taken in response to such information. Continued use of a product after a warning or recall has been issued exposes health care professionals and the organization to liability for adverse outcomes.

Catheter Reuse

A matter of concern addressed by several catheterization laboratory professionals is the reuse of catheters and other intravascular lines. Some individuals are being asked or required to reuse catheters by administrators or physician directors in the interest of cost containment. This equipment is expensive, and reimbursement is continually being reduced by government and private payers.

The dangers inherent in this practice cannot be overemphasized. First, if the packaging states "single use only" or similar wording, any reuse is contrary to manufacturer's instructions. Repeated use is probably unsafe, and if an adverse event occurs subsequent to such use, the user and hospital may be exposed to liability for negligence, exacerbated by the fact of reuse.

Although one may argue that a manufacturer's instruction regarding single patient use may be based on a profit motive, one must assume that the directive is based on the fact that it is neither safe nor prudent to reuse equipment so labeled. Amid the fact and the myth of this situation, it is ill advised to reuse catheters and other devices that, by definition, come in prolonged contact with human blood. Another significant contraindication for reuse is the potential for transmission of acquired immunodeficiency syndrome and other infectious disease.

Summary

Professionals must recognize that thorough documentation and communication are essential to providing the patient the safest and highest quality of care, not only through extraordinary skill and expertise, but also with the safest and most effective diagnostic and therapeutic equipment. All should be standard for the patient as part of the cardiac catheterization laboratory experience.

APPENDIXES

A

INVASIVE CARDIOVASCULAR EXAMINATION AND PROCEDURES

Table A-1

Invasive Cardiovascular Examinations and Procedures

1. Selective vessel and heart chamber pressure recording
2. Selective vessel and chamber blood sampling
   a. Oximetry, carboxy, oxyhemoglobin
   b. Blood gas analysis (pH, pCO_2, pO_2)
   c. Electrolyte content (where suitable equipment is available)
   d. Blood sampling for other diagnostic determinations
      (ACT, INR, HCT)
      (1) Renin and angiotensin levels
      (2) Blood cultures
3. Cardiac output studies
   a. Thermodilution
   b. Dye dilution indicators (e.g., green dye)
   c. Fick determinations
4. Oxygen consumption
   a. Flow-through steady state
   b. Closed system steady state or exercise or both
5. Shunt detection studies
   a. Right-sided heart catheterization with multiple oxygen saturations, Qp/Qs
      determination
   b. Dye curves
6. Selective contrast angiography
   a. Coronary artery studies
   b. Left ventriculogram
   c. Selective heart chamber and vessel studies for congenital heart disease
   d. Peripheral vascular angiograms

ACT, Activated clotting time; *HCT,* hematocrit; *INR,* international normalized ratio.

Continued

Table A-1

Invasive Cardiovascular Examinations and Procedures—cont'd

Note: All of the above-listed angiograms may be performed in conjunction with radiographic film devices, including single and biplane cinefluoroscopy, cut-film rapid-sequence angiography, and rapid-sequence spot film cameras (70/105 mm) or digital imaging and are performed with the assistance and direction of a qualified physician.

7. Electrophysiologic studies
   a. Intracardiac atrial and ventricular pacing for zonal refractory periods, activation times, arrhythmia inducibility, arrhythmia, and accessory bypass tract detection
   b. Intracardiac mapping
8. Temporary and permanent transvenous pacemaker insertion
9. Pericardiocentesis
10. Drug response studies
    a. Adenosine-acetylcholine coronary artery studies
    b. Pulmonary resistance studies
    c. 100% oxygen inhalation studies
    d. Arrhythmia suppression during electrophysiologic studies
    e. Ergonovine for coronary vasospasm
11. Pulmonary arterial wedge catheter placement
12. Balloon atrial septostomy and atrial septal defect closure
13. Percutaneous transluminal coronary interventions
    a. Coronary arteries and grafts
    b. Peripheral arteries
14. Retrieval of foreign body from the heart or great vessels
15. Transseptal puncture procedures
16. Left ventricular transthoracic punctures
17. Placement of arterial or central venous lines
18. Transluminal septal ablation for HOCM
19. Intraaortic balloon pump counterpulsation
20. Balloon valvuloplasty of pulmonary, mitral, or aortic valves

Any of the previous procedures may be combined with either diagnostic or supportive medications and therapeutic interventions.

HOCM, Hypertrophic obstructive cardiomyopathy.

Table A-2

Orientation to the Holding Area

Areas of Knowledge	Skills Acquired
ECG	
Application of electrodes	_____
12-lead ECG	_____
Operation of Portable Monitors	
Functions	_____
NIBP	_____
ECG	_____
Oximetric	_____
Setting intervals	_____
Alarms	_____
Blood Pressures	
Automatic cuff	_____
Manual cuff	_____
Stethoscope	_____
Assessment of Pulses	
Properly marking pedals	_____
Use of Doppler	_____
Compression of Femoral Artery	
Manual hold	_____
C-clamp	_____
Femo-Stop	_____
Groin Preparation	
Provide privacy for patient	_____
Proper place of towel for draping	_____
Shaving groin area	_____
Razors	_____
Clippers	_____
Location of Emergency Equipment	
Crash cart	_____
O_2	_____
Suction	_____
Defibrillator	_____
Medications kept in holding area	_____
Atropine	_____
Nitroglycerin	_____
Knowledge of CCL Permits	
Surgical consent for cardiac catheterization	_____
History and physical examination for conscious sedation	_____

ECG, Electrocardiogram; *NIBP*, noninvasive blood pressure.

Continued

Table A-2

Orientation to the Holding Area—cont'd

Areas of Knowledge	Skills Acquired
Storage of Supplies	
IV fluids and supplies	_____
Urinals	_____
Bedpans	_____
Dressings	_____
Medications	_____
Band-Aids	_____
Suture removal kits	_____
Cups and straws	_____
Gauze and tape	_____
Linens	_____
Selection of IV Lines	
Diabetic patient	_____
Routine	_____
Laboratory Tests	
CCL standards	_____
Potassium	_____
Creatinine	_____
BUN	_____
Blood glucose	_____
PT	_____
INR	_____
PTT	_____
H&H	_____
Lab req	_____
Enter lab into Meditech	_____
Neurologic Checks	
Speech	_____
Orientation	_____
Pupils	_____
Grasps	_____
Movement	_____
Discharge Criteria	
Vital signs stable	_____
Groin site stable	_____
Patient in stable condition	_____

BUN, Blood urea nitrogen; *CCL,* cardiac catheterization laboratory; *H&H,* hematocrit and hemoglobin; *PT,* prothombin time; *PTT,* partial thromboplastin time.

Table A-3

Cardiac Catheterization Skills Checklist

Name	No Experience	Needs Update	Proficient
Emergency Equipment			
IABP	_____	_____	_____
Intubation equipment	_____	_____	_____
Defibrillator	_____	_____	_____
External pacemaker (Zoll)	_____	_____	_____
Temporary pacemaker	_____	_____	_____
Oxygen and airway	_____	_____	_____
Suction	_____	_____	_____
EMERGENCY MEDICATIONS	_____	_____	_____
CODE MANAGEMENT	_____	_____	_____
HEMODYNAMIC MONITORING	_____	_____	_____
ECG INTERPRETATION	_____	_____	_____
Circulation Position			
Use of Acist injector	_____	_____	_____
Use of cardiac output computer	_____	_____	_____
Familiarity with cardiac catheterization supplies	_____	_____	_____
Charting nurses' notes	_____	_____	_____
Scrub Position			
Use of x-ray equipment	_____	_____	_____
Sterile technique	_____	_____	_____
Sterile field preparation	_____	_____	_____
Panning table-angulation of image intensifier	_____	_____	_____
Recording Position			
Use of hemodynamic monitoring system	_____	_____	_____
Archival System			
General knowledge of cineless processing	_____	_____	_____
Retrieval of patient information	_____	_____	_____

ECG, Electrocardiogram; *IABP*, intraaortic balloon pump.   *Continued*

Table A-3

Cardiac Catheterization Skills Checklist—cont'd

Name	No Experience	Needs Update	Proficient
General			
Compression of arterial punctures	_____	_____	_____
Radiation safety	_____	_____	_____
General infection control	_____	_____	_____
Cardiac anatomy	_____	_____	_____
ACLS certified	_____	_____	_____
BLS certified	_____	_____	_____
Other certifications	_____	_____	_____

ACLS, Advanced cardiac life support; *BLS,* basic life support.

Table A-4

Catheter Size Specifications

French Size	Inches	mm	cm
1.0	0.013	0.33	0.03
2.0	0.026	0.67	0.07
3.0	0.039	1.00	0.10
4.0	0.053	1.33	0.13
5.0	0.066	1.67	0.17
6.0	0.079	2.00	0.20
7.0	0.092	2.33	0.23
8.0	0.105	2.67	0.27
9.0	0.118	3.00	0.30
10.0	0.131	3.33	0.34
11.0	0.144	3.67	0.37
12.0	0.158	4.00	0.40

Note: 1 F = 0.33 mm; 2 F = 0.67 mm; 3 F = 1.00 mm.

HEART DIAGRAMS

Previous   CABG: ____YES ____NO
Previous   PTCA: ____YES ____NO

1. Stable Angina: _____
   CHC   I   II   III   IV

2. Unstable Angina: _____

3. Acute MI: _____

THIS IS A PRELIMINARY ESTIMATE
FROM THE TV SCREEN.
A FINAL FILM ANALYSIS WILL FOLLOW.

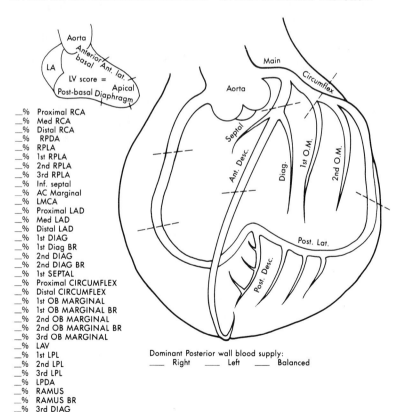

__% Proximal RCA
__% Med RCA
__% Distal RCA
__% RPDA
__% RPLA
__% 1st RPLA
__% 2nd RPLA
__% 3rd RPLA
__% Inf. septal
__% AC Marginal
__% LMCA
__% Proximal LAD
__% Med LAD
__% Distal LAD
__% 1st DIAG
__% 1st Diag BR
__% 2nd DIAG
__% 2nd DIAG BR
__% 1st SEPTAL
__% Proximal CIRCUMFLEX
__% Distal CIRCUMFLEX
__% 1st OB MARGINAL
__% 1st OB MARGINAL BR
__% 2nd OB MARGINAL
__% 2nd OB MARGINAL BR
__% 3rd OB MARGINAL
__% LAV
__% 1st LPL
__% 2nd LPL
__% 3rd LPL
__% LPDA
__% RAMUS
__% RAMUS BR
__% 3rd DIAG

Dominant Posterior wall blood supply:
____ Right   ____ Left   ____ Balanced

Fig. B-1

Name:_____   Date: _____
Age: _____   Cath #:_____
WT: _____
HT: _____
BSA: _____

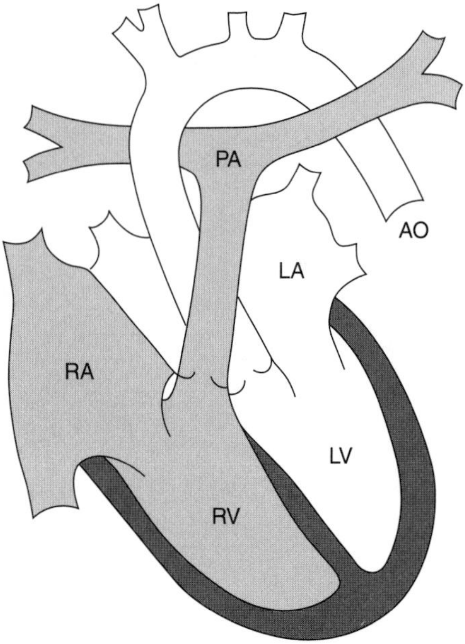

<u>TD:</u>
CO = _____ L/Min
CI = _____ L/Min/M^2

<u>Fick:</u>
CO = _____ L/Min
CI = _____ L/Min/M^2

SVR = _____ dynes/sec/cm^{-5}

PVR = _____ dynes/sec/cm^{-5}

TPG = _____ mm Hg

Fig. B-2

FUNCTIONAL ANATOMY OF THE HEART

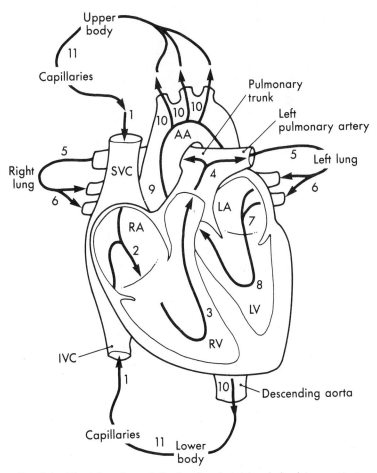

Fig. C-1 Blood flow through the heart and peripheral circulatory system. *AA*, Aortic arch; *IVC*, inferior vena cava; *LA*, left atrium; *LV*, left ventricle; *RA*, right atrium; *RV*, right ventricle; *SVC*, superior vena cava.

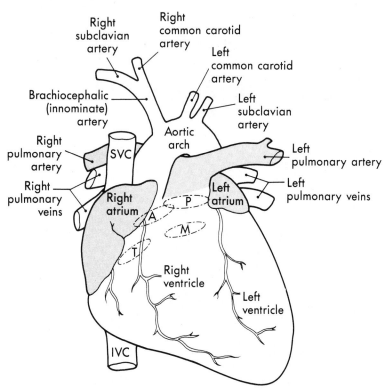

Fig. C-2 Anterior view of the heart and major vessels. *A*, aortic; *IVC*, inferior vena cava; *M*, mitral; *P*, pulmonic; *SVC*, superior vena cava; *T*, tricuspid.

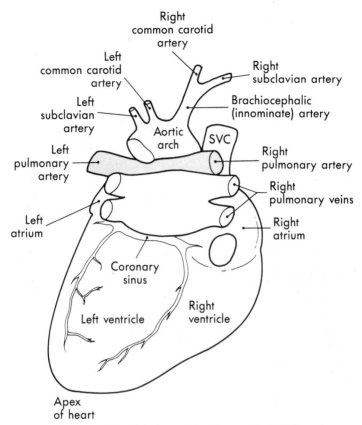

Fig. C-3   Posterior view of the heart and major vessels. *SVC,* Superior vena cava.

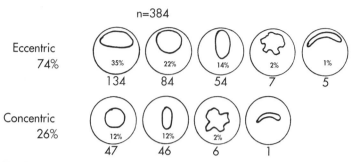

n=384

Eccentric
74%

Concentric
26%

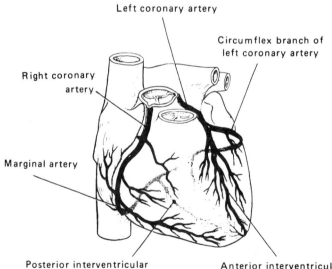

Fig. C-4   Distribution and configuration of coronary stenoses. (From Santamore WP, Corin WJ: *Trends Cardiovasc Med* 2:189-196, 1992.)

Fig. C-5   Coronary anatomy. (From Langley LL, et al: *Dynamic anatomy and physiology,* ed 5, New York, 1980, McGraw-Hill.)

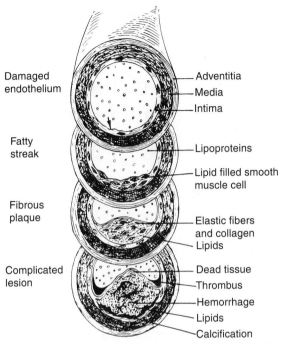

Damaged endothelium

- Adventitia
- Media
- Intima

Fatty streak

- Lipoproteins
- Lipid filled smooth muscle cell

Fibrous plaque

- Elastic fibers and collagen
- Lipids

Complicated lesion

- Dead tissue
- Thrombus
- Hemorrhage
- Lipids
- Calcification

Fig. C-6 Evolution of an atherosclerotic coronary plaque. (From Lewis SM, Collier IC: *Medical-surgical nursing: assessment and management of clinical problems,* St Louis, 1996, Mosby.)

TABLES OF UNITS, CALCULATIONS, AND CONVERSIONS

Table D-1

Guidelines for Location of Catheter Tip for Zero Leveling

Fraction of the AP Distance (from back to front)	Catheter Tip Location Within the Chest
0.75	Right ventricle and apex of the left ventricle
0.70	Anterior wall of the left ventricle
0.65	Middle of the left ventricle and the right atrium
0.60	Posterior wall of the left ventricle
0.55	Mitral valve, superior vena cava, pulmonary trunk
0.50	Left atrium

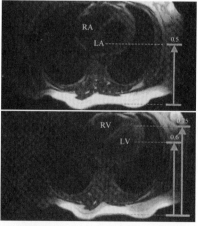

Fig. D-1 Computed tomography of chest demonstrating position of heart chambers. *RA,* Right atrium; *RV,* right ventricle; *LA,* left atrium; *LV,* left ventricle. (From Brown LK, Goff DC, Hamilton CA, et al: *Am J Cardiol* 86:121, 2000.)

Table D-2

Normal Left Ventriculogram Ejection Phase Indexes

	Average	SE	Range
Sinus Beat			
Ejection fraction*	0.71	0.01	0.64-.077
Ejection fraction†	67.3	1.0	62-72
Ejection vector*	1.19	0.03	1.28-1.07
End diastolic volume (ml/m^2)	70.4	3.9	54-89
End systolic volume (ml/m^2)	20.3	0.7	17-24
Postextrasystolic Potentiation Beat			
Ejection fraction*	0.82	0.01	0.76-0.85
Ejection fraction†	69.9	1.9	64-79
Ejection vector*	1.39	0.03	1.26-1.50
End diastolic volume (ml/m^2)	78.5	3.2	68-90
End systolic volume (ml/m^2)	14.2	0.7	11-17

From Pujadas G: *Coronary angiography in the medical and surgical treatment of ischemic heart disease*, New York, 1980, McGraw-Hill.
*As fraction of end-diastolic volume.
†Percentage of total stroke output is 50.

Table D-3

Oxygen Consumption Per Body Surface Area in (ml/min)m² by Sex, Age and Heart Rate

Age (yr)	Heart Rate (beats/min)												
	50	60	70	80	90	100	110	120	130	140	150	160	170
Male Patients													
3				155	159	163	167	171	175	178	182	186	190
4			149	152	156	160	163	168	171	175	179	182	186
6		141	144	148	151	155	159	162	167	171	174	178	181
8		136	141	145	148	152	156	159	163	167	171	175	178
10	130	134	139	142	146	149	153	157	160	165	169	172	176
12	128	132	136	140	144	147	151	155	158	162	167	170	174
14	127	130	134	137	142	146	149	153	157	160	165	169	172
16	125	129	132	136	141	144	148	152	155	159	162	167	
18	124	127	131	135	139	143	147	150	154	157	161	166	
20	123	126	130	134	137	142	145	149	153	156	160	165	
25	120	124	127	131	135	139	143	147	150	154	157		
30	118	122	125	129	133	136	141	145	148	152	155		
35	116	120	124	127	131	135	139	143	147	150			
40	115	119	122	126	130	133	137	141	145	149			

Female Patients

3				150	153	157	161	165	169	172	176	180	183
4			141	145	149	152	156	159	163	168	171	175	179
6		130	134	137	142	146	149	153	156	160	165	168	172
8		125	129	133	136	141	144	148	152	155	159	163	167
10	118	122	125	129	133	136	141	144	148	152	155	159	163
12	115	119	122	126	130	133	137	141	145	149	152	156	160
14	112	116	120	123	127	131	134	133	143	146	150	153	157
16	109	114	118	121	125	128	132	136	140	144	148	151	
18	107	111	116	119	123	127	130	134	137	142	146	149	
20	106	109	114	118	121	125	128	132	136	140	144	148	
25	102	106	109	114	118	121	125	128	132	136	140		
30	99	103	106	110	115	118	122	125	129	133			
35	97	100	104	107	111	116	119	123	127	130			
40	94	98	102	105	109	112	117	121	124	128			

From LaFarge CG, Meittinen OS: The estimation of oxygen consumption, *Cardiovasc Res* 4:23, 1970.

Table D-4

Dimensions and Units of Some Commonly Used Physical Quantities

Physical Quantity	Definition	Common Units	Dimensions
Mass	Not defined	gram (g)	M
Length	Not defined	centimeter (cm)	L
Time	Not defined	second (sec)	T
Area	Length squared	cm^2	L^2
Volume	Length cubed	cm^3	L^3
Density	Mass per unit of volume	g/cm^3	ML^{-3}
Velocity	Length per unit of time	cm/sec	LT^{-1}
Acceleration	Velocity per unit of time	cm/sec^2	LT^{-2}
Flow	Volume per unit of time	cm^3/sec	L^3T^{-1}
Force	Mass times acceleration	dyne or $g/cm/sec^2$	MLT^{-2}
Pressure	Force per unit of area	$dyne/cm^2$ or $g/cm/sec^2$	$ML^{-1}T^{-2}$
Resistance to flow	Pressure drop across a hydraulic segment per unit of flow	dyne sec cm^{-5}	$ML^{-5}T$
Work	Force times distance	erg or dyne cm or $g\ cm^2/sec^2$	ML^2T^{-2}
Power	Work per unit of time	dyne cm/sec or $g\ cm^2/sec^3$	ML^2T^{-3}

From Yan SS: *From cardiac catheterization data to hemodynamic parameters*, ed 3, Philadelphia, 1987, FA Davis.

Table D-5

Conversion Factors and Constants (Decimal Factors)

Multiples	Designation	Symbol	Submultiples	Designation	Symbol
10^{12}	tera-	T	10^{-12}	pico-	p
10^{9}	giga-	G	10^{-9}	nano-	n
10^{6}	mega	M	10^{-6}	micro-	μ
10^{3}	kilo	K	10^{-3}	milli-	m
10^{2}	hecto-	h	10^{-2}	centi-	c
10		dk	10^{-1}		d

Length

1 meter (m) = 10 decimeters = 100 centimeters (cm) = 1000 millimeters (mm) =
1.0936 yards (yd) = 3.2808 feet (ft) = 39.37 inches (in)

1 kilometer (km) = 1000 m = 0.6214 mile (mi)

1 cm = 0.3937 in

1 in = 2.54 cm

1 ft = 30.48 cm = 0.3048 m

1 mi = 1.6093 km = 1609.3 m = 1760 yd = 5280 ft

1 micron (m) = 0.000001 m = 10^{-6} m

1 millimicron (mm) = 0.000000001 m = 10^{-9} m

Weight

1 pound (lb) = 0.454 kilogram (kg)

1 kg = 2.204 lb

Temperature

$$C = \frac{5°(F-32°)}{9}$$

$$F = \frac{(C \times 9) + 32°}{5}$$

Pressure

1 atmosphere = 760 mm Hg = 14.6 pounds/in^2

1 cm $H_2O \times 0.735$ = 1 mm Hg

1 cm Hg $\times 1.36$ = 1 cm H_2O

C, Celsius; *F,* Fahrenheit

Table D-6

Normal Pressures in Heart and Great Vessels*

Pressure (mm Hg)	Average	Range
Right Atrium		
Mean	2.8	1-5
a wave	5.6	2.5-7
c wave	3.8	1.5-6
x wave	1.7	0-5
v wave	4.6	2-7.5
y wave	2.4	0-6
Right Ventricle		
Peak systolic	25	17-32
End-diastolic	4	1-7
Pulmonary Artery		
Mean	15	9-19
Peak systolic	25	17-32
End-diastolic	9	4-13
Pulmonary Artery Wedge		
Mean	9	4.5-13
Left Atrium		
Mean	7.9	2-12
a wave	10.4	4-16
v wave	12.8	6-21
Left Ventricle		
Peak systolic	130	90-140
End-diastolic	8.7	5-12
Brachial Artery		
Mean	85	70-105
Peak systolic	130	90-140
End-diastolic	70	60-90

*Reference level = 10 cm above the spine of a recumbent subject.

Table D-7

Normal Average Values for Left Ventricular Parameters by Angiocardiography

Angiographic Method	No. Patients	Age Group	End-diastolic Volume (ml/m^2)	End-systolic Volume (ml/m^2)	Ejection Fraction	Wall Thickness (mm)
Biplane modified Arvidsson	3	Adults	95	36	0.63	7.7
Biplane Dodge area-length	16	Adults	70	24	0.67	10.9
Biplane Dodge area-length	6	Adults	79	29	0.67	8.5
Biplane modified Dodge	6	Adults	71	30	0.58	
Single plane cineangiogram (right anterior oblique)	5	Adults	104	31	0.70	
Biplane Arvidsson	9	Children	88	32	0.64	
Biplane cineangiographic	19	Children younger than 2 yr	42		0.68	
Biplane cineangiographic	37	Children older than 2 yr	73		0.63	

E

RADIOLOGIC CONFIGURATION
OF PROSTHETIC HEART VALVES

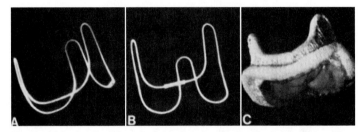

Fig. E-1 Carpentier-Edwards SupraAnnular Bioprosthesis. Aortic position: **A,** posteroanterior radiograph; **B** and **C,** left lateral view radiograph and photograph. One continuous narrow wireform outlines each of the three stents and that portion of the base ring between stents. Although superficially similar to the radiographic silhouettes of the Carpentier-Edwards Bioprosthesis, in the SupraAnnular model the change of shape of the wireform as it shifts from base ring to stent is more gradual, giving the wire a gently curving appearance rather than a right-angle appearance. (From Mehlman DJ: *Circulation* 69:102, 1984.)

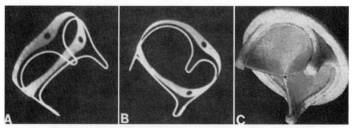

Fig. E-2 Carpentier-Edwards pericardial valve prosthesis. Mitral position: **A,** posteroanterior radiograph; **B** and **C,** left lateral radiograph and photograph. The base ring is marked by a flattened circular ring with three holes. The flattened ring does not extend into the stents as is seen in the Ionescu-Shiley xenograft. In addition, a narrow wireform outlines each of the three stents and the base ring between the stents. The wire curves gently between stent and base ring, similar to the Carpentier-Edwards SupraAnnular Bioprosthesis. (From Mehlman DJ: *Circulation* 69:102, 1984.)

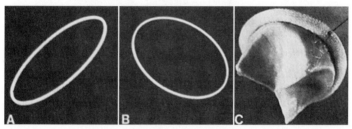

Fig. E-3 Hancock pericardial heart valve. Mitral position: **A,** posteroanterior radiograph; **B** and **C,** left lateral radiograph and photograph. The base ring is a narrow, circular, wirelike form. The remainder of the valve is radiolucent. The radiographic silhouette is similar to that of the Hancock porcine xenograft. (From Mehlman DJ: *Circulation* 69:102, 1984.)

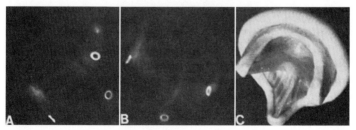

Fig. E-4 Hancock II porcine xenograft. Mitral position: **A,** posteroanterior radiograph; **B** and **C,** left lateral radiograph and photograph. The base ring and stents are radiolucent. Three tiny circular rings mark the distal external aspects of the three stents. (From Mehlman DJ: *Circulation* 69:102, 1984.)

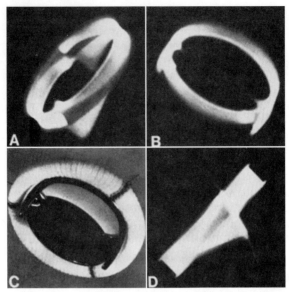

Fig. E-5 Omniscience prosthetic heart valve. Mitral position: **A,** postero-anterior radiograph; **B** and **C,** left lateral radiograph and photograph; **D,** oblique radiograph demonstrating disc on edge. Emerging from the wide base ring are two low-profile struts that are fastened to the base ring along their length. Although reminiscent of the silhouette of the Lillehei-Kaster prosthesis, the struts are shorter and form a much lower profile. On routine chest radiographs the disc is likely to be radiolucent. The disc of the Omniscience prosthesis (unlike the Lillehei-Kaster) is radiopaque when viewed on edge. (From Mehlman DJ: *Circulation* 69:102, 1984.)

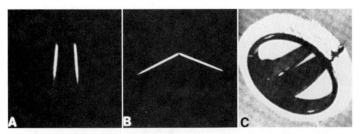

Fig. E-6 St. Jude Medical Valve. Mitral position: **A,** oblique radiograph demonstrating both discs on edge in the open position; **B,** oblique radiograph demonstrating both discs on edge in the closed position; **C,** left lateral photograph. On routine chest radiographs the St. Jude Medical Valve is likely to be radiolucent. When viewed on edge, the discs are radiopaque. The base ring is radiolucent. (From Mehlman DJ: *Circulation* 69:102, 1984.)

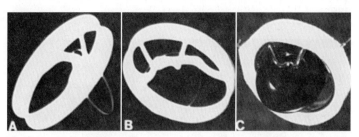

Fig. E-7 Bjork-Shiley cardiac valve prosthesis with ConvexoConcave disc. Mitral position: **A,** posteroanterior radiograph; **B** and **C,** radiograph and photograph. The radiographic silhouette is essentially the same as the Bjork-Shiley prosthesis with straight disc and incorporated disc marker. The flattened base ring is encircled by a groove. Emerging from the base ring toward its center are two eccentrically located U-shaped structures of unequal size. The radiolucent disc contains a narrow circular radiopaque disc marker that is seen from any projection. (From Mehlman DJ: *Circulation* 69:102, 1984.)

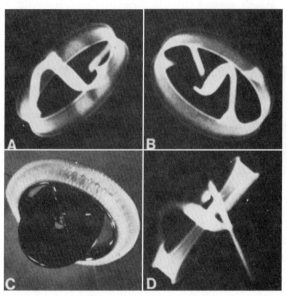

Fig. E-8 Medtronic Hall (formerly called Hall-Kaster) prosthetic heart valve. Mitral position: **A,** posteroanterior radiograph; **B** and **C,** left lateral radiograph and photograph; **D,** oblique radiograph demonstrating disc on edge. Four projections emerge from the base ring toward the center of the ring. Two short straight projections of equal size are on opposing sides of the base ring. A longer straight projection is perpendicular to the short projections. A large hooklike projection is opposite the long straight projection. On routine chest radiographs, the disc is likely to be radiolucent. When viewed on edge, the disc is radiopaque. (From Mehlman DJ: *Circulation* 69:102, 1984.)

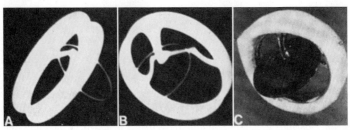

Fig. E-9 Bjork-Shiley integral monostrut cardiac valve prosthesis. Mitral position: **A,** posteroanterior radiograph; **B** and **C,** left lateral radiograph and photograph. The radiographic silhouette is similar to that of the Bjork-Shiley ConvexoConcave and Straight disc valves. The flattened base ring is encircled by a groove. Emerging from the base ring toward its center is a wide U-shaped structure. Perpendicular to the flattened portion of the U is a short straight projection with a very small hook or bulge on its end. The radiolucent disc contains a narrow circular radiopaque disc marker that is seen from any projection. (From Mehlman DJ: *Circulation* 69:102, 1984.)

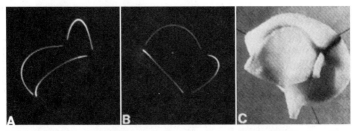

Fig. E-10 Ionescu-Shiley low profile pericardial xenograft. Mitral position: **A,** posteroanterior radiograph; **B** and **C,** left lateral radiograph and photograph. The base ring consists of three narrow wireform arcs, each length approximately one-third the circumference of the base ring. Adjoining arcs are separated by small radiolucent areas. The stents are radiolucent. (From Mehlman DJ: *Circulation* 69:102, 1984.)

F

BASIC ELECTROCARDIOGRAPHY

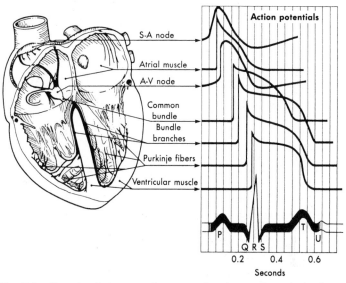

Fig. F-1 Genesis of electrocardiogram and pathways through the heart. (Modified from the CIBA Collection of Medical Illustrations, Vol. 5.)

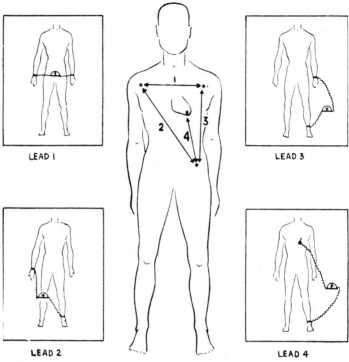

Fig. F-2 Standard limb leads and one precordial lead. (From Marriott HLJ: *Practical electrocardiography,* ed 7, Baltimore, 1983, Williams and Wilkins.)

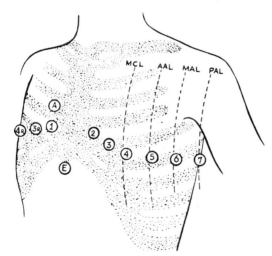

Fig. F-3 Precordial points for chest leads. (From Marriott HLJ: *Practical electrocardiography,* ed 7, Baltimore, 1983, Williams and Wilkins.)

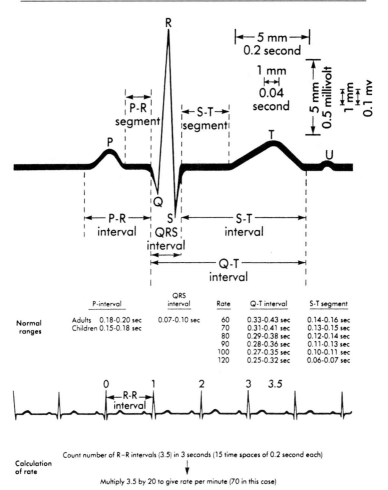

Fig. F-4 Components of the electrocardiogram demonstrating normal intervals. (Modified from the CIBA Collection of Medical Illustrations, Vol. 5.)

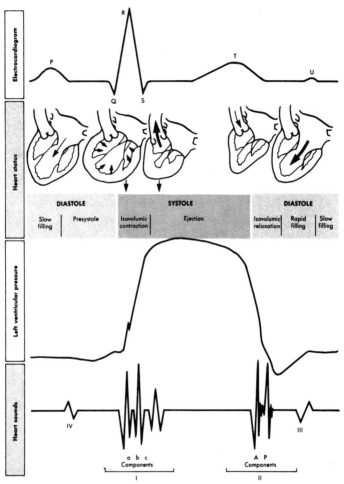

Fig. F-5 Electrical and mechanical activity sequence of the heart. (Modified from the CIBA Collection of Medical Illustrations, Vol. 5.)

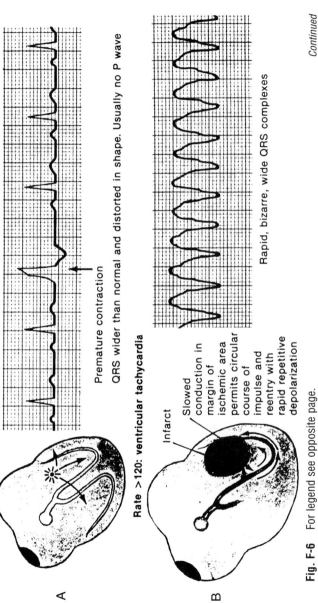

Premature contraction

QRS wider than normal and distorted in shape. Usually no P wave

Rate >120: ventricular tachycardia

Rapid, bizarre, wide QRS complexes

Infarct

Slowed conduction in margin of ischemic area permits circular course of impulse and reentry with rapid repetitive depolarization

A

B

Continued

Fig. F-6 For legend see opposite page.

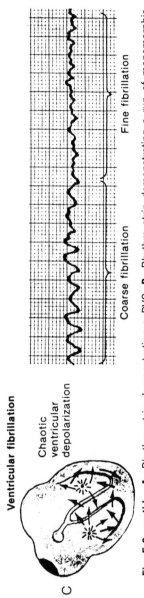

Ventricular fibrillation

Chaotic
ventricular
depolarization

Coarse fibrillation

Fine fibrillation

Fig. F-6, cont'd   A, Rhythm strip demonstrating a PVC. **B,** Rhythm strip demonstrating a run of monomorphic ventricular tachycardia. **C,** Rhythm strip demonstrating ventricular fibrillation. (Adapted from Scheidt S: *Clinical Symposia* 35(2):37, 1983; 36(6):29, 1984.)

Infarction

1. Injury = elevated ST segment

elevation

- Signifies an acute process, ST returns to baseline with time.
- If T wave is also elevated off baseline, suspect pericarditis.
- Location of injury may be determined similar to infarction location.
- If ST depression, suspect digitalis effect or subendocardial infarction.

2. Ischemia = inverted T wave

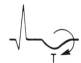

- Inverted T wave is symmetrical.
- T waves are usually upright in leads, I, II, and V_2-V_6, so check these leads for T wave inversion.

3. Infarction = Q wave

Q

- Small Qs may be normal in V_5 and V_6.
- Abnormal Q must be one small square (*.04 sec*) wide.
- Also abnormal if Q wave depth is greater than $\frac{1}{3}$ of QRS height in lead III.

Anterior infarction

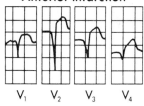

V_1 V_2 V_3 V_4

1. ST elevation with/without abnormal Q wave.

2. Usually associated with occlusion of the left anterior descending branch of the left coronary artery.

Fig. F-7 Electrocardiographic changes seen during myocardial injury, ischemia, and infarction. (Courtesy of Genentech, Inc., South San Francisco, Calif.)

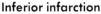

Inferior infarction

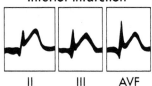

II   III   AVF

1. ST elevation with/without abnormal Q wave.

2. Usually associated with right coronary artery (RCA) occlusion.

Lateral infarction

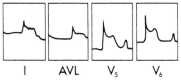

I   AVL   V₅   V₆

1. ST elevation with/without abnormal Q wave.

2. May be a component of a multiple site infarction.

3. Usually associated with obstruction of left circumflex artery.

Posterior infarction

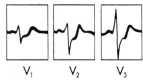

V₁   V₂   V₃

1. Tall R wave and ST depression in V_1 and V_2 (reciprocal changes).

2. May be a component of a multiple site infarction.

3. Usually associated with obstruction of RCA and/or left circumflex coronary artery.

Fig. F-8   Electrocardiographic changes in which acute inferior, lateral, and posterior infarction are demonstrated. (Courtesy of Genentech, Inc., South San Francisco, Calif.)

G

Methods for Common Drugs

Table G-1

Converting Infusion Rates

Converting desired dose (µg/min) to infusion rate (ml/min or ml/hr)

$$\frac{\text{Desired dose (µg/min)}}{\text{Drip concentration (µg/ml)}} = \text{ml/min}$$

If using a volume infusion pump that uses a ml/hr format such as an IVAC Model 560, convert µg/min to mg/hr

$$\frac{\text{Desired dose (µg/min)}}{\text{Drip concentration (µg/ml)} \times 60} = \text{ml/hr}$$

Converting desired dose (mg/min) to infusion rate (ml/min or ml/hr)

$$\frac{\text{Desired dose (µg/min)}}{\text{Drip concentration (µg/ml)}} = \text{ml/min}$$

If using a volume infusion pump that uses a ml/hr format such as an IVAC Model 560, convert µg/min to µg/hr

$$\frac{\text{Desired dose (mg/min)}}{\text{Drip concentration (mg/ml)} \times 60} = \text{ml/hr}$$

Automatic Infusion Pump, IVAC Corporation, Minneapolis, Minn.

Table G-2

Infusion Methods of Potent Drugs

Drug dosages given in different units

mg/min	μg/kg/min	μ/min	U/hr
Lidocaine	Dopamine	Nitroprusside	Heparin
Procainamide	Dobutamine	Nitroglycerin	
Bretylium	Amrinone		
Aminophylline	Levophed		
Hydralazine			
Amiodarone			

Common concentrations

Nitroprusside (50 mg/250 ml) = 200 μg/ml
Nitroglycerin (50 mg/250 ml) = 200 μg/ml
Norepinephrine (8 mg/250 ml) = 32 μ/ml
Dobutamine (1 g/250 ml) = 4000 μ/ml
Dopamine (800 mg/250 ml) = 3200 μg/ml
Hydralazine (100 mg/100 ml) = 1 mg/ml
Lidocaine (2 g/250 ml) = 8 mg/ml
Heparin (2500 U/250 ml) = 100 U/ml

Converting desired dose (in μg/kg/min) to infusion rate (in ml/hr):

1. Weight (in kg) × desired dose/kg/min = μg/min

2. $\dfrac{\mu g/ml}{60}$ = μg/ml/min

3. $\dfrac{\mu g/min}{\mu g/ml/min}$ = ml/hr infusion rate

Example: Dopamine (assume 70 kg at 3 μg/kg/min)

1. Compute dose for weight
   70 × 3 = 210 μg/min
2. Compute drug concentration per minute (from common concentrations)
   $\dfrac{320\ \mu g/ml}{60^*}$ = 53.3 μg/ml.min
3. When using IVAC delivery in ml/hr, compute dose of IVAC
   $\dfrac{210\ \mu g/min}{53.3\ \mu g/ml/min}$ = 3.9* ml/hr

*Round off to nearest whole number when setting infusion pump.

Continued

Table G-2

Infusion Methods of Potent Drugs—cont'd

Converting infusion rates (ml/hr) to dose (µg/min)

$$\frac{\text{Rate (ml/hr)} = \text{µg/ml}}{60} = \text{µg/min}$$

Converting infusion rate (ml/hr) to dose for weight (µg/kg/min)

$$\frac{\text{Rate (ml/hr)} \times \text{µg/ml}}{60} = \text{µg/min}$$

$$\frac{\text{µg/min}}{\text{kg weight}} = \text{µg/kg/min}$$

Automatic Infusion Pump, IVAC Corporation, Minneapolis, Minn.

Table G-3

Quick Millereau Method

1 µg/kg/min = 1 ml/hr
Drug dose (mg = 3 × body weight kg in 50-ml solution)

Example 1: Dobutamine for 50-kg patient

3 × 50 kg = 150 mg in 50 ml
         = 1 ml/hr
         = 1 µg/kg/min
(If 0.1 µg/kg/min is needed, use 0.3 × body weight.)

Example 2: Norepinephrine for 80-kg patient

Need range of 0.1 to 3 µg/kg/hr, use 0.3 × body weight
0.3 × 80 = 24 mg in 50 ml
        = 0.1 µg/kg/min
        = 1 ml/hr
If infusion rate = 2.5 ml/hr, dose infused = 0.25 µg/kg/min

From Millereau M: Dilution of potent drugs, *Am J Cardiol* 68:418, 1991.

INDEX

Page numbers followed by f indicate figures; t, tables; and b, boxes.

601

Vieussens pulse = Corrigans pulse or water hammer pulse in A.I.

Vieussens ring = Collateral connection from LAD to conus branch of the RCA